Precancer: Biology, Importance and Possible Prevention

CANCER SURVEYS

Precancer: Biology, Importance and Possible Prevention

SERIES EDITOR: J Tooze
Consulting Editor: L M Franks
Editorial Assistant: C E Sinclair

Associate Editors

W Bodmer	A Harris	J Ponten
V Beral	NR Lemoine	B Stillman
H Calvert	P Nurse	N Wright
C Dickson	MJ Owen	J Wyke
	T Pawson	

Published for the

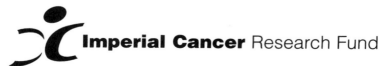

Imperial Cancer Research Fund

Precancer: Biology, Importance and Possible Prevention

Guest Editor
J Pontén

COLD SPRING HARBOR LABORATORY PRESS 1998

CANCER SURVEYS
Precancer: Biology, Importance and Possible Prevention
Volume 32

All rights reserved
Copyright 1998 by Imperial Cancer Research Fund
Published by Cold Spring Harbor Laboratory Press
Printed in the United States of America
ISBN 0-87969-540-4
ISSN 0261-2429
Library of Congress Catalog Card Number: 98-72543

Cover and book design by Leon Bolognese & Associates, Inc.

Authorization to photocopy items for internal or personal use, or the internal or personal use of specific clients, is granted by Cold Spring Harbor Laboratory Press provided that the appropriate fee is paid directly to the Copyright Clearance Center (CCC). Write or call CCC at 222 Rosewood Dr., Danvers, MA 01923 (508-750-8400) for information about fees and regulations. Prior to photocopying items for educational classroom use, contact CCC at the above address. Additional information on CCC can be obtained at CCC Online at http://www.copyright.com/

All Cold Spring Harbor Laboratory Press publications may be ordered directly from Cold Spring Harbor Laboratory Press, 10 Skyline Drive, Plainview, New York 11803-9729. Phone: Continental US & Canada 1-800-843-4388; all other locations (516) 349-1930. FAX: (516) 349-1946. All other locations: (516) 349-1930. FAX: (516) 349-1946. E-mail: cshpress@cshl.org. For a complete catalog of all Cold Spring Harbor Laboratory Press publications, visit our World Wide Web Site http://www.cshl.org/

Contents

v

Introduction

J PONTÉN

Department of Pathology, University of Uppsala, S-751 85 Uppsala

Experimental information about human cancer has to a large extent concerned tumours in advanced stage or as long term tissue culture lines. Our concepts and dogmas about carcinogenesis are largely founded on such observations. But such biological entities as advanced cancers and established tissue culture lines inevitably represent late stages in a dynamic process and will tell us very little about the events that led up to malignant transformation and subsequent selection of the typical mixture of subclones that will present as clinical cancer.

Pathologists have described precancers in great microscopic detail. This has, however, only rarely been complemented by somatic genetic and molecular analysis. Relations between precancer and invasive cancer have often been inferred on rather loose observational grounds. This volume is an attempt to bridge the gap between morphology and modern molecular biology in precancer. The past few years have seen a widening interest in investigations of precancer. Formal proof is starting to come to light about genetic links between putative precancers and invasive cancer. And, more importantly, research is beginning to unravel the critical extra events that seem to be essential for transition from precancer to cancer. A key question is whether very early steps on a long winding road to cancer can be detected. Such detection would decisively help to eradicate cancer before it has had time to develop.

The field of precancer contains some fascinating riddles. One concerns spontaneous regression. Although it is well established that at least a proportion of microscopically distinguishable precancers have permanent mutations and signs of chromosome damage, they do not progress to invasiveness. This stands in sharp contrast to invasive cancers which, if left untreated, virtually always continue to multiply and eventually kill their host. The cause of this striking difference is unknown and has attracted little scientific interest. Vague reference has been made to immortalization, but mortality has not been studied in precancerous cells. Unsuccessful attempts have been made to find clinically important markers that could single out precancers with no or low probability of progression to cancer. A solution to this problem will probably require deep insight into the mechanisms that govern proliferation control both in precancer and in cancer. This problem is particularly relevant in prostatic cancer, where the incidence of precancer is very high and presents an important problem in clinical management. Establishment of genetic links between precancer, small subclinical adenocarcinomas and clinically important cancer of the prostate is in its infancy but should greatly facilitate understanding of important tumour biological problems, as discussed in this volume. Oesophageal cancer was long neglected by tumour biologists. But the discovery of Barrett's oesophagus and new aetiological clues have reversed this picture as outlined in this volume.

Two human precancers stand out, because their essential aetiology seems to have been revealed. For precancer of the skin ultraviolet light energy is a major cause. This has been successfully explored, and remarkable insight into the pathogenesis of precancer has been obtained. One advantage is that ultraviolet light leaves a characteristic mark on DNA by mutations at dipyrimidine sites, especially CC →TT double transitions. Use of this marker has helped to elucidate clonal relations between precancer and cancer and has also revealed facts about the role of the tumour suppressor gene *TP53* in carcinogenesis. But in spite of much effort, the precise role of mutated *TP53* remains to be elucidated. Does it act only indirectly, because DNA repair and/or apoptosis does not proceed properly or does it also have a more direct role in the control of stem cell number and clonal expansion of precancers?

The second human complex of precancer related to a well characterized agent is dysplasia and carcinoma in situ of the cervix. This disease offers the same experimental advantage as skin cancer, because it is common and often biopsied. The first quite recent attempts to establish genetic links between precancer and cancer are reviewed in this volume, as is the complex relation between morphological response and infection by different types of human papillomavirus. Apart from their considerable theoretical tumour biological interest, early observations in this field hint at methods for singling out precancers with no or only very small likelihood of progression to invasive cancer and so for avoiding unnecessary surgery.

Precancers also enter prominently into the field of bioassays of carcinogenetic properties of chemical compounds. Their study provides not only insights into mechanisms of malignant transformation but also a possible avenue for more rapid testing of suspect compounds.

The current volume puts much emphasis on analysis rather than description of a variety of precancerous lesions. The importance of somatic mutations has been particularly stressed. Precancers offer special advantages in elucidating whether hypermutability is a feature of malignant neoplasia. The use of acquired variations in length of microsatellites as a biological clock in precancer of the colon points to methods by which colon polyps may be assessed with respect to their age and their tendency to develop heterogeneity. The answer to the question of hypermutability may well be different depending on cancer type.

The field has been plagued by lack of suitable techniques for analysis of small samples. This has, however, been remedied by the utilization of well controlled microdissection with careful elimination of contaminating normal cells and the development of increasingly robust methods for in situ hybridization, immunohistochemistry and direct sequencing of polymerase chain reaction amplified DNA. A picture, which this volume critically overviews, has emerged of the roots from which clinical cancers grow. This knowledge should not only be of theoretical interest but should also be important for prevention, early diagnosis and effective therapy.

Cell Biology of Precancer

JAN PONTÉN

Department of Pathology, University of Uppsala, S-751 85 Uppsala, Sweden

Introduction
Definitions
Clonality and cell lineage: relevance for precancer
Are all cancers preceded by precancer?
    Oligohit neoplasia
    Precancer in a multihit scenario
    Dynamics of multihit lineages
    Precancer and hypermutability
Overview

INTRODUCTION

The scientific study of cancer has its roots in the clinic. No definition of cancer is entirely satisfactory from a cell biological point of view despite the fact that cancer is essentially a cellular disease. Whereas clinicians and pathologists, who usually encounter cancer at a biologically late stage, have had no principal doubts about a qualitative difference between malignant, ie cancer, and benign overgrowths, modern tumour biology has emphasized a quantitative model by which cells undergo gradual "progressive" alterations, taking them from normal via less well understood proliferative or even inflammatory/degenerative intermediate stages to benign neoplasia to cancer-in-situ to locally invasive cancer to metastasizing "frank" malignancies. In this scheme, borders between hyperplasia, regeneration, precancer and cancer become rather arbitrary.

A discussion about precancer will lack substance unless a qualitative transition is assumed between precancer and cancer, at which a cell undergoes a permanent change which takes it to an irreversible state where there is not only net proliferation but also the kind of "asocial" behaviour which makes the cells grow without formation of functionally or morphologically normal tissue. This will eventually lead to impairment of vital functions incompatible with life of the host organism. The transition to the malignant phenotype is conventionally termed "malignant transformation".

There is indirect evidence of malignant transformation in a qualitative sense. An enormous amount of empirical morphological evidence has been amassed showing that a malignant cell, or at least an assembly of such cells, can be distinguished in the microscope on the basis of cellular atypia and growth

Cancer Surveys Volume 32: *Precancer: Biology, Importance and Possible Prevention*
© 1998 Imperial Cancer Research Fund. 0-87969-540-4/98. $5.00 + .00

patterns distinct from those displayed by cells in hyperplasia, embryonic development, or inflammation. This largely holds true also in vitro, with its strong correlation between focal non-inhibited irregular growth (Pontén, 1975; Abercrombie and Heaysman, 1976) and malignant behaviour upon transplantation to syngeneic hosts. It is remarkable that the best predictor of malignancy in vivo was cellular atypia in a study of spontaneous transformation of mouse fibroblasts (Barker and Sanford, 1970; Sanford *et al*, 1970). The cellular or molecular biology behind the characteristic features of cellular atypia have hardly been discussed or investigated. They are of importance for any understanding of precancer and will therefore be dealt with here despite meagre experimental data.

Our task is to illuminate steps before malignant transformation, ie to attempt to understand precancer in cell biological or molecular rather than clinical or pathological terms. The emphasis will be on human cells, not only because of practical implications but also because of inherent genetic problems of animal cells, particularly those of rodent origin.

Crucial questions for any understanding of precancer are: Are all cancers preceded by precancer? Is a precancer cell lineage characterized by hypermutability? Is there a direct DNA lineage from precancer to cancer, and if so how long is it and how many mutations have been added as a function of number of DNA generations? Related questions concern the phenotypic changes that occur in a precancer–cancer lineage. Can they be morphologically and/or functionally discerned? Are basic features such as degree of aggressiveness and differentiation laid down already in precancer, ie before malignant transformation, or are such features added during progression after malignant transformation? Is precancer reversible? Can analysis of precancer provide a short cut to assessment of carcinogenic risk? Answers to these questions will differ from cancer to cancer and be dealt with in the relevant chapters of this volume. This introductory chapter will explore possibilities of understanding precancer at a more general level and highlight unexplained phenomena. Until now there has been such a heavy emphasis on cancer that we are only at a beginning in understanding precancer.

DEFINITIONS

Precancer is defined as any morphologically distinguishable (cellular atypia and impaired differentiation) proliferative lesion that statistically is known to be followed by cancer with significant likelihood. This likelihood is often below 100%. The formal proof, ie that a precancer lineage contains cells on a direct path to cancer, is rarely delivered.

Within the broad category of precancer, the following terms are applicable.

Carcinoma-in-situ is defined as a condition confined to epithelial cancers (carcinomas) with all morphological criteria of cancer except signs of invasive growth. There will consequently always be a degree of disorder among the constituent cells. In the breast and other exocrine glands intraductal carcinoma is synonymous with carcinoma-in-situ. A few non-epithelial cancers have analogous terms, for example melanoma-in-situ. Solid mesenchymal tumours, leukaemias and lymphomas do not have recognized analogues to carcinoma-in-situ. Malignant gliomas do not have any recognized counterparts to carcinoma-in-situ, possibly because of their peculiar pathology. The possibility that high grade astrocytomas are analogous to carcinoma-in-situ will however, be discussed in the chapter by Collins.

Dysplasia is an epithelial lesion with a degree of cellular atypia and disturbed differentiation. It is conventionally graded mild, moderate or severe. In contrast to carcinoma-in-situ, constituent cells are still ordered along physiological lines.

CLONALITY AND CELL LINEAGE: RELEVANCE FOR PRECANCER

A useful way to look at development of precancer and cancer is to concentrate on numbers of generations of newly synthesized cellular DNA rather than the cells themselves, which from a genetic point of view can be regarded as temporary phenotypic costumes of variable appearance, which the genome will modify and use as it multiplies.

At the very beginning there will be one diploid genome of the fertilized egg. During development of the individual, branching chains or lineages of DNA will arise, all of which belong to the same clone and therefore carry along any mutations or polymorphisms delivered by the paternal and maternal haploid genomes. For lack of markers and the impossibility of experimental manipulation this maze of lineages and relay of genomes will presumably never be as completely disentangled as in the nematode worm *Caenorhabditis elegans* (Kornfeld, 1997; Sommer, 1997), but some main principles can be formulated for mammals, including humans.

DNA lineages of variable lengths measured in number of rounds of DNA replication will unfold. These lineages should not be defined in phenotypic terms but rather according to genotype, in order to facilitate understanding of, for instance, "hypermutability" and "multihit", as these terms are used in precancer and cancer. Lineages will have a very variable fate. Some will continuously propagate their DNA via rounds of replication throughout the lifetime of the individual, others will die out. Others will remain in limbo until reactivated by a call for regeneration, and still others will persist in an irreversible dormant stage from the point of view of potential to enter new rounds of DNA synthesis. Some may even continue as cripples with occasional new rounds of DNA synthesis.

The lineages of tumour biological interest are those that lead up to a point where precancer can be spotted or where malignant transformation of a single cell starts the growth of a cancer.

Fig. 1 surveys some general principles. Lineages are traced from the zygote to single cells in the peripheral semicircle, which either have transformed to invasive cancer (black centres), in situ cancer (dark purple centres) or dysplasia (light purple centres) or remained untransformed (unfilled centre). The snapshot is taken when the first malignantly transformed cell appears in certain lineages. All lineages are depicted as running through developmental stages where embryonic cells, stepwise by epigenetic mechanisms, irreversibly lose their potency to differentiate into a multitude of directions (Hendrich and Willard, 1995). The light green lineage, for instance, passes through rounds of omnipotence (bright red) via generations of multipotence (dark green) to monopotence (light green). DNA synthesis followed by asymmetrical divisions will create a genomic chain schematically depicted as containing 14 rounds until dysplasia ensues. After six further rounds of DNA synthesis, carcinoma-in-situ develops in the light green lineage, in which after three additional rounds, one in situ cell transforms to invasive cancer. Each cell on the light green route will, as hinted at by two clusters of cells, give off numerous lineages that end with terminal differentiation after a few rounds. The dark blue lineage illustrates the possibility that in situ cancer develops without being preceded by dysplasia. It also demonstrates the possibility that daughter cells rapidly disappear in apoptosis. Single precancer cells may then continue multiplying without any increase in the size of the cell population. The purple line leads straight to dysplasia and the orange one straight to carcinoma-in-situ. The dysplastic and in situ cells on their respective lineages divide symmetrically and thus give rise to subclones with an increasing number of cells with retained "stemcellness". In the purple lineage an in situ clone is seen to have emerged. The figure illustrates the important point that neoplastic lineages (orange and purple) may split into parallel lineages because more than half of the daughter cells retain stem cell character, ie are capable of infinite propagation of the property of self renewal. The implications of symmetrical and asymmetrical cell divisions in precancer lineages are thoroughly discussed in the chapter by Shibata.

Fig. 1 also portrays the importance of point of time of any mutation. The purple, light blue and dark blue lineages show (arrows) how lineages may branch away from each other at stages before monopotence is reached. The earlier a mutation occurs the more lineages will carry it.

Fig. 2 shows estimates of the lengths of lineages measured as numbers of rounds of DNA synthesis. Units of such a lineage are referred to as stem cells, functionally defined by "stemcellness", that is a capacity of the cellular genome, at each round of DNA synthesis, to give rise to at least one new genome which still possesses the original proliferative capacity to an undiminished degree. Fig. 2 demonstrates that human cancer can have variable but never very many rounds of cellular DNA synthesis before malignant transformation. For such a constantly regenerating tissue as epidermis 4000 rounds of DNA synthesis are computed at age 55, including a stretch from precancer to cancer corresponding to about 1000 rounds from age 40. In this case, which may be representa-

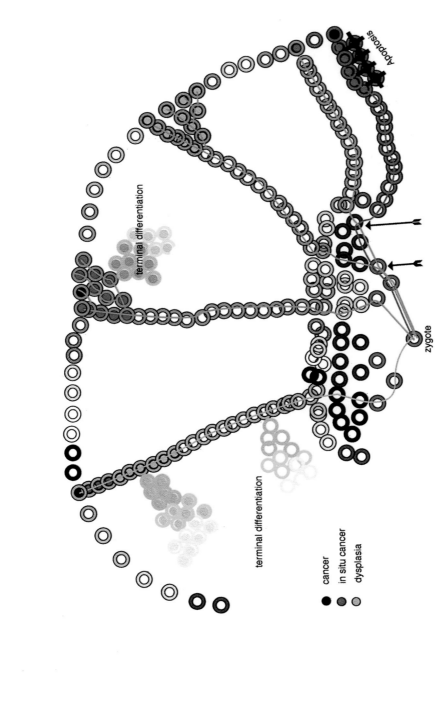

Fig. 1. Principles of cell lineage formation. For details see text

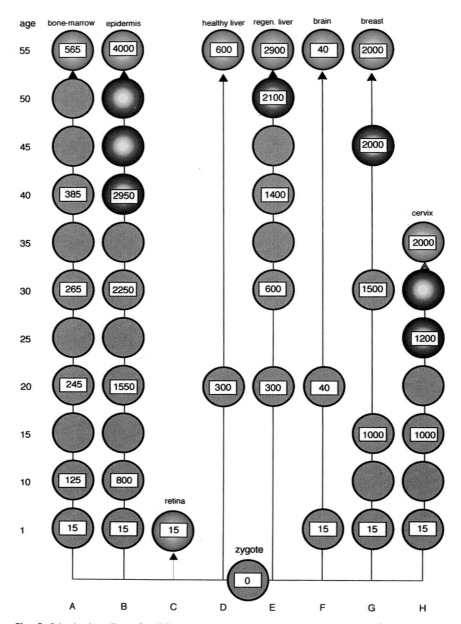

Fig. 2. Principal outline of cell lineages leading towards transformation to precancer (purple with yellow centre) and cancer (orange with yellow centre). A–H represent the tracks of rounds of genomic DNA synthesis among stem cells which end by malignant transformation in bone marrow, epidermis, retina, healthy liver, regenerating liver (eg in cirrhosis), brain, breast and cervix. Assumptions about the number of rounds of DNA synthesis (white labels) are expounded in the text. Age of an individual in the column to the left

tive also of gut epithelium, an average stem cell cycle time of about five days is assumed (Potten, 1981). A retinoblastoma may have been preceded by as few as 15 rounds of DNA synthesis to fit with recorded rates of incidence and number of retinoblasts at risk (Hethcote and Knudson, 1978). Estimates of intervals between rounds of DNA synthesis in bone marrow stem cells illustrate the extreme difficulty of obtaining reliable results. The definition of stem cells is not unequivocal, but several investigators regard them as quiescent because of lack of evidence of ongoing DNA synthesis, and one estimate of murine bone marrow stem cells gave a value of one month. Fig. 2 is based on about 35 days. In the healthy liver, where cellular turnover is slow (Michalopoulos and DeFrances, 1997), there may be only 600 rounds before the first hepatocellular cancer cell makes its appearance at age 55. As a corollary, the influence of chronic liver cell regeneration is illustrated by the guess that 2900 rounds of DNA synthesis may constitute the lineage that ends with malignant transformation. Breast and cervix take intermediate positions, whereas astrocytes of the brain may have undergone only 40 rounds before malignant transformation, as suggested by the virtual absence of DNA synthesis in putative precursor cells.

The estimates of number of cell cycle rounds of Fig. 2 are rough, based on imperfect data and intended only to illustrate principles. But they show that the genetic hits generally considered necessary for malignant transformation need to occur more frequently than intuitively expected. This paradox is, however, only apparent, because the number of potential lineages leading to malignant transformation is large in an individual. The denominator of risk of precancer (and cancer) is the total number of genomes at risk of crucial mutations on lineages able to end by transformation. The numerator will be the number of lineages that actually have ended in precancer and cancer, respectively. The latter is in turn reflected by incidence figures, as recorded in cancer registries. The essence of malignant transformation of a single cell is that its lineage has suffered mutations of crucial genes at a high rate. Below follows a discussion of whether this is so because of hypermutability (Loeb, 1996) or whether it can be explained on the basis of a normal rate of spontaneous mutations in combination with selection (Tomlinson *et al*, 1996).

A model of precancer and cancer can be formulated from the concept of genomic lineages and single cell origin of neoplasia. The following factors will determine whether any given cell will undergo transformation. (1) Frequency of fixed genetic "hits" per round of DNA synthesis necessary to accomplish transformation, ie a progressive count of hits in alleles necessary to forge the "malignant phenotype". This implies not only a defined set of genes (oncogenes, tumour suppressor genes and other, unidentified genes) as targets but also that the hits occur at codons that alter encoded proteins in a critical manner. For most adult cancers the number of necessary rate limiting hits before malignant transformation of a cell lineage is conjectured to be of the order of 4–6. For carcinoma-in-situ it may be one fewer, ie 3–5 and for dysplasia two fewer ie 2–4. Most data indicate that the order by which the hits accumulate is not important. If a mutation leads to genetic instability this will be reflected as an increased rate of hits. (2) Number of DNA rounds in the lineage that undergoes transformation. This number will vary depending on the proliferative status of the lineage and here is estimated to be between 15 and 4000 (Fig. 2). The more rounds of DNA synthesis the more likely that the necessary hits will accumulate. (3) Number of lineages susceptible to transformation. This number will vary considerably within an individual. For human bone marrow it may be as large as 10^8, in contrast to the cervix, where a narrow transformation zone is the target with perhaps as few as 1000 lineages (see the chapter by Pontén and Guo). The number of lineages may be modified during embryonic, fetal and childhood development, for example by selective action of steroid hormones (Ekbom *et al*, 1992) or by regeneration. (4) The time pattern of acquisition of hits. Early hits will affect a larger number of lineages than late hits (Knudson, 1992). (5) The effect of the hits on the likelihood of self renewal. If a mutation increases the probability of self renewal (symmetrical mitoses with preserved "stemcellness") it will by branching increase the number of lineages and thus increase the number of target cells primed for transformation. (6) The effect of competing hits, ie the numerous mutations which in excess of the transforming ones affect the remaining genome. The majority are neutral, but a fraction will cause changes in metabolism, cell structure and so on, often with a negative effect on viability but sometimes, instead, rendering a positive selective value. The importance of this component has to a large extent been neglected. (7) The phenotype of the target lineage. Certain cells such as retinoblasts, haemopoietic stem cells, mesenchymal cells and endocrine and neuroendocrine epithelia behave as if they require fewer hits than the bulk of epithelial stem cells. (8) Species derivation of target cells. Certain factors co-operate, according to an obscure scheme, to ensure that a correlation exists between the lifespan of a species and the length of the cell lineage until malignant transformation occurs. In a comparison between species the probability of cancer is roughly the same per individual but vastly different per target cell or lineage.

ARE ALL CANCERS PRECEDED BY PRECANCER?

Oligohit Neoplasia

It is commonly assumed that all cancers are preceded by precancer. The reason for our failure sometimes to detect putative precancers would then be explained by the selective growth advantage of cancer cells, which permits them to overgrow and destroy any precursors.

Retinoblastoma was the first clear example of a human two hit malignancy depending on homozygous obliteration of the function of both alleles of a tumour suppressor gene (Knudson, 1971; Cavenee *et al*, 1985). The tumour serves as a convincing demonstration of the qualitative nature of malignant transformation, the importance of correct target cells and absence of precancer in a two hit suppressor gene scenario.

In Fig. 3, from a fictitious hereditary case of retinoblastoma, all cell lineages carry a non-functional *RB* allele. Lineages A–D have by epigenetic mechanisms differentiated to retinoblasts in the embryo. By chance, and with a likelihood

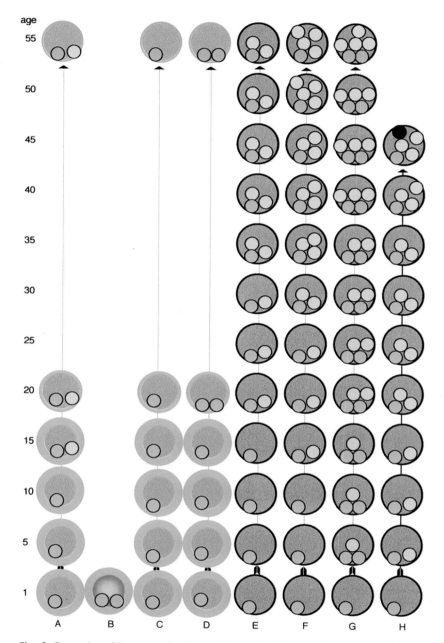

Fig. 3. Examples of lineages of cellular DNA synthesis in spontaneous retinoblastoma compared with non-transformed lineages. Thick blue rings denote retinoblasts. Orange-red indicates malignant transformation to retinoblastoma. Mutations are indicated by small circles. blue=*RB* allele, yellow=neutral allele, black=lethal allele

estimated at about 10^{-7} mutations per locus per round of DNA synthesis (Knudson, 1971; Hethcote and Knudson, 1978; Moolgavkar and Venzon, 1979), a second *RB* mutation has occurred in lineage B. The retinoblast responds by

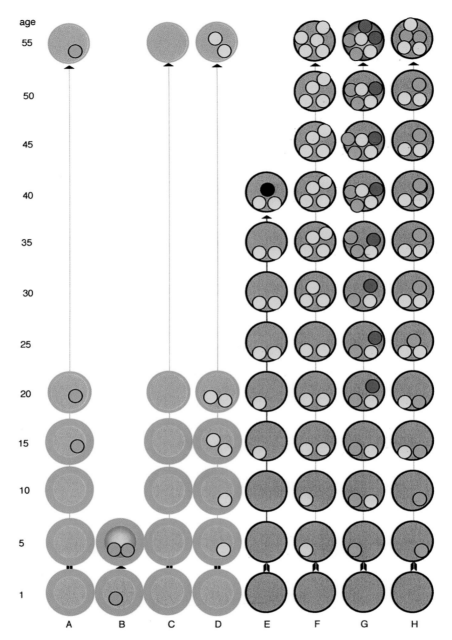

Fig. 4. Examples of lineages of cellular DNA synthesis in spontaneous retinoblastoma compared with non-transformed lineages. Thick blue rings denote retinoblasts. Organge-yellow indicates malignant transformation. Mutations are indicated by small circles: blue=*RB* allele, yellow=neutral allele, black=lethal allele, red=suppressor gene

malignant transformation, in this particular kind of tumour predominantly characterized by profound inhibition of differentiation with rapid proliferation of blast cells. Some tumour cells may undergo sufficient numbers of rounds of

DNA synthesis to accumulate more mutations (not illustrated). But there is no direct evidence that the mutation rate is increased in retinoblastoma, even if some reports have claimed that loss of *RB* function will in a moderate manner influence genetic stability negatively (Reznikoff *et al*, 1994; Almasan *et al*, 1995; Donehower, 1997). By and large retinoblastomas behave in a uniform manner both morphologically and clinically, supporting the notion that the two original hits are sufficient to explain their neoplastic properties.

There is no indication that destruction of the function of only one *RB* allele has any phenotypic effect ie that precancers exist. Retinoblasts in a child who has inherited a defective *RB* gene perform normally, ie the classical suppressor gene scenario is displayed. This part of the *RB* story is recapitulated in genetically manipulated mice, with the unexplained difference that pituitary adenomas rather than retinoblastomas are created after a second *RB* hit (Jacks *et al*, 1992; Hu *et al*, 1994).

Fig. 3 illustrates some other consequences of Knudson's two hit model. It is not excluded that the second *RB* mutation will occur after the retinoblasts have left their stem cell stage to become irreversibly committed to terminal differentiation. Then a few mature retina cells may carry homozygously destroyed *RB* genes but will fail to develop retinoblastoma (lineage D)—a prediction fully compatible with virtual absence of retinoblastoma once childhood is over.

A second possibility (not illustrated) is that cells resting in G_0 may acquire permanent mutations. Although interesting extrapolations from bacteria have been discussed (Bridges, 1996), there is no convincing evidence that this ever happens in mammalian cells, at least on a scale of importance when DNA repair is untouched. The reasons for low or no mutability in resting cells are (a) that repair will have sufficient time to be effective and (b) that mutations caused by error prone DNA polymerase cannot happen (Minnick and Kunkel, 1996).

Epithelial stem cells outside of the retinoblastoma lineages (E–H, Fig. 3) will, according to theory, accumulate *RB* mutations at the same rate of 10^{-7} per DNA synthesis round. This will cause some lineages to suffer the same two *RB* hits as the retinoblast founder of a malignant eye tumour. No excessive risk for any tumours other than mesenchymal tumours, particularly osteosarcomas has been established for carriers of *RB* mutations (Draper *et al*, 1986). This suggests that the stem cells involved in epithelial cancers can have homozygous destruction of two important suppressor genes without adverse effects. The earlier this happens the more cells will carry doubly defective *RB* alleles, because the homozygous state will be transmitted to larger numbers of daughter stem cells. One explanation for the inference that *RB* gene lesions can behave as neutral mutations might be that retinoblasts (and osteoblasts etc.) cannot substitute for loss of *RB*, in contrast to other cells, which may be provided with backup systems and therefore require more than disruption of *RB* to undergo malignant transformation, as indicated by lineage G in Fig. 3, which remains normal in spite of two *RB* and four other mutations.

Fig. 4 illustrates the difference between hereditary and spontaneous retinoblastoma. For the latter to occur two spontaneous hits will have to inactivate both *RB* loci. This will take more rounds of DNA synthesis than the single second hit needed in hereditary cases. The likelihood of such a combination will be 10^{-14}, based on the standard figure of 10^{-7} (Hethcote and Knudson, 1978). To accommodate this a large number of retinoblast lineages have to be at risk, ie spontaneous retinoblastoma will become a rare disease at the population level. Lineage H illustrates that non-retinoblastoma cells may suffer homozygous mutational inactivation of *RB* without undergoing transformation. Lineage G shows the possibility that malignant transformation may, at least theoretically, be irrelevant in a non-retinoblastoma cell, which in this case was transformed because of mutations of two other suppressor genes (red dots).

Basal cell cancer (BCC) has always puzzled observers by its apparent absence of precursors. This stands in sharp contrast to squamous cell cancer and melanoma, which have well recognized precursors to be dealt with in the chapter by Brash.

Recent results point at possibilities to explain the absence of "pre-BCC" along the same lines as in retinoblastoma. The gene defect that causes a hereditary BCC syndrome with early onset of tumours was shown to involve the gene *patched*. This gene, which has a homologue in fruit flies and mice, is part of the "hedgehog" signalling pathway, which regulates embryonic patterning, including the development of the nervous system (Tabata and Kornberg, 1994; Bokor and DiNardo, 1996; Goodrich *et al*, 1996; Hahn *et al*, 1996a; Marigo *et al*, 1996). Homozygous genetically based inhibition of the function of *patched* (*ptc*) may, from still limited data, be a sine qua non for development of hereditary and acquired BCC, which would then qualify as a two hit tumour without any need to postulate a precursor (Gailani *et al*, 1996; Hahn *et al*, 1996b; Johnson *et al*, 1996; Undén *et al*, 1996). The hereditary form is transmitted via point mutations or small deletions within *ptc*. In the tumours the other allele will somatically be subject to inactivation typically detected as loss of heterozygosity (LOH) at chromosome 9q22.3, ie the site of *ptc*. Recent data suggest the possibility that *Gli1* (overexpression or mutation?) may substitute for damaged *ptc* (Damane *et al*, 1997)—a not unreasonable proposition in view of the involvement of both genes in the same control system.

Hereditary BCCs usually become manifest during the third or fourth decade, and the acquired form in the seventh or eighth decade. About 10^7 or 10^{14} interphase genomes at risk, respectively, would be required for accumulation of homozygous mutations in *patched*, in analogy with retinoblastoma. Spontaneous BCC would arise from a type of lineage indicated by B in Fig. 2. According to the model, 5500 rounds of DNA synthesis would be completed before malignant transformation to BCC at age 70, compared with only 15 for a retinoblastoma in a one year old child. Such age of onset difference would be conceivable if the number of stem cell lineages for BCC were few compared with retinoblastoma lineages. In reality, a much higher incidence of BCC than of retinoblastoma suggests the opposite. These theoretical deliberations strongly suggest that more than two hits are required for BCC. The possibility that a

TP53 gene mutation is one of them will be discussed in the chapter by Brash and Pontén.

Sequencing of mutated *ptc* has, surprisingly, only shown the typical ultraviolet (UV) light involvement of dipyrimidines in one third of the cases, in contrast to the spectrum of *TP53* mutations in the same tumours, which is of the order of 80% py-py involvement, hinting at indirect mechanisms for *ptc* damage by UV light (Hahn *et al*, 1996b; Gailani and Bale, 1997).

From cytogenetic data there is evidence that morphological absence of precancer in sarcoma, leukaemia, lymphoma and myeloma could be explained as a result of a requirement for only few hits to accomplish malignant transformation (Mitelman, 1995; Johansson, 1996). The existence of leukaemia/lymphoma/sarcoma already in childhood hints at two hit neoplasia. Karyotypic and molecular analysis, particularly of chronic myelogenous leukaemia and follicular lymphoma, is compatible with a requirement of only a few hits. Since they are not childhood tumours it could—in analogy with the reasoning about BCC above—be suggested that the number has to be at least three.

Most forms of cancers in endocrine glands resemble mesenchymal malignancies by conforming to a concept of genetic stability. They are usually diploid or near diploid in DNA content and karyotypes (Mitelman, 1995; Johansson, 1996). Studies of extent of global point mutations do not seem to have been carried out. Endocrine cancers follow the pattern of most other epithelial cancers by having clearly defined precancers. This has been extensively studied in intestinal carcinoids, where one typically will see multiple precancers morphologically termed "adenomas" without invasion, which often individually undergo malignant transformation to invasive metastasizing carcinoids. Endocrine cancers look like oligohit, but in their case a single hit may have phenotypic effects as precancer in the form of hyperplasia and/or adenoma. Sequential genetic analyses of lineages from normal via precancer to (neuro)endocrine cancer could be extremely rewarding.

Precancer in a Multihit Scenario

The multihit concept of cancer and precancer has developed gradually. An early indication came through plotting incidence of cancer as a function of age. A log–log plot will form a straight line. The necessary number of rate limiting hits can be derived from its slope (Nordling, 1953). This model was extended and elaborated on by Armitage and Doll, who concluded that four to six hits were required for clinical cancer to develop (Armitage and Doll, 1954). Such statistics will reflect the combination of all cancers and cannot give any deeper insight into events at the single cell level. This is conspicuously illustrated by the fact that a similar curve for cancers in the rat, which of course develop within just a few years compared with eight human decades, has the same slope. To accommodate this it is necessary to assume that the rate at which hits accumulate in the rat is very much higher than in the human—something for which no evidence exists (see Holliday, 1996).

Demonstration of complete multihit sequences at the single cell level has not succeeded. Stringent experiments, which would require sequential addition of defined mutations on a stable genetic background until the endpoint of pre-cancer or malignant transformation is reached (Pontén, 1974), have not been feasible to devise.

Murine cells in culture were originally employed in pioneering discoveries of oncogenes. After transfection with mutated *RAS*, 3T3 cells responded by malignant transformation as if this single hit was sufficient—a finding that seemed to violate the multihit theory of cancer (Krontiris and Cooper, 1981; Murray *et al*, 1981; Weinberg, 1989; Cooper, 1992). Later research has made it likely that 3T3 and other similar cell lines are already primed for malignant transformation by several genetic hits. Transfection of mutated *RAS* will there-fore supply only the last of a number of necessary hits and in this way give the false impression of being sufficient. Established lines such as 3T3 should be regarded as "precancer" in a cell biological sense.

In spite of numerous attempts it has never been possible to achieve malig-nant transformation of normal human cells in analogy with the *RAS*-3T3 system (see Pontén, 1971; Holliday, 1996). The explanation rests with the vast differ-ence in sensitivity to transformation between the two species. One estimate claims that mouse fibroblasts are 10^9 times more susceptible to transformation than their human counterparts (Peto *et al*, 1986). Such a huge difference has not been explained. Differences in mutability, DNA repair, effects of non-dis-junction (chromosome error propagation), quality of cell cycle checkpoints, epi-genetic changes concerning methylation and telomere maintenance are the most commonly cited factors (see Holliday, 1996; Harley and Sherwood, 1997).

A remarkable biological phenomenon with profound influence on our understanding of precancer, cancer and ageing still searches for an explanation. From the point of view of understanding precancer and progression to cancer extrapolation from findings in mice to human beings (and vice versa) will always be uncertain. This probably also applies to knockout mice and other forms of genetic manipulation, where, additionally, omnipresent tumourigenic retro-viruses may inadvertently be activated, as incidentally suggested by the com-mon development of lymphomas rather than the intended malignancies.

Dynamics of Multihit Lineages

The cellular biology of multihit precancer (and cancer) has turned out to be complex and much more difficult to understand than the principally simpler oligohit models provided foremost by retinoblastoma (Knudson, 1987, 1992).

To prove that precancer is a precursor of cancer it is necessary to show that a stable marker in precancer prevails after malignant transformation to cancer, ie that the lineage to cancer passes through a recognizable stage of precancer (lineages B, E, G and H in Fig. 2). This approach would ideally require serial sampling from the same lesion—clearly unattainable in humans and hardly ever tried in experimental animals. A good substitute is, however, provided by genetically probing synchronously present precancer and cancer. A marker found in precancer that is also consistently present in a clone of cancer cells will prove that the cancer cells belong to a lineage already present in precancer.

Markers suitable for clonality determination operate at different levels. Historically they were all linked to inactivation of the X chromosome in females (Lyon, 1972; Fialkow, 1976). Inactivation occurs in a way that, in most organs, produces a stable mosaic mixture of cells with suppression of either the paternal or maternal X. Inactivation is accompanied by methylation of genes, which alters their restriction enzyme cleavage pattern. In informative cases, where the two alleles of a particular gene differ in length, gel electrophoresis after enzyme cleavage will reveal whether an allele is intact, ie has not undergone methylation associated with inactivation. Three patterns are possible (a) partial disappearance of both alleles, (b) disappearance of the paternal allele and (c) disappearance of the maternal allele. The two last patterns are interpreted as indicative of sampling a monoclonal cell population, whereas the first indicates polyclonality.

The clonal nature of colonic precancer (adenoma) was originally suggested by an X chromosome marker. Polyps consistently had either the paternal or the maternal X chromosome inactivated (Fearon *et al*, 1987). But these early results could not exclude the possibility that the adenomas were derived from crypts with identical X chromosome inactivation (Griffiths *et al*, 1988). Subsequent studies have with increasing likelihood demonstrated that this, indeed, seems to be the case. One patient with X0/XY mosaicism (estimated to occur by chance in 1 out of 100 million people), also had familial adenomatous polyposis (Novelli *et al*, 1996). Normal crypts were either X0 or XY. The patient's colon was studded by tubular adenomas, either monocryptic or slightly larger "microadenomas". The first variety was monoclonal, but the second scored polyclonal in excess of what could be statistically expected, suggesting a field effect possibly with symbiosis between adjacent originally monoclonal adenomas.

Clonality analysis by X chromosome inactivation is beset with difficulties, mainly founded on inadequate sampling, which reflects the difficulty of identifying proper controls. One needs to exclude the artefact that monoclonality scoring reflects multiple origins from a field of cells with identical X chromosome inactivation—a condition that is hard to meet unless microdissection of normal potential target cells is meticulous. Unfortunately, virtually all published control tissue has been composed of a mixture of epithelial and stroma cells, even including lymphocytes as in the normal gut. We have no way of knowing whether a polyclonal X chromosome inactivation signal in these circumstances reflects a mixture of cells of different developmental origin or a random mixture of X inactivated potential target cells for transformation.

If significant contamination by normal cells can be excluded, the finding of polyclonality in neoplasia convincingly indicates that the population in question must have originated by malignant transformation of at least two separate cells. Recording of a monoclonal type of electrophoretic X chromosome inactivation will, on the other hand, never be equally convincing because of the possibility of derivation from a cluster of cells with identical X chromosome inactivation, the possibility of statistical coincidence caused by origin from two cells with the same paternal or maternal X inactivation or the possibility that selection of one clone from an original mixture of several transformed clones had taken place before the time of sampling. This will be further discussed in connection with cervical cancer, where precursors were found to score either as clonal or poly-clonal cell populations.

No direct genetic link seems to have been proven between individual adenomas and cancer in the colorectum. The possibility remains that precancer (adenoma) develops independently, governed by its particular set of mutations, and that adenocarcinoma may develop de novo from a normal cell lineage, which has developed another set of mutations before malignant transformation. That set may never have forced cells to evolve the phenotype of adenoma-precancer cells.

There have been recent studies where clonality was based on somatic marker mutations rather than X chromosome inactivation. For skin and cervix a few cases with direct genetic linkage between synchronous dysplasia, in situ and invasive cancer have been established (Pontén, 1996; Ren *et al*, 1997), but the issue is not yet settled. Detailed discussion will be found in the chapters on specific precancers.

From a practical point of view it will only be meaningful to eradicate individual precancers if such lesions are known precursors of invasive cancer and not separate neoplastic lesions that arise as parallel phenomena. The extent to which invasive cancers arise without visible precursors still remains to be elucidated.

Precancer and Hypermutability

The concept of hypermutability has its root in microbiology, where it is rather straightforward to establish a "mutator phenotype". Increased formation of colonies in suitable selective media measures a mutation frequency above background. Mutations can be analysed at the level of the individual base pair. Analogous in vitro methods are of only limited value for animal cells. Normal cells are generally unsuitable, because plating efficiency is too low. They will also be heterogeneous with respect to number of divisions remaining until the Hayflick senescence limit is reached (Hayflick and Moorehead, 1961; Hayflick, 1965) and thus carry an unknown number of chromosome lesions and point mutations. In such circumstances cells may be unable to form a colony even if the index mutation has occurred. For these reasons most research has been based on established lines with high plating efficiency and endless capacity for proliferation. But such results may not be trustworthy or possible to generalize from, because the cells do not possess normal genotypes and could easily have unidentified defects in DNA repair. Use of diploid lymphoblastoid lines may provide a solution to estimating background mutation rate in normal human cells (Chen and Thilly, 1996), but the method has not yet been widely used.

Genetic Instability in Human Cancer Cells

The usual starting point has been analysis of cell populations from longstanding cancers, where, as techniques have become increasingly sensitive, there have been striking instances of a multitude of alterations at all levels of genetic analysis.

Thanks to monumental work by Mitelman and collaborators a catalogue (Mitelman, 1994; Mertens et al, 1997) of karyotypic abnormalities in human cancer exists, which abundantly shows how common various forms of heteroploidy are and how vast the heterogeneity found particularly in epithelial cancers of non-endocrine origin on a background of non-random development of karyotypic stem lines (Mertens et al, 1997; Mitelman et al, 1997). Mechanisms behind aneuploidization, which according to old data may be preceded by tetraploidization, are not well understood, but a host of possibilities have been supported, such as mutations in genes that control spindle formation and function of centromeres, leading to non-disjunction. Reduction of telomeric length has been suggested, since this would create unstable chromosomes (Wright and Shay, 1992; Shay and Wright, 1996; Engelhardt et al, 1997). Other possibilities include defunct cell cycle checkpoints in either G_1 or G_2 or a disturbed stoichiometry among histones (Holliday, 1989; see also Holliday, 1996; Harley and Sherwood, 1997).

By use of two dimensional electrophoretic analysis of DNA fragments obtained after digestion with restriction enzymes an overall picture of deviations from the normal may be obtained. Cancer tissue has then shown a multitude of aberrantly sized fragments that can only be explained by presence of numerous mutations (Hovig et al, 1992, 1993; Verwest et al, 1994). Normal tissue, on the other hand, will show no significant deviations from a "standard" human profile.

Taken at face value, these results suggest that the number of mutations including structural chromosome changes, in many cancer cell populations could run into the hundreds or even thousands. There are caveats, however. Mitelman's group has interpreted its findings of a large number of "clonal" karyotypes to indicate that epithelial cancers are of polyclonal origin (Gorunova et al, 1995a,b; Pandis et al, 1995). In that case analysis of large populations of cancer cells may reflect different sets of genetic lesions in parallel cancer lineages rather than genetic instability in each. It cannot, furthermore, be excluded that large global findings of a multitude of base changes in a population of cancer cells at least partly reflect heterogeneity caused by "senescence" in neoplastic and/or normal cells known to be accompanied by aneuploidy (Saksela and Moorehead, 1963). Conclusions about genetic instability based solely on genetic heterogeneity in a large cancer cell population may be spurious. It would be important to find ways to specifically analyse stem cells known to be on the lineage path to precancer or cancer (Figs. 1 and 2) in order to settle this controversial issue.

Results from all types of cancer have not been equally clear-cut. Many leukaemias, lymphomas and sarcomas, particularly of high differentiation, do not show heteroploidy (Mertens *et al*, 1997; Mitelman *et al*, 1997). The same seems to be true for well differentiated endocrine neoplasms, such as carcinoids of the gut and thyroid carcinoma. There do not seem to be sufficient data on restriction fragment length polymorphism to permit conclusions about the overall numbers of point mutations in these subcategories of cancer.

Numerical Estimates of Mutation Frequencies in Human Cells

Since no direct way of determination of mutation frequency in vivo is at hand, one has to rely on uncertain indirect estimates.

There are still large gaps in our understanding of DNA synthesis and repair, but an outline that agrees with most data for eukaryotic cells from higher animals including humans may be presented as a framework for discussion and hypotheses. It will no doubt be changed and refined in the future.

Cells resting in G_0 or moving forward in G_1 are subject to spontaneous base alterations, including depurination, hydrolytic deamination, oxidation and methylation (Lindahl, 1993). These are repaired predominantly by a base excision repair pathway, which is considered efficient enough to leave few if any base changes behind, even if speculations to the contrary have been voiced (Bridges, 1996). The rate of base changes will be strongly elevated by several insults, of which mutagenic chemicals, reactive oxygen radicals and UV light deserve most attention from a precarcinogenetic point of view. The base excision repair pathway is then aided by a nucleotide excision repair (NER) system, that is particularly important for lesions that cause more serious distortion of DNA than for instance depurination, and a mismatch repair system (MMR), which takes care of larger lesions, mainly heteroduplexes. Cyclobutane pyrimidines and 6-4 pyrimidine-pyrimidones after UV require NER to be mended (Sancar, 1994), as do bulky DNA adducts caused for instance by benzopyrene (in tobacco smoke) and cisplatin. Methylated bases, including the commonly occurring O^6–methylguanine induced by alkylating agents, may use MMR (Karran and Hampson, 1996).

An inevitable drawback of NER is that it fails to distinguish between the correct DNA strand and the strand carrying the single base pair alteration that caused the mismatch. This will by chance in up to 50% of instances result in misincorporation in the correct strand and thus a permanent mutation instead of proper repair. NER in human cells is not completely understood. A 27–29 unit long oligonucleotide is excised, including the damaged bases, and replaced by the correct bases. It requires at least 17 polypeptides, including those that are mutated in the different types of xeroderma pigmentosum (XP).

NER is triggered partly by interrupted transcription, which explains preferential repair of the transcribed strand (Hanawalt, 1994). Even within transcribed genes those parts not predestined to become hot spots are preferentially repaired (Tornaletti and Pfeifer, 1994).

MMR is under control of at least 4 different genes in the human. These are all of suppressor type ie only after homozygous incapacity will microsatellite instability ensue (Jiricny, 1996).

G_0/G_1 will have to be sufficiently long to permit repair to be finished after a burst of base damage. *TP53* retards G_1 after primary DNA damage. This will prevent fixation of mutations arising from replication of mutated single strand DNA (Lane, 1992).

It is not certainly known how many base pair changes a normal cell is burdened with at the end of G_1, but this number should be a reflection of the length of G_1. In untouched stem cells on lineages towards malignant transformation, with their slow rate of multiplication this number may approach zero in view of the efficiency with which base, nucleotide and mismatch excision repair pathways are presumed to operate. If, on the other hand, the rate of damage is increased by orders of magnitude, for instance in UV exposed epidermis, numbers of changed base pairs become templates for DNA polymerases during S phase. Particularly if repair is defunct, this number becomes very large, as dramatically shown in XP, where even such a tiny fraction of the genome as a few exons of *TP53* showed abundant missense mutations (Williams *et al*, in press).

During S phase any remaining misincorporated base pairs or other nucleotide alteration is copied and transmitted to one daughter cell as a permanent mutation. Additional mutations are created because of imperfections in the DNA synthesis machinery centred around five DNA polymerases and a number of accessory proteins. The resultant of two opposite forces will determine the final number of misincorporated bases, which will show up as mutations in G_2 and subsequent cell generations. This number is believed to form the major determinant of the spontaneous mutation rate. During extension of the nucleotide chain, insertion of the correct base has an estimated likelihood of about 10^5 compared with misincorporation. If this was not counteracted, each round of DNA synthesis would generate 60 000 base pair changes. But excision by $3'-5'$ exonucleases will remove misincorporations and thus reduce error frequency. The efficiency of this proofreading is not accurately known, but it cannot be expected to eliminate all misincorporated bases, as suggested by the observed spontaneous mutation rate of about 10^{-7} in human B cells (Keohavong and Thilly, 1989; Cha *et al*, 1992; Chen and Thilly, 1996).

The second type of error introduced during S phase derives from the tendency to create mismatches, particularly of repeated nucleotide sequences, where so called slippage will increase or decrease the number of repeats. This need not have any functional consequences because most repeats are found outside of genes and other functionally important parts of DNA. Those few repeats found in introns are, however, a potential risk, because slippage here would easily create frameshift mutations with dire consequences. The importance of creation of repeats (microsatellites) is profoundly discussed elsewhere in this issue by Shibata. Mutations of MMR genes may create hundreds or even thousands of abnormal length repeats.

Not much is known about mutations and their repair in G_2. It seems reasonable to assume that the same mechanisms as in G_0/G_1 have a role also here.

Mitosis—the next phase of the cell cycle—is prone to mistakes, but the error rate has not been determined (Meeks-Wagner and Hartwell, 1986). Endomitosis, non-disjunction, sister chromatid exchanges, other types of recombinations and deletions (LOH) have been observed in normal cells (see Heim and Mitelman, 1995). There is also suggestive evidence from DNA measurements of instances of unequal distribution of DNA at mitosis (Widell *et al*, 1993; Macieira Coelho and Puvion Dutilleul, 1985). Since such gross effects will result from any chromosomal rearrangement, most mistakes can be expected to result in non-viable progeny. Certain abnormalities will, however, be stable and could at least theoretically become part of a precancerous genotype.

For unclear reasons certain chromosome configurations are unstable in the sense that continuous creation of new karyotypes takes place from which there will often be a selection of stem lines with reduced heterogeneity (Holliday, 1989). Such instability is a hallmark particularly of the bulk of epithelial cancers, where it has been regarded as more important than accumulation of point mutations for creation and maintenance of the malignant phenotype (Cairns, 1975).

Chromosomal instability has repeatedly been associated with progression of precancer to cancer. Direct observation of karyotypes suffers from a quantitative problem of collecting enough metaphases. This method also has to resort to short term cultivation with built in problems of selection (Mitelman, 1995). More extensive data have arisen from cytophotometrical measurements of nuclear DNA content, which in the most penetrating studies have been combined with time lapse filming. For established cancer cell lines rapid restoration of heteroploidy with large intercellular differences between individual cells could be established. It was not possible to isolate stable clones, heteroploidy being recreated as the cells multiplied (Killander, 1965). Similar observations of precancer or dysplastic cells with their nuclear atypia could be rewarding.

It has not been possible to arrive at a firm estimate of the average number of changed base pairs and other genomic lesions that physiologically and inevitably are consequences of each cell cycle. This is in spite of rapidly increasing insight into molecular aspects of DNA damage and its repair. This number will almost certainly vary, but for any understanding of the road to precancer and cancer it would be particularly valuable to have an estimate for stem cells on a lineage towards malignant transformation (Fig. 1).

It is well established that the diploid human genome has 6×10^9 bp. About 10% of these (6×10^8) are genes, ie they are transcribed. The total number of alleles has been variously estimated, and 2×10^5 will be used here. This gives $6 \times 10^8/2 \times 10^5 = 3 \times 10^3$ bp as an average size of an allele. Two thirds of these may constitute introns, giving 1 kb as the average size of the translated exons per allele. Hence, $10^3 \times 2 \times 10^5 = 2 \times 10^8$ bp suffice to encode all exons. The remaining base pairs are partly repeats and partly perform functions as promoters, enhancers and so on. The number of base pairs that do not participate in any function is unknown, but they form an important platform for neutral mutations. As a basis for subsequent calculations 50×10^8 bp are assumed to serve no function. The result is that 60×10^8 bp are divided into three major classes: (a) exon coding 2×10^8; (b) other functions 8×10^8; and (c) no function 50×10^8. By definition mutations in (c) are neutral, whereas mutations in (a) or (b) are neutral or of positive or negative selective value. All in (a) and (b) have phenotypic effects.

Imperfect DNA polymerase function seems to be the major conveyor of base pair errors to daughter genomes. The intricacies of the fidelity by which DNA synthesis is carried out are still to a large extent unknown. Estimates centre around an error rate of 10^{-5} (Keohavong and Thilly, 1989), which may vary considerably depending on such factors as alternate use of different polymerases, imbalance within dNTP pools and availability of accessory proteins (for review see Minnick and Kunkel, 1996). Then $10^{-5} \times 6 \times 10^9 = 60\,000$ bp would be permanently altered at each round of DNA synthesis. They are divided into three classes: exons 2000 bp, other functions 8000 bp, no function 50 000 bp. This is a maximum figure, and speculatively DNA repair could reduce it by two orders of magnitude, in which case 20, 80 and 500 bp, respectively, would be mutated.

Table 1 summarizes forecasts of the mutational load. The minimum number of fixed bp changes corresponds to a mutation rate of 5×10^{-5} computed as functional changes per allele. This figure is about 100 times higher than Knudson's figure for neuroblastoma (Hethcote and Knudson, 1978). In view of the uncertainties in both the current and Knudson's estimates this is not inexplicable. A substantial proportion of the "mutations" in retinoblastoma are severe chromosome rearrangements (Cavenee *et al*, 1985; see also Heim and Mitelman, 1995). These are expected to be less common than base pair misincorporations. The calculations in Table 1 do not take selective advantage into

TABLE 1. Estimates of average mutation rates for three categories of human DNA. See text for explanation of categorization and enumeration of alleles and rationale behind calculation of minimal and maximal values.

Type of DNA	Altered bp[a]	No. mutations[b]	Mutation rate[c]
Exons	20–2000	10–1000	$5 \times 10^{-5} - 5 \times 10^c$
Other functions	80–8000	80–8000	$4 \times 10^{-4} - 0.4$
Neutral	500–50 000		
Total	600–60 000	90–9000	

[a] Computed per round of DNA synthesis
[b] Only 50% of bp changes predicted to give a significant functional disturbance
[c] Computed from $2 \times 100\,000$ alleles/human genome

consideration, whereas the *RB* mutations, to have a visible phenotypic effect, necessarily have to permit clonal expansion after malignant transformation. The calculations in Table 1 may be way off in terms of guesses about efficiency of repair.

It is not improbable that the human genome, because of physiological and biochemically unavoidable imperfections in synthesis and repair of DNA, endures a high load of mutagenic base pair changes. Their prevalence in lineages leading to precancer and cancer will vary from case to case, depending on the selective value of the respective mutations. Lethal mutations would at any stage interrupt a lineage. But neutral base pair alterations would accumulate at each cell cycle. In one example shown in Fig. 2, 4000 rounds of DNA synthesis in epidermal stem cells could be expected to result in between 2×10^6 and 2×10^8 changed base pairs without any impact on the cell phenotype at the age of 55. The latter figure corresponds to 4% of all "functionless" base pairs at risk.

If a heavy genetic load suggested in Table 1 is created per somatic cell, it comes as no surprise that, for instance, old skin shows many signs of profound pathology, such as focal hyperpigmentation, depigmentation, basal cell papillomas, senile lentigo, atrophy and some precancers (melanoma-in-situ, squamous cell dysplasia). This is particularly true after exposure to ultraviolet (UV) light, which may increase the number of mutations by one to several orders of magnitude.

That human cells are able to sustain heavy loads of mutations is suggested by findings in xeroderma pigmentosum (XP). In a case of XP, subgroup C, studied by Williams *et al*, in press, 29 different mutations were found in exons 5–8 of *TP53*. This corresponded to an amazing 17% of all possible UV characteristic Py-Py mutations of the non-transcribed strand. To become detectable the mutations, virtually all missense, had to be accompanied by selective clonal cell expansion. They were also clustered at known hotspots. By extrapolation, and since there is no reason to assume any particular hypersensitivity to UV in the *TP53* gene, the conclusion is that each average allele must have suffered a number of mutations. The dynamics of this striking scenario is not understood, but the findings support that the human somatic genome is able to sustain a substantial number of point mutations.

Is a Precancer Lineage Characterized by Hypermutability?

This difficult question has never been approached directly. Indirect evidence is, however, provided by analysis of aneuploidy in precancer, mainly in colon, cervix and lung. The most extensive data come from cytometrical measurements of DNA content in adenoma, dysplasia and adenocarcinoma-in-situ of the colorectum. The overall picture has been rather consistent. Normal mucosa surrounding neoplastic lesions is diploid. A large majority of adenomas have near diploid profiles (Quirke *et al*, 1986; Giaretti *et al*, 1988; Enblad and Glimelius, 1989). With increasing degree of dysplasia the proportion of aneuploid nuclei increased (Goh and Jass, 1986; Petrova *et al*, 1986; Saraga *et al*, 1997). Aneuploidy was more prevalent, together with villous rather than tubular morphology (van den Ingh *et al*, 1985). About 80% of invasive cancers were DNA aneuploid (Enblad *et al*, 1985; Giaretti and Santi, 1990).

A sequence of changes has been proposed from an early start with development of nuclei with near diploid (particularly hypodiploid) DNA content, followed by tetraploidization, followed by subtetraploid aneuploidy (Giaretti, 1994), where aneuploidization roughly coincides with appearance of severe dysplasia. Individual departures from this scheme are considerable.

One attempt has been made to bring rough measurements of DNA content into cell biological context (Mulder *et al*, 1992). Computerized quantitative image analysis of nuclei in colorectal tumours confirmed the time honored cytopathological observation that nuclear "atypia" increases with progression along the adenoma→invasive cancer axis. There was no correlation, however, between *RAS* mutations and allelic loss on 5q, 18q and 17p either alone or in combination with nuclear texture (atypia). The important implication by this finding is that genetic alterations, generally considered "hits" responsible for creation of the malignant phenotype (Fearon and Vogelstein, 1990; Vogelstein and Kinzler, 1993; Fearon, 1997), could not explain the individual characteristics of atypia, ie one diagnostic hallmark of malignancy. A dose–response relation was, however, suggested between certain atypical morphological features and number of genetic "hits".

In all essential respects results from cervical and bronchial cancer are compatible with the scheme provided by colorectal cancer (Kashyap *et al*, 1990; Steinbeck *et al*, 1995; Smith *et al*, 1996). The same also seems to be true for experimentally induced skin cancer in the mouse (Aldaz *et al*, 1987).

The conclusion would be that there is no proof that genetic instability/hypermutability is required for the development of precancer. Many precancers, such as adenomas in endocrine glands or the gut, do not show the conspicuous genetic or chromosomal heterogeneity quoted as the major argument for genetic instability. Whether transition to invasive cancer is preceded or even caused by acquisition of genetic instability is unresolved, although this is suggested by development of heteroploidy and considerable alterations of restriction fragment lengths at least in the majority of human cancer types. Careful analysis of clonally related precancers and cancers would stand a good chance of illuminating this dark but important corner of tumour biology. Lineages of non-transformed cells with comparable lengths to transformed ones have to be analysed genetically to provide a reliable estimate of mutability. This has to be done on a single cell basis, and pooling of many lineages will randomly dilute any mutations only found in one lineage. Polymerase chain reaction analysis of single microdissected cells was recently introduced (Pontén *et al*, 1997) for *TP53* and may be further developed to cover many potential sites of mutations.

Is Precancer Reversible?

Dysplasia and carcinoma-in-situ are characterized by cytological atypia. In at least a proportion of cases genomic alterations have been noted, ranging from abnormal amounts of DNA via chromosome aberrations to defined mutations. Against such a background it would not be unreasonable to assume that the population of precancerous cells is "transformed" to irreversible commitment to continued net increase. But there exists good evidence that a proportion of pre-cancers are reversible. In the case of cervical cancer the much higher incidence of carcinoma-in-situ than of invasive cancer cannot be explained unless one accepts that a proportion of the former will never appear as invasive cancers (Gustafsson and Adami, 1989; van Oortmarssen and Habbema, 1991). Statistical-epidemiological evidence has been supported by direct observation of regression without intervention (Kottmeier, 1955; Nasiell *et al*, 1983). The likelihood of spontaneous regression has been conservatively estimated at about 30% (Koss, 1993), but other estimates have landed at 80% (Gustafsson and Adami, 1989).

The principal tumour biological significance of regression in cervical cancer can be questioned, mainly because unusual immunological responses could be expected in view of the common involvement of papillomavirus (zur Hausen, 1988), but also in skin cancer there is evidence for spontaneous regression. About 25% of dysplasias disappeared during continuous observation (Marks *et al*, 1986). Reversibility was also demonstrated in bronchial cell atypia (Auer *et al*, 1982).

The mechanism by which regression is instigated has hardly been studied apart from vague speculations about immunity and increased apoptosis (Cole, 1976; Firminger, 1976). Its cellular biology may, however, be very important to elucidate, particularly since an absolute difference may exist to invasive cancer, where spontaneous regression is extremely rare if it exists at all (Challis and Stam, 1990).

Existence of reversibility in precancer shows furthermore that early hits on a lineage to cancer can give phenotypic effects in the form of atypia but that these hits need to be followed by a decisive last hit to prevent regression and accomplish malignant transformation. Attempts to distinguish between precancer likely to progress or regress are discussed in the chapter by Pontén and Guo.

Can Precancer Be Epigenetic?

Experimental carcinogenesis in rat liver has revealed a rather clear sequence of events (Farber, 1976). The main difficulty has been to construct a system where non-specific influence of toxicity and reactive cell proliferation can be avoided or at least controlled. On a morphological level it seems by now well established that the initiation–promotion path towards cancer after application of a variety of chemical carcinogens begins with multiple focal hepatocellular changes. These foci will then, after a phase of mitotic inhibition, rather synchronously begin to show increased rates of cell division. A few will later show cellular dysplasia and grow expansively as "adenomas". At some stage a minority of these foci will transform into rapidly growing nodules considered in-situ cancers, because of their high probability of further development into invasive hepatocellular cancer.

Application of the current dogma that cancer arises via sequential addition of somatic genetic changes and selection would explain this as a result of original mutations in a large number of stem cells, which then would acquire additional mutations until a few of them by chance had accumulated a set that caused malignant transformation and selection as hepatocellular carcinomas. Precancer would take up an intermediate position with rather few mutations, which, however, would have distinct phenotypic consequences.

This view has been challenged. It has been observed that the earliest foci are characterized by metabolic alterations explicable by increased local exposure (or sensitivity) to insulin which, in turn, would lead to abnormal glycogen metabolism partly involving mitochondrial systems. Similar foci are produced in a variety of ways, including intrahepatic transplantation of Langerhans islets, hepatitis virus and chemicals, which cannot be expected to cause an identical initial causative mutation (Bannasch, 1988). It has therefore been suggested that irreversible epigenetic mechanisms akin to forces driving embryonic development are active (Bannasch *et al*, in press; Kopp-Schneider *et al*, in press). Attempts to search for *RAS* mutations and other oncogenes/suppressor genes have yielded only negative results in the early histochemically detected foci.

Epigenetic mechanisms are responsible for essentially irreversible well ordered embryonic development with appearance of "new" phenotypes. The speculation is that similar mechanisms may, in reverse, by dedifferentiation, create foci of cells that now have acquired a low but definite likelihood of undergoing progression, possibly because unknown promoters are acting on a phenotype hypersensitive to malignant transformation. The challenge to the somatic genetic dogma of carcinogenesis has been given a general formulation (Prehn, 1994).

OVERVIEW

The field of precancer has been and still is plagued by ambiguous terminology and confusion about definitions of precursors of invasive cancer. This chapter presents a cell and tumour biological approach based on the idea that precancer, in conformity with cancer, should be understood as a result of a chain of mutations (the term being taken in a wide sense and possibly mixed with irreversible epigenetic changes) affecting an uninterrupted cell lineage. The phenotypic consequences of this genotypic progression will vary from case to case and type to type of cancer. In some instances exemplified by endocrine and neuroendocrine tumours, mutations en route to malignant transformation may change the phenotype predictably from hyperplasia to adenoma to carcinoma-in-situ to invasive cancer. The other extreme is exemplified by retinoblastoma, basal cell cancer and probably also some forms of lymphoma/leukaemia, where only the final mutation will lead to a phenotypic change in the form of cancer. The vast majority of precancers/cancers are intermediate. Some will develop via recognizable forms of dysplasia and/or in-situ cancer, others will appear without any traces of precursors. Current evidence indicates a stochastic process by which crucial mutations/chromosomal rearrangements are added to the genotype. These mutations are drawn from several hundred oncogenes/suppressor genes. The mutational spectrum and the specifically involved oncogenes/suppressor genes, together with the additional effect of mutations in non-oncogenic genes, will fashion a phenotype that may be unique. Inherent in such a unique genotype lineage is a possibility that all essential features determining subsequent clinical malignancy are laid down in the precancer and held in abeyance until the final hit that causes invasive growth. Such clandestine hits may determine degree of differentiation, amplification of oncogenes, capacity for invading vessels and so on. Other genotypes in precancer may not have a stable selective advantage, for example because telomere shortening is not stopped or self renewal of stem cells is insufficient and will therefore die out and score as regressors. Determinants of malignant transformation are summarized in Table 2.

Genetic links have usually not been established between precancers and invasive cancers. Formal evidence for direct transition is thus generally lacking, but circumstantial morphological and epidemiological evidence supports the time honoured notion that precancers develop into cancer via selection of fit

TABLE 2. Genetic determinants of malignant transformation

Rate of transforming mutations per round of DNA synthesis	This is a function of total rate of mutations (background + actively acquired). The frequency is increased by deficient repair, decreased fidelity of DNA synthesis and exposure to mutagens
No. of DNA rounds in the lineage which ends in transformation	This will vary between a few hundred and several thousands depending on the tissue
No. of lineages susceptible to transformation	This number reflects number of stem cells. It will vary widely within an individual depending on embryological development of the respective types of cells
Time of mutation	Mutations in a lineage possessing symmetrical stem cell divisions will affect more progeny than mutations in lineages with only asymmetric divisions
Effects of competing mutations	Mutations outside oncogenes and suppressor genes outnumber transforming mutations by a wide margin. Sublethal/lethal mutations may indirectly give a transforming lineage selective advantage
Phenotype of lineage	Certain cell types require fewer hits than others
Species derivation of target lineages	Human cells are more resistant to malignant transformation than murine cells after an equal number of externally inflicted mutations

[a]Mutation = genetic change with significant impact on encoded protein. Transforming mutation = mutation, which in combination with other transforming mutations, causes transformation to precancer or cancer. Genes subject to transforming mutations are either oncogenes or suppressor genes

genotypes. Elimination of precancer will prevent cancer only if it indeed can be proven that cancer develops from the same lineage as precancer.

Existence of hypermutability in precancer has never been substantiated except in colonic adenomas in the mismatch repair deficiency syndrome. If hypermutability (genetic instability) is functionally important it may be so only after malignant transformation, and then not as a regular or necessary trait.

References

Abercrombie M and Heaysman JEM (1976) Invasive behavior between sarcoma and fibroblast populations in cell culture. *Journal of the National Cancer Institute* **56** 561-570

Aldaz CM, Conti CJ, Klein Szanto AJ and Slaga TJ (1987) Progressive dysplasia and aneuploidy are hallmarks of mouse skin papillomas: relevance to malignancy. *Proceedings of the National Academy of Sciences of the USA* **84** 2029–2032

Almasan A, Linke S, Paulson T, Huang L-C and Wahl G (1995) Genetic instability as a consequence of inappropriate entry into and progression through S phase. *Cancer and Metastasis Reviews* **14** 59–73

Armitage P and Doll R (1954) The age distribution of cancer and a multistage theory of carcinogenesis. *British Journal of Cancer* **8** 1–12

Auer G, Ono J, Nasiell M *et al* (1982) Reversibility of bronchial atypia. *Cancer Research* **42** 4241–4247

Bannasch P (1988) In: Iversen OH (ed). *Theories of Carcinogenesis*, Hemishere Publishing Corporation, Washington, DC

Bannasch P, Klimek F and Mayer D (1997) Early bioenergetic changes in hepato carcinogenesis: Preneoplastic phenotypes mimic responses to insulin and thyroid hormone. *Journal of Bioenergetics and Biomembranes* **29** 303–313

Barker BE and Sanford KK (1970) Cytologic manifestations of neoplastic transformation *in vitro*. *Journal of the National Cancer Institute* **44** 39–63

Bokor P and DiNardo S (1996) The roles of hedgehog, wingless and lines in patterning the dorsal epidermis in Drosophila. *Development* **122** 1083–1092

Bridges BA (1996) Mutation in resting cells: the role of endogenous DNA damage. *Cancer Surveys* **28** 155–167

Cairns J (1975) Mutation selection and the natural history of cancer. *Nature* **255** 197–200

Cavenee W, Hansen M, Nordenskjold M *et al* (1985) Genetic origin of mutations predisposing to retinoblastoma. *Science* **228** 501–503

Cha RS, Zarbl H, Keohavong P *et al* (1992) Mismatch amplification mutation assay (MAMA): application to the *c-H-ras* gene. *PCR Methods Applications* **2** 14–20

Challis GB and Stam HJ (1990) The spontaneous regression of cancer: a review of cases from 1900 to 1987. *Acta Oncologica* **29** 545–550

Chen J and Thilly WG (1996) Mutational spectra vary with exposure conditions: benzo[a]pyrene in human cells. *Mutation Research* **357** 209–217

Cole WH (1976) Relationship of causative factors in spontaneous regression of cancer to immunologic factors possibly effective in cancer. *Journal of Surgical Oncology* **8** 391–411

Cooper GM (1992) Oncogenes as markers for early detection of cancer. *Journal of Cellular Biochemistry* (**Supplement 16G**) 131–136

Damane N, Lee J, Robins P *et al* (1997) Activation of the transcription factor Gli1 and the Sonic hedgehog signalling pathway in skin tumours. *Nature* **389** 876–881

Donehower LA (1997) Genetic instability in animal tumorigenesis models. *Cancer Surveys* **29** 329–352

Draper G, Sanders B and Kingston J (1986) Second primary neoplasms in patients with retinoblastoma. *British Journal of Cancer* **53** 661–671

Ekbom A, Trichopoulos D, Adami H-O *et al* (1992) Evidence of prenatal influence on breast cancer risk. *Lancet* **340** 1015–1018

Ellegren H and Fridolfsson A-K (1997) Male-driven evolution of DNA sequences in birds. *Nature Genetics* **17** 182–184

Enblad P and Glimelius B (1989) The DNA content in rectal adenomas. *Anticancer Research* **9** 749–752

Enblad P, Glimelius B, Bengtsson A *et al* (1985) DNA content in carcinoma of the rectum and rectosigmoid. *Acta Pathologica, Microbiologica et Immunologica Scandinavica* **93** 277–284

Engelhardt M, Kumar R, Albanell J *et al* (1997) Telomerase regulation, cell cycle and telomere stability in primitive hematopoietic cells. *Blood* **90** 182–93

Farber E (1976) In: Cameron DALaGPW HM (ed). *Liver Cell Cancer*, pp 243–277, Elsevier, Amsterdam

Fearon ER (1997) Human cancer syndromes: clues to the origin and nature of cancer. *Science* **278** 1043–1050

Fearon ER and Vogelstein B (1990) A genetic model for colorectal tumorigenesis. *Cell* **61** 759–767

Fearon ER, Hamilton SR and Vogelstein B (1987) Clonal analysis of human colorectal tumors. *Science* **238** 193–197

Fialkow PJ (1976) Clonal origin of human tumors. *Biochimica et Biophysica Acta* **458** 283–321

Firminger HI (1976) A pathologist looks at spontaneous regression of cancer. *National Cancer Institute Monographs* **44** 15–8

Gailani MR and Bale AE (1997) Developmental genes and cancer: role of patched in basal cell carcinoma of the skin. *Journal of the National Cancer Institute* **89** 1103–1108

Gailani MR, Leffell DJ, Ziegler A *et al* (1996) Relationship between sunlight exposure and a key genetic alteration in basal cell carcinoma. *Journal of the National Cancer Institute* **88** 349–354

Giaretti W (1994) A model of DNA aneuploidization and evolution in colorectal cancer. *Laboratory Investigation* **71** 904–910

Giaretti W and Santi L (1990) Tumor progression by DNA flow cytometry in human colorectal cancer. *International Journal of Cancer* **45** 597–603

Giaretti W, Sciallero S, Bruno S *et al* (1988) DNA flow cytometry of endoscopically examined colorectal adenomas and adenocarcinomas. *Cytometry* **9** 238–244

Goh HS and Jass JR (1986) DNA content and the adenoma-carcinoma sequence in the colorectum. *Journal of Clinical Pathology* **39** 387–392

Goodrich LV, Johnson RL, Milenkovic L *et al* (1996) Conservation of the hedgehog/patched signaling pathway from flies to mice: induction of a mousepatched gene by Hedgehog. *Genes and Development* **10** 301–312

Gorunova L, Johansson B, Dawiskiba S *et al* (1995a) Massive cytogenetic heterogeneity in a pancreatic carcinoma: fifty-four karyotypically unrelated clones. *Genes Chromosomes and Cancer* **14** 259–266

Gorunova L, Johansson B, Dawiskiba S *et al* (1995b) Cytogenetically detected clonal heterogeneity in a duodenal adenocarcinoma. *Cancer Genetics and Cytogenetics* **82** 146–150

Griffiths DFR, Davies SJ, Williams D *et al* (1988) Demonstration of somatic mutation and colonic crypt clonality by X-linked enzyme histochemistry. *Nature* **333** 461–463

Gustafsson L and Adami H-O (1989) Natural history of cervical neoplasia: consistent results obtained by an identification technique. *British Journal of Cancer* **60** 132–141

Hahn H, Christiansen J, Wicking C *et al* (1996a) A mammalian patched homolog is expressed in target tissues of sonic hedgehog and maps to a region associated with developmental abnormalities. *Journal of Biological Chemistry* **271** 12125–12128

Hahn H, Wiking C, Zaphiropoulos PG *et al* (1996b) Mutations of the human homolog of *Drosophila patched* in the nevoid basal cell carcinoma syndrome. *Cell* **85** 841–851

Hanawalt PC (1994) Transcription-coupled repair and human disease. *Nature* **266** 1957–1958

Harley C and Sherwood SW (1997) Telomerase, checkpoints and cancer. *Cancer Surveys* **29** 263–284

Hayflick L (1965) The limited in vitro lifetime of human diploid cell strains. *Experimental Cell Research* **37** 614–636

Hayflick L and Moorehead P (1961) The serial cultivation of human diploid cell strains. *Experimental Cell Research* **25** 585–621

Heim S and Mitelman F. (1995) *Cancer Cytogenetics, Chromosomal and Molecular Genetic Aberrations of Tumor Cells*, Wiley-Liss, New York

Hendrich BD and Willard HF (1995) Epigenetic regulation of gene expression: the effect of altered chromatin structure from yeast to mammals. *Human Molecular Genetics* **4** 1765–1777

Hethcote HW and Knudson Jr AG (1978) Model for the incidence of embryonal cancers: application to retinoblastoma. *Proceedings of the National Academy of Sciences of the USA* **75** 2453–2457

Holliday R (1989) Chromosome error propagation and cancer. *Trends in Genetics* **5** 42–45

Holliday R (1996) Neoplastic transformation: the contrasting stability of human and mouse cells. *Cancer Surveys* **28** 103–115

Hovig E, Smith Sorensen B, Uitterlinden AG *et al* (1992) Detection of DNA variation in cancer. *Pharmacogenetics* **2** 317–328

Hovig E, Mullaart E, Borresen AL *et al* (1993) Genome scanning of human breast carcinomas using micro- and minisatellite core probes. *Genomics* **17** 66–75

Hu N, Gutsmann A, Herbert D *et al* (1994) Heterozygous Rb-1 delta/+ mice are predisposed to tumors of the pituitary gland with a nearly complete penetrance. *Oncogene* **9** 1021–1027

Jacks T, Fazeli E, Schmitt E *et al* (1992) Effects of an RB mutation in the mouse. *Nature* **359** 295–300

Jiricny J (1996) Mismatch repair and cancer. *Cancer Surveys* **28** 47–68

Johansson B, Mertens F and Mitelman F (1996) Primary vs secondary neoplasia-associated chromosomal abnormalities: balanced rearrangements vs genomic imbalances? *Genes Chromosomes and Cancer* **16** 155–163

Johnson RL, Rothman AL, Xie J *et al* (1996) Human homolog of *patched,* a candidate gene for the basal cell nevus syndrome. *Science* **272** 1668–1671

Karran P and Hampson R (1996) Genomic instability and tolerance to alkylating agents. *Cancer Surveys* **28** 69–85

Kashyap V, Das DK and Luthra UK (1990) Microphotometric DNA analysis in mild and moderate dysplasia of the uterine cervix: a retrospective study. *Indian Journal of Pathology and Microbiology* **33** 30–34

Keohavong P and Thilly WG (1989) Fidelity of DNA polymerases in DNA amplification. *Proceedings of the National Academy of Sciences of the USA* **86** 9253–9257

Killander D (1965) Intercellular variations in generation time and amounts of DNA, RNA and mass in a mouse leukemia population in vitro. *Experimental Cell Research* **40** 21–31

Knudson Jr AG (1971) Mutation and cancer: statistical study of retinoblastoma. *Proceedings of the National Academy of Sciences of the USA* **68** 820–823

Knudson Jr AG (ed). (1987) *A Two-mutation Model for Human Cancer*, Raven Press, New York

Knudson Jr AG (1992) Stem cell regulation, tissue ontogeny and oncogenic events. *Cancer Biology* **3** 99–106

Kopp-Schneider A, Portier C and Bannasch P A model for hepatocarcinogenesis treating phenotypical changes in focal hepatocellular lesions as epigenetic events. *Mathematical Biosciences* (in press)

Kornfeld K (1997) Vulval development in *Caenorhabditis elegans*. *Trends in Genetics* **13** 55–61

Koss LG (1993) In: Marks PA, Türler H and Weil R (eds). *Precancerous Lesions: A Multidisciplinary Approach*, vol 1, pp 5–25, Ares-Serona Symposia Publications, Rome, Italy

Kottmeier HL (1955) Evolution et traitement des épithéliomas. *Revue francais Gynécologie* **56** 821–825

Krontiris T and Cooper G (1981) Transforming activity of human tumor DNAs. *Proceedings of the National Academy of Sciences of the USA* **78** 1181–1184

Lane DP (1992) p53, guardian of the genome. *Nature* **358** 15–16

Lindahl T (1993) Instability and decay of the primary structure of DNA.*Nature* **362** 709–715

Loeb LA (1996) Many mutations in cancers. *Cancer Surveys* **28** 329–342

Lyon MF (1972) X-chromosome inactivation and developmental patterns in mammals. *Biological Reviews* **47** 1–35

Macieira Coelho A and Puvion Dutilleul F (1985) Genome reorganization during aging of dividing cells. *Advances in Experimental Medicine and Biology* **190** 391–419

Marigo V, Scott MP, Johnson RL *et al* (1996) Conservation in hedgehog signaling: induction of a chicken patched homolog by Sonic hedgehog in the developing limb. *Development* **122** 1225–1233

Marks R, Foley P, Goodman G *et al* (1986) Spontaneous remission of solar keratoses: the case for conservative management. *British Journal of Dermatology* **115** 649–655

Meeks-Wagner D and Hartwell LH (1986) Normal stochiometry of histone dimer sets is necessary for high fidelity of mitotic chromosome transmission. *Cell* **44** 43–52

Mertens F, Johansson B, Hoglund M *et al* (1997) Chromosomal imbalance maps of malignant solid tumors: A cytogenetic survey of 3185 neoplasms. *Cancer Research* **57** 2765–2780

Michalopoulos GK and DeFrances MC (1997) Liver regeneration. *Science* **276** 60–66

Minnick DT and Kunkel TA (1996) DNA synthesis errors, mutations and cancer. *Cancer Surveys* **28** 3–20

Mitelman F (1994) *Catalog of Chromosome Aberrations in Cancer*, Wiley-Liss, New York

Mitelman F (1995) *Cancer Cytogenetics*, Wiley-Liss, New York

Mitelman F, Mertens F and Johansson B (1997) A breakpoint map of recurrent chromosomal rearrangements in human neoplasia. *Nature Genetics* 417–474

Moolgavkar SH and Venzon DJ (1979) Two-event model for carcinogenesis: incidence curves for childhood and adult tumors. *Mathematical Biosciences* **47** 55–77

Mulder J-WR, Offerhaus GJA, de Feyter EP *et al* (1992) The relationship of quantitative nuclear morphology to molecular genetic alterations in the adenoma-carcinoma sequence of the large bowel. *American Journal of Pathology* **141** 797–804

Murray M, Shilo B-Z, Shih C *et al* (1981) Three different human tumor cell lines contain different transforming genes. *Cell* **25** 355–361

Nasiell K, Nasiell M and Vaclavinkova V (1983) Behavior of moderate cervical dysplasia during long term follow-up. *Obstetrics and Gynecology* **61** 609–614

Nordling CO (1953) A new theory on the cancer-inducing mechanism. *British Journal of Cancer* **7** 68–72

Novelli MR, Williamson JA, Tomlinson IPM *et al* (1996) Polyclonal origin of colonic adenomas in an XO/XY patient with FAP. *Science* **272** 1187–1190

Pandis N, Jin Y, Gorunova L *et al* (1995) Chromosome analysis of 97 primary breast carcinomas: identification of eight karyotypic subgroups. *Genes Chromosomes and Cancer* **12** 173–185

Petrova AS, Subrichina GN, Tschistjakova OV *et al* (1986) DNA ploidy and proliferation characteristics of bowel polyps analysed by flow cytometry compared with cytology and histology. *Archiv für Geschwultzforschung* **56** 179–191

Pontén J (1971) *Spontaneous and Virus Induced Transformation in Cell Culture*, Springer-Verlag, Vienna and New York

Pontén J (1974) Carcinogenesis in vitro. *Recent Results in Cancer Research* **44** 98–102

Pontén J (1975) In: Becker FF (ed). *Cancer*, vol 4, pp 55–100, Plenum Publishing Company, New York, New York

Pontén F (1996) *Pathology*, pp 64, Uppsala University, Uppsala, Sweden

Pontén F, Williams C, Ling G *et al* (1997) Genomic analysis of single cells from human basal cell using laser-assisted capture microscopy. *Mutation Research Genomics* **382** 45–55

Potten CS (1981) Cell replacement in epidermis (keratopoiesis) via discrete units of proliferation. *International Review of Cytology* **69** 271–318

Prehn RT (1994) Cancer begets mutations *versus* mutations beget cancers. *Cancer Research* **54** 5296–5300

Quirke P, Fozard JB, Dixon MF *et al* (1986) DNA aneuploidy in colorectal adenomas. *British*

Journal of Cancer **53** 477–481

Ren Z-P, Ahmadian A, Pontén F *et al* (1997) Benign clonal keratinocyte patches with p53 mutations show no genetic link to synchronous squamous cell precancer or cancer in human skin. *American Journal of Pathology* **150** 1791–1803

Reznikoff C, Belair C, Savelieva E *et al* (1994) Long-term genome stability and minimal genotypic and phenotypic alterations in HPV16 E7- but not E6-immortalized human uroepithelial cells. *Genes and Development* **8** 2227–2240

Saksela E and Moorehead P (1963) Aneuploidy in the degenerative phase of serial cultivation of human cell strains. *Journal of the National Cancer Institute* **41** 390–395

Sancar A (1994) Mechanisms of DNA excision repair. *Nature* **266** 1954–1956

Sanford KK, Barker BE, Parshad R *et al* (1970) Neoplastic conversion in vitro of mouse cells: cytologic, chromosomal, enzymatic, glycolytic and growth properties. *Journal of the National Cancer Institute* **45** 1071–1096

Saraga E, Bautista D, Dorta G *et al* (1997) Genetic heterogeneity in sporadic colorectal adenomas. *Journal of Pathology* **181** 281–286

Shay JW and Wright WE (1996) Telomerase activity in human cancer. *Current Opinion in Oncology* **8** 66–71

Smith AL, Hung J, Walker L *et al* (1996) Extensive areas of aneuploidy are present in the respiratory epithelium of lung cancer patients. *British Journal of Cancer* **73** 203–209

Sommer RJ (1997) Evolution and development—the nematode vulva as a case study. *Bioessays* **19** 225–231

Steinbeck RG, Heselmeyer KM, Moberger HB *et al* (1995) The relationship between proliferating cell nuclear antigen (PCNA), nuclear DNA content and mutant p53 during genesis of cervical carcinoma. *Acta Oncologica* **34** 171–176

Tabata T and Kornberg TB (1994) Hedgehog is a signaling protein with a key role in patterning *Drosophila* imaginal discs. *Cell* **76** 89–102

Tomlinson IPM, Novelli MR and Bodmer WF (1996) The mutation rate and cancer. *Proceedings of the National Academy of Sciences of the USA* **93** 14800–14803

Tornaletti S and Pfeifer GP (1994) Slow repair of pyrimidine dimers at p53 mutation hotspots in skin cancer. *Science* **263** 1436–1438

Undén A, Holmberg E, Lundh-Rozell B *et al* (1996) Mutations in the human homolog of the *Drosophila patched* in basal cell carcinomas and the Gorlin syndrome. Different in vivo mechanisms of PTC inactivation. *Cancer Research* **56** 4562–4565

van den Ingh HF, Griffioen G and Cornelisse CJ (1985) Flow cytometric detection of aneuploidy in colorectal adenomas. *Cancer Research* **45** 3392–3397

van Oortmarssen GJ and Habbema JDF (1991) Epidemiological evidence for age-dependent regression of pre-invasive cervical cancer. *British Journal of Cancer* **64** 559–565

Verwest AM, de Leeuw WJ, Molijn AC *et al* (1994) Genome scanning of breast cancers by two-dimensional DNA typing. *British Journal of Cancer* **69** 84–92

Vogelstein B and Kinzler KW (1993) The multistep nature of cancer. *Trends in Genetics* **9** 138–141

Weinberg RA (1989) Oncogenes, antioncogenes and the molecular bases of multistep carcinogenesis. *Cancer Research* **49** 3713–3721

Widell S, Auer G, Hast R *et al* (1993) Variation in DNA content of immature normal bone marrow cells. *American Journal of Hematology* **43** 291–2944

Williams C, Pontén F, Ahmadian A *et al* Clones of normal keratinocytes and a variety of simultaneous epidermal lesions contain a multitude of p53 gene mutations in a xeroderma pigmentosum patient. *Cancer Research* (in press)

Wright WE and Shay JW (1992) Telomere positional effects and the regulation of cellular senescence. *Trends in Genetics* **8** 193–197

zur Hausen H (1988) Papillomaviruses in human cancers. *Molecular Carcinogenesis* **1** 147–150

The author is responsible for the accuracy of the references.

Gliomas

V P COLLINS

Division of Tumor Pathology and Ludwig Institute for Cancer Research, Karolinska Hospital, Stockholm, and Department of Histopathology, University of Cambridge, Addenbrooke's Hospital, Cambridge CB2 2QQ

INTRODUCTION

The names given to tumours generally reflect similarities between the tumour cells and differentiated adult cells or cell types found during embryogenesis and organogenesis. The gliomas are a series of tumours thought to arise from the glial cells of brain tissue. Histologically, the tumour cells may resemble astrocytes, oligodendrocytes, ependymocytes (all normal components of differentiated brain) or cells seen during embryogenesis. In some cases they may be so aberrant that it is difficult to see any similarity to a normal cell type—thus terms such as "glioblastoma" have come to be used. There have been many sets of empirically derived rules defining the morphological criteria for the classification and malignancy grading of these tumours. All have the aim of permitting an assessment of the biological aggressiveness of the tumour cell population, estimating prognosis and helping in choosing some form of therapy. The currently most developed and accepted classification system for brain tumours is that of the World Health Organization (Kleihues *et al*, 1993). This classification system will be used in this text.

The true cell of origin is known for some tumours (particularly those where premalignant states are recognized and well defined), but this is not the case with brain tumours. As the spectrum of tumours varies with age, it seems likely that the presence of cells in a particular state of development is a prerequisite for the occurrence of some tumour types. For example primitive neuroectodermal tumours, pilocytic astrocytomas and the ependymomas (see below) occur mainly in childhood and are rare in late and middle age. On the other hand, glioblastomas occur mainly in late middle age, with the incidence increasing into old age. Some of the molecular genetic data support these observations. We will return to this later.

As premalignant states are not recognized, we know little about the earliest changes associated with the development of human brain tumours. Even in the case of chemically induced brain tumours in experimental animals, little or nothing is known. Precursor lesions and the early development of brain tumours are impossible to study in humans, and even animal studies would be difficult. As there are no good animal model systems at present, the study of human lesions is the only alternative. The progression of gliomas may be examined in cases where the tumour is of low malignancy grade at first diagnosis and recurs later as a tumour of higher malignancy grade. Progression of human gliomas was first observed and reported at the end of the last century and studied particularly well by Scherer (1940). The acquisition and study of such material from individual patients is difficult and only a few reports have been published (Reifenberger *et al*, 1996b; Weber *et al*, 1996a).

Studies of large series of astrocytic tumours of all malignancy grades have shown that the more malignant the tumour the greater the number of genetic abnormalities. As will become clear from the description below, the genes coding for proteins involved in certain cellular growth control mechanisms appear to be targeted during progression. The genetic abnormalities identified up to now and their consequences will be described. In considering the premalignant states we can only extrapolate from our knowledge of the progression from the least to the most malignant tumour forms.

The earliest studies of the genome of brain tumours used cytogenetic techniques (Bigner *et al*, 1984, 1990). These investigations were complemented by many studies using molecular genetic techniques. Amplification of the epidermal growth factor receptor (*EGFR*) gene was the earliest finding (Ullrich *et al*, 1984) and the first gene shown to be involved. This was followed by molecular studies identifying the position of many further aberrations in the genome (James *et al*, 1988, 1989; Fujimoto *et al*, 1989). As the genomic maps improved, more and more genes were being identified as being specifically involved in both the development and progression of gliomas. A summary of the regions of the genome and the genes thought to be involved in tumourigeneis or progression either by amplification or loss of the wild type is presented below.

We will deal only with the astrocytic tumour series, since these tumour forms have been most rigorously studied. Only limited data are available for other glioma types.

ASTROCYTIC GLIOMAS

The astrocytic gliomas are divided into four malignancy grades. Grade I is the least malignant and includes one major well defined clinical and histopathological entity, the pilocytic astrocytoma. These tumours most commonly occur in the cerebellum of children but can occur anywhere from the optic nerve to the medulla oblongata. The incidence is increased in patients with neurofibromatosis type 1 (NF1), where these tumours often involve the optic nerve. They are biologically the least aggressive form of astrocytic tumour and are remarkable among the astrocytic tumours in maintaining their grade I status over years and decades. Progression is extremely uncommon.

Astrocytomas (malignancy grade II), anaplastic astrocytomas (malignancy grade III) and glioblastomas (malignancy grade IV) are generally tumours of adulthood. The low grade tumours have a peak incidence between 25 and 50 years, and the glioblastomas have a peak incidence between 45 and 70 years. The glioblastomas are both the most common and the most malignant and have consequently been studied in the greatest numbers. Clinically, glioblastomas can be divided into those that develop from an astrocytoma of lesser malignancy grade and those that appear to develop de novo (Winger *et al*, 1989). The hypothesis that these tumours may develop by a number of pathways is supported by both clinical and the molecular data (James *et al*, 1988; von Deimling *et al*, 1993b; Reifenberger *et al*, 1996b).

Patient survival is an approximate indicator of the relevance of a malignancy grading scheme. Patients with pilocytic astrocytomas have a very good prognosis, and it is uncommon for this form of glioma to be fatal. Average survival of patients with an astrocytoma (malignancy grade II) is around seven years (McCormack *et al*, 1992), while patients with anaplastic astrocytomas survive half that time (Winger *et al*, 1989). Patients with a glioblastoma have a very poor prognosis, with average survival reported between 9 and 11 months (Simpson *et al*, 1993).

Pilocytic Astrocytomas

The genetic aberrations underlying pilocytic astrocytomas (malignancy grade I) are unknown. Very few of these tumours have been studied cytogenetically (Jenkins *et al*, 1989; Karnes *et al*, 1992; Ransom *et al*, 1992a), and attempts at deletion mapping limited numbers of tumours have failed to identify regions of the genome that are consistently lost (James *et al*, 1990; Ransom *et al*, 1992a). Allelic loss on 17q, including the region encompassing the *NF1* (see Table 1) locus, has been reported. This and the increased incidence in NF1 patients strongly suggest that the *NF1* gene might be involved (von Deimling *et al*, 1993a). The retained allele appears to be overexpressed, and no evidence of mutation has yet been found. The *NF1* transcripts expressed appear to be similar to those found in reactive astrocytes and astrocytomas (Platten *et al*, 1996). However, the *NF1* gene with its 59 exons is huge, making mutation analysis difficult. Immunocytochemistry for TP53 may be positive in these tumours, suggesting mutation of the gene resulting in a prolonged half life for the protein. However, there is only one case where a *TP53* mutation has been demonstrat-

TABLE 1. Gene and protein abbreviations used in the text

Gene name	Gene abbreviation	Synonyms
Cyclin dependent kinase inhibitor 2A	CDKN2A	CDKN2, MTS1, p16^{INK4A}
Cyclin dependent kinase inhibitor 2B	CDKN2B	p15^{INK4B}, MTS2
Cyclin dependent kinase 4	CDK4	
Epidermal growth factor receptor	EGFR	
Murine double minutes	MDM2	
Neurofibromatosis type 1	NF1	
Neurofibromatosis type 2	NF2	
Phosphatase and tensin homology deleted on chromosome 10	PTEN	MMAC1
Retinoblastoma 1	RB1	
Sarcoma amplified sequence	SAS	
Tumor protein 53	TP53	p53

ed (Lang *et al*, 1994). The technique of comparative genomic hybridization (Kallioniemi *et al*, 1992) has yet to give clues as to where the genetic aberrations that cause this tumour form are located.

Astrocytomas

Cytogenetic data on the astrocytomas (malignancy grade II) are limited (Jenkins *et al*, 1989; Kimmel *et al*, 1992). Few astrocytomas have been subjected to comparative genomic hybridisation (Weber *et al*, 1996a). Studies using molecular genetic techniques have defined regions of the genome with loss of alleles in these tumours. The most frequent regions include 13q, 17p and 22q (el-Azouzi *et al*, 1989; James *et al*, 1989; Fults *et al*, 1990, 1992; von Deimling *et al*, 1992; Wu and Darras 1992; Ohgaki *et al*, 1993; Kraus *et al*, 1994; Liang *et al*, 1994; Rasheed *et al*, 1994; Ichimura *et al*, 1996). Both 13q and 22q show loss of alleles in around 30% of the tumours, whereas losses of alleles on 17p are more frequent, occurring in around 45% of astrocytomas. There is no evidence to suggest that loss of one *RB1* allele is associated with mutation of the retained allele at 13q14 in astrocytomas, although this does occur in glioblastomas (see below and Ichimura *et al*, 1996). Hereditary retinoblastoma patients have one wild type allele and have not been reported to show an increase in the incidence of astrocytomas. The *NF2* tumour suppressor gene on 22q has been suggested as a candidate tumour suppressor gene, but no evidence has been presented to support this (Hoang-Xuan *et al*, 1995).

Loss of alleles on 17p is associated in the majority of cases with mitotic recombination and reduplication, which explains the lack of cytogenetic evidence for 17p losses (James *et al*, 1989). However, the loss of one *TP53* allele (17p) is associated with mutation of the remaining allele (albeit two mutated copies) in the majority of cases (von Deimling *et al*, 1992; Ohgaki *et al*, 1993; Rasheed *et al*, 1994).

Infrequent losses of alleles have been found on 9p (common in the more malignant astrocytic tumours). However, reverse-transcriptase polymerase chain reaction (RT-PCR) expression studies indicate that approximately a third of astrocytomas may not be expressing transcripts for the *CDKN2A* gene (which inhibit *CDK4*) (Schmidt *et al*, 1997). Deletion mapping of chromosome 10 shows preferential loss of the distal end of 10p in around one-third of astrocytomas (Ichimura *et al*, 1998). No genes have been consistently reported amplified in astrocytomas (Ekstrand *et al*, 1991; Hoang-Xuan *et al*, 1995; Reifenberger *et al*, 1995; Ichimura *et al*, 1996). Some examples of the patterns of genetic changes found in individual astrocytomas are shown in Fig. 1.

Anaplastic Astrocytomas

These tumours have been studied cytogenetically in reasonable numbers (Jenkins *et al*, 1989; Kimmel *et al*, 1992; Ransom *et al*, 1992b). The use of the term "malignant gliomas" to denote both anaplastic astrocytomas and glioblastomas can make interpretation of some published data difficult. A number of comparative genomic hybridization (CGH) studies have included these tumours (Schröck *et al*, 1994; Weber *et al*, 1996a). The cytogenetic and CGH findings show that in addition to the losses on 13q and 22q, occurring at similar frequencies as in the astrocytomas, sites of amplification (12q) and new sites of loss of genetic material (e.g. 9p) are found. Many of the comparative genomic hybridization findings have confirmed the results of molecular analysis carried out during the past eight years, but some indicate new regions for investigation.

In a study of 50 anaplastic astrocytomas, 16% had homozygous deletions encompassing the *CDKN2A* gene (see Table 1 for synonyms), located at 9p21 (Ichimura *et al*, 1996). A further 4% had no wild type gene, owing to loss of one allele and mutation of the retained allele, specifically implicating the *CDKN2A* gene (Ichimura *et al*, 1996; Schmidt *et al*, 1997). This makes a total of 20% tumours with no wild type *CDKN2A* gene. Loss of one allele with retention of one wild type allele was seen in 24% (Ichimura *et al*, 1996). The *CDKN2B* gene and the *CDKN2A* gene, located within 25kb of one another, were generally deleted simultaneously. No point mutations of *CDKN2B* have been detected in tumours retaining one allele (Schmidt *et al*, 1997). RT-PCR did not detect expression of *CDKN2A* transcripts in some of the cases with loss of one allele and in some cases retaining two alleles. Thus evidence was presented suggesting the absence of the wild type protein in a total 50% of the tumours (Ichimura *et al*, 1996; Schmidt *et al*, 1997).

Amplification of genes on 12q occurs in about 14% of anaplastic astrocytomas (Reifenberger *et al*, 1994, 1996a). In the majority of cases the *CDK4* and

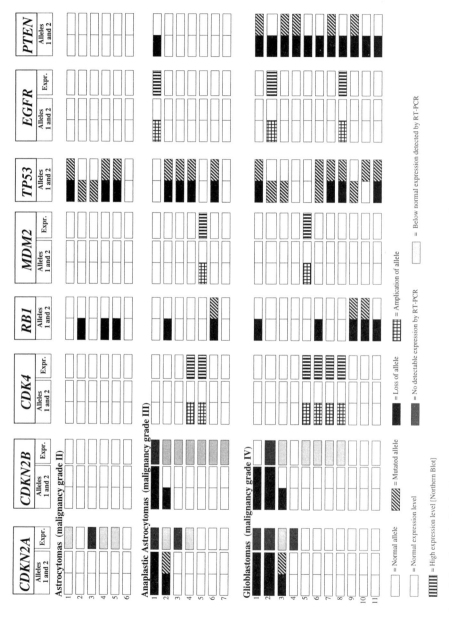

Fig. 1. Examples of data from individual human gliomas. For each gene shown two columns represent the two alleles present under normal circumstances. Explanations of the patterns are given under the table. For the *CDKN2A*, *CDKN2B*, *CDK4*, *MDM2*, and *EGFR* genes a third column (*right*) shows the levels of transcript expression detected

SAS genes are involved (distance between genes approximately 10kb). The *MDM2* gene is also amplified in 10% of tumours (physical distance between *CDK4* and *MDM2* 3–4Mb). Although amplification of *MDM2* generally occurs only in tumours with amplification of *CDK4* and *SAS*, amplicon mapping has shown that part of the region between these genes is not included in any amplicon, excluding the possibility of a target gene in this region. The amplicons in some tumours are extremely large and encompass several genes. Only some of the amplified genes are consistently over-expressed, and these include *CDK4*, *SAS* and *MDM2* (Reifenberger *et al*, 1994, 1996a). The combined mapping and expression studies strongly suggest that *MDM2* and *CDK4/SAS* are the genes targeted by the amplification process. In addition to the gap of non-amplified DNA between *MDM2* and *CDK4/SAS*, further gaps of normally contiguous DNA have been found in the amplicons (Reifenberger *et al*, 1994). While the *EGFR* gene is frequently amplified in glioblastomas, in a series of 50 anaplastic astrocytomas we have found amplification of *EGFR* in only 8% of cases.

Anaplastic astrocytomas with loss of one allele of *RB1* retain one wild type allele in the vast majority of cases. This contrasts with the glioblastomas, where the retained *RB1* allele is often mutated. Loss of wild type *CDKN2A* (homozygously deleted or hemizygously deleted with mutation of the retained allele) and amplification of *CDK4* were mutually exclusive abnormalities and never occurred in the same anaplastic astrocytoma (Ichimura *et al*, 1996). The single tumour with loss of one allele of the *RB1* gene and mutation of the other allele had no abnormalities of the *CDKN2A* or *CDK4* genes. When lack of evidence for expression is added to the above, 68% of the series of 50 anaplastic astrocytomas lacked normal components of the G_1–S phase cell cycle control mechanism. However, 32% showed none of these abnormalities (Ichimura *et al*, 1996).

Our current understanding of the anaplastic astrocytomas suggests that they fall into two subgroups, one that shows similarities to the astrocytomas and one that shows abnormalities of the G_1–S phase cell cycle control mechanisms similar to the glioblastomas (Fig. 1).

Glioblastomas

The greatest number of genetic abnormalities have been identified in the glioblastomas (malignancy grade IV). Cytogenetically they are the best studied primary tumour of the brain. Common findings include losses of chromosomes 6, 10, 13 and Y, gain of chromosomes 7 and 19 and structural abnormalities of chromosomes 1 and 9 (Rey *et al*, 1987; Bigner *et al*, 1988; Jenkins *et al*, 1989). Double minute chromosomes have also been frequently reported, indicating the presence of amplified genes (Bigner *et al*, 1988a,b, 1990). Studies using comparative genomic hybridization have confirmed these findings and identified a number of amplified regions (Muleris *et al*, 1994; Mohapatra *et al*, 1995; Weber *et al*, 1996a). Glioblastomas have also been studied extensively with molecular genetic techniques. Losses of alleles in regions similar to those identified in the anaplastic astrocytomas are seen (Schmidt *et al*, 1994; Ichimura *et al*, 1996). The incidences of losses are found to increase in some areas (for example on 9p) and in others decrease (for example on 17p) (Rasheed *et al*, 1994; Ichimura *et al*, 1996).

The incidence of homozygous deletions on 9p encompassing the *CDKN2A* gene increases from 16% in anaplastic astrocytomas to 39% in glioblastomas (Ichimura *et al*, 1996). The incidence of loss of one allele at loci on 9p shows no significant increase. Point mutations of a single retained allele of *CDKN2A* are also found at the same frequency as in anaplastic astrocytomas. Thus approximately 41% of glioblastomas in total have no wild type *CDKN2A* gene and a further 14% show no or very low levels of transcript by RT-PCR, despite retention of one or even two wild type copies (Schmidt *et al*, 1997). Methylation of the 5′ CpG islands of the *CDKN2A* gene have been shown to be associated with repression of expression (Gonzalez-Zulueta *et al*, 1995; Herman *et al*, 1995; Merlo *et al*, 1995). We examined methylation of the 5′ end of *CDKN2A* and have only been able to demonstrate partial methylation in only a small proportion of tumours. In total, 61% of glioblastomas do not or cannot express wild type CDKN2A protein (Schmidt *et al*, 1997). Other reports have found correlations between methylation and the absence of expression of the *CDKN2A* gene (Costello *et al*, 1996; Fueyo *et al*, 1996).

Amplifications of the 12q14 region occur at a similar frequency as in anaplastic astrocytomas and involve the same genes, *CDK4*, *SAS* and *MDM2* (Reifenberger *et al*, 1994, 1996a; Ichimura *et al*, 1996).

Loss of alleles on 13q is more common among the glioblastomas (43%) than the anaplastic astrocytomas (22%). The *RB1* gene is involved almost always. Lack of a wild type *RB1* gene due to homozygous deletion or loss of one allele and mutation of the retained allele is reported in 14% of glioblastomas. This is a marked increase when compared with the very low incidence among anaplastic astrocytomas (Ichimura *et al*, 1996).

Around 80% of glioblastomas have abnormalities affecting one or other of the *CDKN2A*, *RB1* and *CDK4* genes (Ichimura *et al*, 1996; Ueki *et al*, 1996). Non-expression of a wild type protein from the *CDKN2A* gene occurs in 55% of glioblastomas through loss of both copies of the genes, mutation or methylation. An additional 11% overexpress CDK4 and a further 14% have no wild type RB1 protein. Such alterations will result in the tumour cells lacking protein components controlling progression from G_1 to the S phase of the cell cycle (Hunter and Pines, 1994; Sherr, 1994; Morgan, 1995; Sherr and Roberts, 1995; Weinberg, 1995, 1996).

Release of the E2F/DP1 transcription factors from the RB1 protein on its phosphorylation is considered to be a key event in preparation for entry into the S phase of the cell cycle (Weinberg, 1995; Weinberg, 1996). Thus loss of wild type RB1 or any cellular aberration resulting in uncontrolled phosphorylation of RB1 may result in uncontrolled entry into the S phase. Phosphorylation of RB1 may be executed by a heterodimer of CDK4 and cyclin D1. The activity of the CDK4/cyclin D1 heterodimer can be blocked by CDKN1 binding to the

CDK4/cyclin D1 complex. The expression of CDKN1 is controlled by the TP53 protein. Availability of CDK4 for heterodimerization with cyclin D1 will increase with overexpression owing to *CDK4* amplification and in the absence of CDKN2A and CDKN2B proteins that bind CDK4 and inhibit the formation of the heterodimer. CDKN2A and B are normally expressed in response to different growth inhibitory signals.

This illustrates the fact that different genetic aberrations may target different components of a single cellular control mechanism, all of which can be expected to result in a similar phenotype.

These are far from the only genetic abnormalities seen in glioblastomas. Amplification and overexpression of the *EGFR* gene (located on 7p11-12) was one of the first molecular genetic abnormalities reported in these tumours (Libermann *et al*, 1985). At the same time rearrangement of the amplified gene was suggested. This was later demonstrated to occur and the most common rearrangement shown to result in a transcript that is aberrantly spliced, yet remains in frame (Humphrey *et al*, 1990; Sugawa *et al*, 1990; Wong *et al*, 1992). The aberrant transcript codes for a mutated *EGFR* that has lost 267 aminoacids of its extracellular domain and does not bind ligand (Ekstrand *et al*, 1994; Nishikawa *et al*, 1994). This mutated EGFR is constitutively activated (Ekstrand *et al*, 1994; Nishikawa *et al*, 1994). Other rearrangements of the amplified *EGFR* gene occur less frequently and may result in abnormalities of the cytoplasmic domain (Ekstrand *et al*, 1992).

The most common finding in glioblastomas is loss of one copy of chromosome 10 (James *et al*, 1988; Fujimoto *et al*, 1989; Ransom *et al*, 1992b; Rasheed *et al*, 1992, 1995; Fults and Pedone, 1993; Karlbom *et al*, 1993; Albarosa *et al*, 1996; Kimmelman *et al*, 1996; Ichimura *et al*, 1998). Attempts to identify a smaller region of the chromosome have indicated a number of regions consistently lost (Ichimura *et al*, 1998). A region at chromosome 10q23-24 was shown to contain a tumour suppressor gene, designated *PTEN* or *MMAC1* (Li *et al*, 1997; Steck *et al*, 1997). The gene has been shown to be a dual specificity phosphatase (necessary for its ability to function as a tumour suppressor) and to show homology to the cytoskeletal protein tensin (Myers *et al*, 1997). However, the fact that one entire copy of chromosome 10 is generally lost would suggest that more than one gene is involved, and deletion mapping results also support this (Ichimura *et al*, 1998). Mutations of *PTEN/MMAC1* have been documented in glioblastomas (Rasheed *et al*, 1997; Wang *et al*, 1997).

MOLECULAR PATHWAYS TO GLIOBLASTOMA

It is tempting to try to sort these findings into a series of events explaining the development and progression of astrocytic tumours. The earliest findings seen in the astrocytomas are the loss of both wild type alleles of *TP53*, most commonly by loss of one and mutation of the other. In addition, loss of alleles on 13q, including one copy of *RB1* with retention of a wild type copy, is seen. The significance of this is unclear. Furthermore, losses of alleles from the distal end of 10p have been reported (Kimmelman *et al*, 1996; Ichimura *et al*, 1998). However, approximately a third of our series of 20 astrocytomas lack, as yet, demonstrable genetic lesions.

The anaplastic astrocytomas are different, showing a broader spectrum of abnormalities as well as few cases lacking genetic aberrations (only 8% of 50 cases). Amplification of genes is seen for the first time—mainly of the 12q14 region but even of *EGFR* in single cases. The most striking supplementary findings are those affecting the cell cycle control systems. The losses on 13q, including one copy of *RB1* with retention of a wild type copy and the lack of a wild type copy of *TP53*, occur at a slightly lower frequency than in the astrocytomas.

Among a series of 121 glioblastomas we have only one case with no genetic abnormality. This case, for unknown reasons, does not express a *CDKN2A* transcript detectable by RT-PCR and thus lacks CDKN2A. Abnormalities of the cell cycle control genes are more common in glioblastomas than in the anaplastic astrocytomas. The incidence of loss of one allele on 17p and mutation of the retained *TP53* allele is not as common in glioblastomas (26%) as in astrocytomas (50%) or anaplastic astrocytomas (42%) (Rasheed *et al*, 1994; Reifenberger *et al*, 1996b; Weber *et al*, 1996b; and unpublished data). Even if *MDM2* amplification and overexpression is considered equivalent to *TP53* mutation, it occurs in merely 7% of glioblastomas. This would bring the total targeting of the *TP53* pathway in glioblastomas up to only 33% (*MDM2* amplification is exclusively seen in combination with wild type p53 alleles [Reifenberger *et al*, 1993]).

Amplification of the *EGFR* gene appears to be more common in de novo glioblastomas than in those known to arise from a pre-existing astrocytoma (Rasheed *et al*, 1994; Reifenberger *et al*, 1996b; Weber *et al*, 1996b). On the other hand, loss of the ability to produce wild type TP53 is more common in the latter. This suggests that whereas some glioblastomas may arise from anaplastic astrocytomas not all do so, and that there is an alternative route not involving the *TP53* gene likely taken by the de novo tumours (von Deimling *et al*, 1993b, 1995). However, there is quite a degree of overlap between the groups when clinically defined.

CONCLUSIONS

We knew almost nothing about the genetic basis of human gliomas 15 years ago. During the past decade we have made significant advances in our understanding of the molecular mechanisms involved in their development. We are beginning to realize that these tumours originate as a result of a series of complex derangements of normal cellular functions. The almost bewildering number of genetic abnormalities is becoming intelligible as we discover that different genes coding for components of the same mechanisms are being targeted in individual tumours and that failure of different components of the same pathway may result in a single phenotype. Understanding the anomalous molecular mechanisms involved should give us the opportunity of finding ways to specifically target the glioma cell. However, we have much to learn before we can say we understand the earliest events involved in the development of human brain tumours.

SUMMARY

Gliomas are thought to arise from the glial cells of brain tissue. The spectrum of tumours varies with age, implying that cells in a particular state of development are a prerequisite for the occurrence of some tumour types. Premalignant states are not recognized, so we know little about the earliest events in oncogenesis. However, progression of gliomas has been examined by studying large series of tumours of different malignancy grades and by following cases where the tumour is of low malignancy grade at first diagnosis and recurs later as a tumour of higher malignancy grade. When considering premalignant states we can only extrapolate from our knowledge of progression from the least to the most malignant tumour forms. The best studied variants are the astrocytic tumours. There are no consistent genetic aberrations known to characterize the most benign variant of astrocytoma, the pilocytic astrocytoma (malignancy grade I), which occurs mainly in children. Astrocytomas (malignancy grade II) show loss of alleles at 13q, 17p and 22q and occur mainly in early middle age. Loss of one *TP53* allele (17p) is associated with mutation of the remaining allele. Loss of one *RB1* allele is not. Anaplastic astrocytomas (malignancy grade III) have in approximately 50% of cases aberrations of genes coding for proteins involved in the control of entry into the S phase of the cell cycle, as well as other genetic defects affecting unknown genes. The greatest number of genetic abnormalities is seen in glioblastomas (malignancy grade IV), which have a peak incidence in late middle age. Around 80% of glioblastomas can be shown to have genetic alterations resulting in aberrant control of progression from G_1 to the S phase of the cell cycle, and many show amplification of growth factor receptor genes as well as other abnormalities. The bewildering number of genetic anomalies becomes intelligible as we discover that different components of the same cellular control mechanisms are being targeted in individual tumours resulting in a similar phenotype.

References

Albarosa R, Colombo BM, Roz L *et al* (1996) Deletion mapping of gliomas suggest the presence of two small regions for candidate tumor-suppressor genes in a 17-cM interval on chromosome 10q. *American Journal of Human Genetics* **58** 1260–1267

Bigner SH, Mark J, Mahaley JMS and Bigner DD (1984) Patterns of the early gross chromosomal changes in malignant human gliomas. *Hereditas* **101** 103–113

Bigner SH, Burger PC, Wong AJ *et al* (1988a) Gene amplification in malignant human gliomas: clinical and histopathologic aspects. *Journal of Neuropathology and Experimental Neurology* **47** 191–205

Bigner SH, Mark J, Burger PC *et al* (1988b) Specific chromosomal abnormalities in malignant human gliomas. *Cancer Research* **48** 405–411

Bigner SH, Mark J and Bigner DD (1990) Cytogenetics of human brain tumors. *Cancer, Genetics and Cytogenetics* **47** 141–154

Costello JF, Berger MS, Huang HS and Cavenee WK (1996) Silencing of p16/CDKN2 expression in human gliomas by methylation and chromatin condensation. *Cancer Research* **56** 2405–2410

Ekstrand AJ, James CD, Cavenee WK *et al* (1991) Genes for epidermal growth factor receptor, transforming growth factor alpha, and epidermal growth factor and their expression in human gliomas in vivo. *Cancer Research* **51** 2164–2172

Ekstrand AJ, Sugawa N, James CD and Collins VP (1992) Amplified and rearranged epidermal growth factor receptor genes in human glioblastomas reveal deletions of sequences encoding portions of the N- and/or C-terminal tails. *Proceedings of the National Academy of Sciences of the USA* **89** 4309–4313

Ekstrand AJ, Longo N, Hamid ML *et al* (1994) Functional characterization of an EGF receptor with a truncated extracellular domain expressed in glioblastomas with EGFR gene amplification. *Oncogene* **9** 2313–2320

el-Azouzi M, Chung RY, Farmer GE *et al* (1989) Loss of distinct regions on the short arm of chromosome 17 associated with tumorigenesis of human astrocytomas. *Proceedings of the National Academy of Sciences of the USA* **86** 7186–7190

Fueyo J, Gomez-Manzano C, Bruner JM *et al* (1996) Hypermethylation of the CpG island of p16/CDKN2 correlates with gene inactivation in gliomas. *Oncogene* **13** 1615–1619

Fujimoto M, Fults DW, Thomas GA *et al* (1989) Loss of heterozygosity on chromosome 10 in human glioblastoma multiforme. *Genomics* **4** 210–214

Fults D and Pedone C (1993) Deletion mapping of the long arm of chromosome 10 in glioblastoma multiforme. *Genes, Chromosomes and Cancer* **7** 173–177

Fults D, Pedone CA, Thomas GA and White R (1990) Allelotype of human malignant astrocytoma. *Cancer Research* **50** 5784–5789

Fults D, Brockmeyer D, Tullous MW, Pedone CA and Cawthon RM (1992) p53 mutation and loss of heterozygosity on chromosomes 17 and 10 during human astrocytoma progression. *Cancer Research* **52** 674–679

Gonzalez-Zulueta M, Bender CM, Yang AS *et al* (1995) Methylation of the 5' CpG island of the p16/CDKN2 tumor suppressor gene in normal and transformed human tissues correlates with gene silencing. *Cancer Research* **55** 4531–4535

Herman JG, Merlo A, Mao L *et al* (1995) Inactivation of the CDKN2/p16/MTS1 gene is frequently associated with aberrant DNA methylation in all common human cancers. *Cancer Research* **55** 4525–4530

Hoang-Xuan K, Merel P, Vega F *et al* (1995) Analysis of the NF2 tumor-suppressor gene and of chromosome 22 deletions in gliomas. *International Journal of Cancer* **60** 478–481

Humphrey PA, Wong AJ, Vogelstein B *et al* (1990) Anti-synthetic peptide antibody reacting at the fusion junction of deletion-mutant epidermal growth factor receptors in human glioblastoma. *Proceedings of the National Academy of Sciences of the USA* **87** 4207–4211

Hunter T and Pines J (1994) Cyclins and cancer. II: Cyclin D and CDK inhibitors come of age. *Cell* **79** 573–582

Ichimura K, Schmidt EE, Goike HM and Collins VP (1996) Human glioblastomas with no alterations of the CDKN2A (p16INK4a, MTS1) and CDK4 genes have frequent mutations of the retinoblastoma gene. *Oncogene* **13** 1065–1072

Ichimura K, Schmidt EE, Miyakawa A, Goike HM and Collins VP (1998) Distinct patterns of deletion on 10p and 10q suggest involvement of multiple tumor suppressor genes in the development of astrocytic gliomas of different malignancy grades. *Genes, Chromosomes and Cancer* **22** 9–15

James CD, Carlbom E, Dumanski JP *et al* (1988) Clonal genomic alterations in glioma malignancy stages. *Cancer Research* **48** 5546–5551

James CD, Carlbom E, Nordenskjold M, Collins VP and Cavenee WK (1989) Mitotic recombination of chromosome 17 in astrocytomas. *Proceedings of the National Academy of Sciences of the USA* **86** 2858–2862

James CD, He J, Carlbom E *et al* (1990) Loss of genetic information in central nervous system tumors common to children and young adults. *Genes, Chromosomes and Cancer* **2** 94–102

Jenkins RB, Kimmel DW, Moertel CA *et al* (1989) A cytogenetic study of 53 human gliomas. *Cancer Genetics and Cytogenetics* **39** 253–279

Kallioniemi A, Kallioniemi OP, Sudar D *et al* (1992) Comparative genomic hybridization for molecular cytogenetic analysis of solid tumors. *Science* **258** 818–821

Karlbom AE, James CD, Boethius J *et al* (1993) Loss of heterozygosity in malignant gliomas involves at least three distinct regions on chromosome 10. *Human Genetics* **92** 169–174

Karnes PS, Tran TN, Cui MY *et al* (1992) Cytogenetic analysis of 39 pediatric central nervous system tumors. *Cancer Genetics and Cytogenetics* **59** 12–19

Kimmel DW, O'Fallon JR, Scheithauer BW *et al* (1992) Prognostic value of cytogenetic analysis in human cerebral astrocytomas. *Annals of Neurology* **31** 534–542

Kimmelman AC, Ross DA and Liang BC (1996) Loss of heterozygosity of chromosome 10p in human gliomas. *Genomics* **34** 250–254

Kleihues P, Burger PC and Scheithauer BW (1993) *Histological Typing of Tumors of the Central Nervous System*, Springer-Verlag, New York

Kraus JA, Bolln C, Wolf HK *et al* (1994) TP53 alterations and clinical outcome in low grade astrocytomas. *Genes, Chromosomes and Cancer* **10** 143–149

Lang FF, Miller DC, Pisharody S, Koslow M and Newcomb EW (1994) High frequency of p53 protein accumulation without p53 gene mutation in human juvenile pilocytic, low grade and anaplastic astrocytomas. *Oncogene* **9** 949–954

Li J, Yen C, Liaw D *et al* (1997) PTEN, a putative protein tyrosine phosphatase gene mutated in human brain, breast, and prostate cancer. *Science* 275 1943–1947

Liang BC, Ross DA, Greenberg HS, Meltzer PS and Trent JM (1994) Evidence of allelic imbalance of chromosome 6 in human astrocytomas (erratum *Neurology* [1994] **44** 1190). *Neurology* **44** 533–536

Libermann TA, Nusbaum HR, Razon N *et al* (1985) Amplification, enhanced expression and possible rearrangement of EGF receptor gene in primary human brain tumours of glial origin. *Nature* **313** 144–147

McCormack BM, Miller DC, Budzilovich GN, Voorhees GJ and Ransohoff J (1992) Treatment and survival of low-grade astrocytoma in adults—1977–1988. *Neurosurgery* **31** 636–642 and 642

Merlo A, Herman JG, Mao L *et al* (1995) 5′ CpG island methylation is associated with transcriptional silencing of the tumour suppressor p16/CDKN2/MTS1 in human cancers. *Nature Medicine* **1** 686–692

Mohapatra G, Kim DH and Feuerstein BG (1995) Detection of multiple gains and losses of genetic material in ten glioma cell lines by comparative genomic hybridization. *Genes, Chromosomes and Cancer* **13** 86–93

Morgan DO (1995) Principles of CDK regulation. *Nature* **374** 131–134

Muleris M, Almeida A, Dutrillaux AM *et al* (1994) Oncogene amplification in human gliomas: a molecular cytogenetic analysis. *Oncogene* **9** 2717–2722

Myers MP, Stolarov JP, Eng C *et al* (1997) P-TEN, the tumor suppressor from human chromosome 10q23, is a dual-specificity phosphatase. *Proceedings of the National Academy of Sciences of the USA* **94** 9052–9057

Nishikawa R, Ji XD, Harmon RC *et al* (1994) A mutant epidermal growth factor receptor common in human glioma confers enhanced tumorigenicity. *Proceedings of the National Academy of Sciences of the USA* **91** 7727–7731

Ohgaki H, Eibl RH, Schwab M *et al* (1993) Mutations of the p53 tumor suppressor gene in neoplasms of the human nervous system. *Molecular Carcinogenesis* **8** 74–80

Platten M, Giordano MJ, Dirven CM, Gutmann DH and Louis DN (1996) Up-regulation of specific NF 1 gene transcripts in sporadic pilocytic astrocytomas. *American Journal of Pathology* **149** 621–627

Ransom DT, Ritland SR, Kimmel DW *et al* (1992a) Cytogenetic and loss of heterozygosity studies in ependymomas, pilocytic astrocytomas, and oligodendrogliomas. *Genes, Chromosomes and Cancer* **5** 348–356

Ransom DT, Ritland SR, Moertel CA *et al* (1992b) Correlation of cytogenetic analysis and loss of heterozygosity studies in human diffuse astrocytomas and mixed oligo-astrocytomas. *Genes, Chromosomes and Cancer* **5** 357–374

Rasheed BK, Fuller GN, Friedman AH, Bigner DD and Bigner SH (1992) Loss of heterozygosity for 10q loci in human gliomas. *Genes, Chromosomes and Cancer* **5** 75–82

Rasheed BK, McLendon RE, Herndon JE *et al* (1994) Alterations of the TP53 gene in human gliomas. *Cancer Research* **54** 1324–1330

Rasheed BK, McLendon RE, Friedman HS *et al* (1995) Chromosome 10 deletion mapping in human gliomas: a common deletion region in 10q25. *Oncogene* **10** 2243–2246

Rasheed BKA, Stenzel TT, McLendon RE *et al* (1997) Pten gene mutations are seen in high-grade but not in low-grade gliomas. *Cancer Research* **57** 4187–4190

Reifenberger G, Liu L, Ichimura K, Schmidt EE and Collins VP (1993) Amplification and over-expression of the MDM2 gene in a subset of human malignant gliomas without p53 mutations. *Cancer Research* **53** 2736–2739

Reifenberger G, Reifenberger J, Ichimura K, Meltzer PS and Collins VP (1994) Amplification of multiple genes from chromosomal region 12q13-14 in human malignant gliomas: preliminary mapping of the amplicons shows preferential involvement of CDK4, SAS, and MDM2. *Cancer Research* **54** 4299–4303

Reifenberger G, Reifenberger J, Ichimura K and Collins VP (1995) Amplification at 12q13-14 in human malignant gliomas is frequently accompanied by loss of heterozygosity at loci proximal and distal to the amplification site. *Cancer Research* **55** 731–734

Reifenberger G, Ichimura K, Reifenberger J *et al* (1996a) Refined mapping of 12q13-q15 amplicons in human malignant gliomas suggests CDK4/SAS and MDM2 as independent amplification targets. *Cancer Research* **56** 5141–5145

Reifenberger J, Ring GU, Gies U *et al* (1996b) Analysis of p53 mutation and epidermal growth factor receptor amplification in recurrent gliomas with malignant progression. *Journal of Neuropathology and Experimental Neurology* **55** 822–831

Rey JA, Bello MJ, de Campos JM *et al* (1987) Chromosomal patterns in human malignant astrocytomas. *Cancer Genetics and Cytogenetics* **29** 201–221

Scherer HJ (1940) Cerebral astrocytomas and their derivatives. *American Journal of Cancer* **40** 159–198

Schmidt EE, Ichimura K, Reifenberger G and Collins VP (1994) CDKN2 (p16/MTS1) gene deletion or CDK4 amplification occurs in the majority of glioblastomas. *Cancer Research* **54** 6321–6324

Schmidt EE, Ichimura K, Messerle KR, Goike HM and Collins VP (1997) Infrequent methylation of CDKN2A(MTS1/p16) and rare mutation of both CDKN2A and CDKN2B(MTS2/p15) in primary astrocytic tumours. *British Journal of Cancer* **75** 2–8

Schröck E, Thiel G, Lozanova T *et al* (1994) Comparative genomic hybridization of human malignant gliomas reveals multiple amplification sites and nonrandom chromosomal gains and losses. *American Journal of Pathology* **144** 1203–1218

Sherr CJ (1994) G1 phase progression: cycling on cue. *Cell* **79** 551–555

Sherr CJ and Roberts JM (1995) Inhibitors of mammalian G1 cyclin-dependent kinases. *Genes and Development* **9** 1149–1163

Simpson JR, Horton J, Scott C *et al* (1993) Influence of location and extent of surgical resection on survival of patients with glioblastoma multiforme: results of three consecutive Radiation Therapy Oncology Group (RTOG) clinical trials. *International Journal of Radiation Oncology, Biology, Physics* **26** 239–244

Steck PA, Pershouse MA, Jasser SA *et al* (1997) Identification of a candidate tumour suppressor gene, MMAC1, at chromosome 10q23.3 that is mutated in multiple advanced cancers. *Nature Genetics* **15** 356–362

Sugawa N, Ekstrand AJ, James CD and Collins VP (1990) Identical splicing of aberrant epidermal growth factor receptor transcripts from amplified rearranged genes in human glioblastomas. *Proceedings of the National Academy of Sciences of the USA* **87** 8602–8606

Ueki K, Ono Y, Hensen JW *et al* (1996) Cdkn2/p16 or rb alterations occur in the majority of glioblastomas and are inversely correlated. *Cancer Research* **56** 150–153

Ullrich A, Coussens L, Hayflick JS *et al* (1984) Human epidermal growth factor receptor cDNA sequence and aberrant expression of the amplified gene in A431 epidermoid carcinoma cells. *Nature* **309** 418–425

von Deimling A, Eibl RH, Ohgaki H *et al* (1992) p53 mutations are associated with 17p allelic loss in grade II and grade III astrocytoma. *Cancer Research* **52** 2987–2990

von Deimling A, Louis DN, Menon AG *et al* (1993a) Deletions on the long arm of chromosome 17 in pilocytic astrocytoma. *Acta Neuropathologica* **86** 81–85

von Deimling A, von Ammon K, Schoenfeld D *et al* (1993b) Subsets of glioblastoma multiforme defined by molecular genetic analysis. *Brain Pathology* **3** 19–26

von Deimling A, Louis DN and Wiestler OD (1995) Molecular pathways in the formation of gliomas. *Glia* **15** 328–338

Wang SI, Puc J, Li J *et al* (1997) Somatic mutations of pten in glioblastoma multiforme. *Cancer Research* **57** 4183–4186

Weber RG, Sabel M, Reifenberger J *et al* (1996a) Characterization of genomic alterations associated with glioma progression by comparative genomic hybridization. *Oncogene* **13** 983–994

Weber RG, Sommer C, Albert FK, Kiessling M and Cremer T (1996b) Clinically distinct subgroups of glioblastoma multiforme studied by comparative genomic hybridization. *Laboratory Investigation* **74** 108–119

Weinberg RA (1995) The retinoblastoma protein and cell cycle control. *Cell* **81** 323–330

Weinberg RA (1996) E2F and cell proliferation: a world turned upside down. *Cell* **85** 457–459

Winger MJ, Macdonald DR and Cairncross JG (1989) Supratentorial anaplastic gliomas in adults. The prognostic importance of extent of resection and prior low-grade glioma. *Journal of Neurosurgery* **71** 487–493

Wong AJ, Ruppert JM, Bigner SH *et al* (1992) Structural alterations of the epidermal growth factor receptor gene in human gliomas. *Proceedings of the National Academy of Sciences of the USA* **89** 2965–2969

Wu JK and Darras BT (1992) Loss of heterozygosity on the short arm of chromosome 17 in human astrocytomas. *Neurological Research* **14** 39–44

The author is responsible for the accuracy of the references.

Molecular Precursor Lesions in Oesophageal Cancer

R MONTESANO • P HAINAUT

Unit of Mechanisms of Carcinogenesis, International Agency for Research on Cancer, 150 Cours Albert-Thomas, 69372 Lyon, Cedex 08, France

Introduction
Loss of alleles at multiple chromosomal loci
Alterations of the *TP53* gene
Alterations in cell cycle regulatory genes
Clonality and multiple primary cancers
Molecular epidemiology
    Increased prevalence of *TP53* mutations in smokers
    Distinct *TP53* mutation spectra in squamous cell carcinoma and adenocarcinoma
Perspectives
Summary

INTRODUCTION

Tumour progression has been described by Foulds (1975) as "neoplastic development by way of irreversible change in one or more of the characters of neoplastic cells". The same author, in discussing the complexity and the limitations of definitions of the various stages of tumour progression, considered that one should "deliberately avoid the term precancerous on the ground that it is inadequately descriptive and unreliably predictive". More recently, Correa (1996) used the term "precursors" to avoid the implication that these early lesions inevitably become cancer. This issue on terminology is not simply a semantic one, since the availability of reliable cellular or molecular precursor lesions predictive of cancer progression may have a direct and important bearing on the implementation of preventive measures, the clinical management of the disease and the evaluation of the efficacy of intervention studies.

In the case of both squamous cell carcinoma (SCC) and adenocarcinoma (ADC) of the oesophagus, histological and cytological criteria to define precursor lesions related to cancer have been proposed. In SCC, it was suggested (Muñoz, 1997) that the natural history is as follows: chronic oesophagitis to atrophy to dysplasia to cancer. In ADC specialized intestinal metaplasia is recognized as a precursor lesion (Spechler, 1997). The early occurrence of such lesions has often been defined on the basis of retrospective studies and/or analysis of lesions occurring in "non-cancerous" mucosa adjacent to the cancer (Correa, 1982; Spechler, 1997; Kim *et al*, 1997).

Similarly, the majority of the studies examining the presence of various genetic alterations in normal tissue, metaplastic and dysplastic lesions and cancer tissue have been of a descriptive nature, with the assumption that these lesions are representative of the natural history of oesophageal cancer. A better assessment of the significance of these lesions as precursors of cancer development should be provided by the analysis of cellular and genetic changes, for which there is sound biological evidence for their relevance to cancer, in well designed prospective studies with clearly characterized pathologies.

It is estimated that in 1996 the number of deaths due to oesophageal cancer world wide amounted to some 450 000 out of a total of 7.1 million cancer deaths, making oesophageal cancer the fifth most frequent cause of cancer death world wide (World Health Organization, 1997). More than 85% of the cases, particularly SCC, occur in developing countries, and there are significant variations in incidence between regions of the world and between areas and ethnic groups within countries (Day and Varghese, 1994). ADC is less frequent and occurs mainly in developed countries (Kim *et al*, 1997). For both of these types of oesophageal cancer the efficacy of treatment is rather poor, with a survival rate at 5 years of less than 10% (Berrino *et al*, 1995).

The molecular changes occurring in the natural history of these cancers have been neglected until now and only recently have studies been undertaken to elucidate the temporal occurrence of cellular and genetic alterations in this type of cancer. These studies are reviewed here and their relevance to the implementation of primary prevention and of early diagnosis is discussed.

Although they have an equally bad prognosis and cure rate, SCC and ADC represent distinctly defined histopathological entities. SCC arises from the oesophageal squamous epithelium undergoing chronic inflammation, atrophy and dysplastic changes. ADC generally arises in the context of a metaplasia of the lower third of the oesophagus, in which the normal squamous epithelium is replaced by metaplastic, columnar cells of the intestinal type. However, both types of cancer share at least two essential molecular characteristics. The first is that they generally display a high frequency of allelic losses (>40%) at various loci on chromosomes 5q, 9p, 13q, 17q and 18q (Table 1). The second is that they both show a relatively high frequency of alterations (mutations and loss of alleles) in the *TP53* gene located on chromosome 17p13 (see below).

LOSS OF ALLELES AT MULTIPLE CHROMOSOMAL LOCI

Most of the studies on genetic alterations in oesophageal cancers have analysed the involvement of a single or a limited number of chromosomal sites. Loss of alleles has been detected at high frequency at several loci containing known tumour suppressor genes, such as *APC* (5q21), *RB1* (13q14), *DCC* (18q23.3), *DPC4* (18q 21.1) and *MLH1* (3p 21.3) (Montesano *et al*, 1996). However, muta-

TABLE 1.Allelic losses in oesophageal cancers

Chromosome	Minimal area of loss	Candidate genes	Mutations
3p[a]	3p21.3	MLH1	
4q[b]	4q21-qtr		
5q	5q21.2	APC/MCC	Very rare
9p	9p22	CDKN2A	0 <> 40%
9q[a]	9q31-32	ESS1	
13q	13q14.1	PRB1	None
17p	17p13	TP53	>60%
17q	17q21.3	BRCA1	
	17q11.2-q12	ERBB2, CSF3	
		NF1, ITGB4	
18q	18q23.3	DCC	Rare
	8q21.1	DPC4	None

[a] SCC only

[b] ADC only

From Mori *et al*, 1994; Miura *et al*, 1995; Barrett *et al*, 1996a,b,c; Hammoud *et al*, 1996; Montesano *et al*, 1996; Wang *et al*, 1996; Zhuang *et al*, 1996; Hayashi *et al*, 1997; Maesawa *et al*, 1997; Muzeau *et al*, 1997b.

tion of the remaining allele of these genes is highly infrequent, and the consequence of loss of heterozygosity at these loci on tumour development is poorly understood. Moreover, it is probable that these chromosomal regions may contain other, not yet identified, tumour suppressor genes that are involved in oesophageal cancers. Loss of heterozygosity is also common at the *TP53* locus (17p13) and at the *CDKN2A* locus (9p22). For these two genes, there is strong evidence that the remaining allele can also be inactivated by mutation or by other mechanisms. Point mutations in *TP53* are detected in 40 to 60% of oesophageal cancers (see paragraph below). Missense or nonsense mutations in *CDKN2A* have been reported in 10 to 20% of SCC (Esteve *et al*, 1996; Montesano *et al*, 1996). Moreover, expression of *CDKN2A* can also be down-regulated by other mechanisms, such as hypermethylation of promoter or coding regions (see below).

Two recent studies (Aoki *et al*, 1994; Barrett *et al*, 1996a) have extensively analysed loss of heterozygosity at multiple loci in oesophageal cancers. They show that most tumours have alterations at multiple chromosomal sites (from 5 to 20). In a recent study of six SCC and six ADC by comparative genomic hybridization (CGH) (Henn T, Barnas C, Tanière P , Haas OA, Hainaut P, and Montesano R, unpublished), it was observed that there is a correlation between tumour stage/grade and the number of chromosomal sites affected. This is in agreement with the notion that tumour progression is associated with the sequential accumulation of genetic lesions. However, the data available are too limited to determine which of these events may occur at an early stage of tumour development. Recent studies in ADC suggest that alteration of the *CDKN2A* gene may represent an early event (Barrett *et al*, 1996b).

Although differences between the frequencies of losses at particular loci have been reported, the areas of losses are similar in SCC and ADC. However, CGH studies (Henn T, Barnas C, Tanière P, Haas OA, Hainaut P and Montesano R, unpublished) reveal that loss of material of chromosome 4q may be more frequent in ADC than in SCC. This observation also confirms earlier loss of heterozygosity studies showing a relatively frequent involvement of chromosome 4q in ADC (Hammoud *et al*, 1996). These observations raise the possibility that chromosome 4q contains one or several unknown suppressor genes that are involved in ADC.

ALTERATIONS OF THE *TP53* GENE

The *TP53* gene is the best analysed of all genes involved in oesophageal cancers. Mutations were first described in SCC by Hollstein *et al* (1990) and in ADC by Casson *et al* (1991) and have since been confirmed by numerous independent studies in cancers from various geographical areas (for review, see Montesano *et al*, 1996). To date, more than 350 *TP53* mutations have been described in oesophageal cancers, and these are compiled in the IARC *TP53* mutation database (Hainaut *et al*, 1998). Analysis of these mutations provides valuable information on the aetiology and pathogenesis of oesophageal cancers.

Mutations in *TP53* appear to be an early event in the development of oesophageal cancer. In the case of SCC the evidence of early occurrence of *TP53* mutation is based on the detection of TP53 protein and/or *TP53* mutations in the basal layer of normal or dysplastic oesophageal mucosa in patients with SCC (Bennett *et al*, 1992; Gao *et al*, 1994; Sarbia *et al*, 1994; Mandard *et al*, 1997). These findings, although suggestive, do not constitute direct evidence that these molecular alterations and the associated pathologies are clonal precursors of the SCC. The evidence that this is the case is much stronger in Barrett's ADC, as shown by the elegant studies of Reid and collaborators (Neshat *et al*, 1994; Galipeau *et al*, 1996). Patients with Barrett's oesophagus were followed up by periodic endoscopies, allowing the prospective examination of the sequential occurrence of genetic and cell cycle alterations occurring during neoplastic progression. These studies show that inactivation of the *TP53* tumour suppressor gene, by point mutations and 17p allelic loss, already detected in Barrett's metaplastic epithelial cells, leads to an increase in the 4N (G$_2$/tetraploid) cell populations, which are the target of subsequent development of aneuploidy and other genetic alterations. In addition, in the sequential endoscopies obtained from one patient the same *TP53* mutation and allelic loss were detected, indicating that a *TP53* mutation occurs at an early stage and that this clonal population of cells with a specific *TP53* mutation is the target for further genetic alterations. These observations are consistent with the observation by Nowell (1976) that cancer is the result of accumulation of multiple genetic changes in a given cell and of the clonal evolution of this cell population.

The clinical significance of *TP53* mutations in oesophageal cancer is still unclear. Several studies aimed at determining whether the presence of a mutation in *TP53* may represent an additional marker of poor prognosis have yielded conflicting results. However, many of these studies are based on the histochemical examination of *TP53* accumulation rather than on the actual identification of the mutation (Sarbia *et al*, 1994; Wang DY *et al*, 1994; Wang LD *et al*, 1994; Chanvitan *et al*, 1995). Recently, it has been suggested that in breast and colon cancers the exact nature and position of *TP53* mutations may affect the outcome of the disease (Goh *et al*, 1995; Aas *et al*, 1996; Borresen-Dale *et al*, 1997). Indeed, all TP53 mutant proteins are not functionally equivalent and some of them may retain a significant degree of wild type activity (Ory *et al*, 1994). Further studies are needed to better determine the type(s) of *TP53* mutation present in the precursor lesions that are critical in the neoplastic progression of oesophageal cancer.

Analysis of TP53 mutations also provides valuable information to differentiate pathological lesions at the gastro-oesophageal junction. From the histopathological point of view, ADC of the oesophagus is difficult to distinguish from ADC of the gastric cardia, a type of cancer that occurs at the gastro-oesophageal junction and sometimes extends into the lower third of the oesophagus. Using strict criteria to select ADC of the gastric cardia (ie tumours located in the cardiac area, without microscopic or macroscopic evidence of Barrett's mucosa and without any documented evidence of prior metaplasia at endoscopy), we have found that TP53 mutations were much less frequent in these tumours (25%) than in ADC of the oesophagus (71%) or in ADC of the distal stomach (40%) (Tanière P, Martel-Planche G, Lombard-Bohas C, Berger F, Takahashi S, Montesano R and Hainaut P, unpublished). Furthermore, most of the tumours tested were overexpressing the MDM2 protein (Fig. 1), sometimes in association with gene amplification. *MDM2* encodes a protein that binds to TP53 and inactivates its transcriptional activity (Levine, 1997). In contrast, we found that overexpression of MDM2 was rare in oesophageal and gastric ADC. These results suggest that ADC of the cardia represents a distinct pathological entity, in which TP53 could be frequently inactivated by an indirect mechanism (MDM2 overexpression) instead of a TP53 mutation.

ALTERATIONS IN CELL CYCLE REGULATORY GENES

The *TP53* gene encodes a multifunctional protein that plays regulatory roles in cell cycle control, DNA repair, apoptosis and differentiation (Levine, 1997). The TP53 protein shares common molecular pathways with other genes that are also commonly affected in oesophageal cancers, such as *CDKN2A, CCND1* and *PRB1*. All these molecules cooperate in the regulation of the G_1/S checkpoint in response to various growth control or stress stimuli. The picture emerging from several independent studies is that inactivation of one or more of these

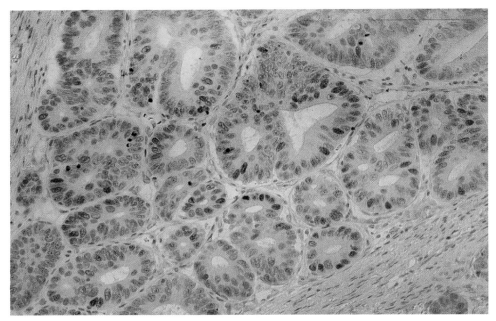

Fig. 1. MDM2 immunostaining in a well-differentiated cardia adenocarcinoma. More than 50% of the tumoural cells show positive nuclear staining with variable intensity (×160)

genes is essential for the occurrence and/or progression of oesophageal cancers.

The *RB1* locus is often the target of loss of heterozygosity (see above). *CCND1* is frequently overexpressed (Jiang *et al*, 1993), often as a result of amplification of a large chromosomal stretch encompassing the *CCND1* locus on chromosome 11q and which may also contain other genes contributing to oesophageal carcinogenesis. The *CDKN2A* locus is more complex. Inactivation of the *p16* gene may occur by loss of alleles, by missense or nonsense mutations or by loss of expression through hypermethylation of promoter or coding (exon 1) regions. The CDKN2A protein is a cell cycle inhibitor that negatively controls the kinases regulated by *CCND1*. An alternative transcript from the same locus has been identified (Stone *et al*, 1995). This transcript, initiated from a different promoter than the CDKN2A transcript, encodes CDKN2B, another protein with cell cycle inhibitory properties. Moreover, the area of loss on chromosome 9p often extends to *CDKN2B*, a close homologue of *CDKN2A*. Thus, alterations on 9p may also involve more than one gene.

The analysis of cell lines derived from human oesophageal cancers provides further evidence for a role of cell cycle regulatory genes. All cell lines studied to date have at least one alteration in either TP53, CDKN2A, CCND1 or PRB1 (Igaki *et al*, 1994; Barnas *et al*, 1997; Kitahara *et al*, 1997; Tanaka *et al*, 1997). In the TE-1 cell line, we have recently identified a mutant TP53 (with a valine instead of alanine at codon 272) that encodes a protein with temperature sensitive properties. This cell line reversibly undergoes G_1/S cell cycle arrest under culture at the restrictive temperature (32°C), expresses the CDKN2A and

CCND1 proteins but lacks detectable PRB1 expression. This unique cell line may represent an interesting cellular model for the analysis of the functional consequences of alterations of G_1/S regulatory genes in oesophageal cancers (Barnas C, Montesano R and Hainaut P, unpublished).

CLONALITY AND MULTIPLE PRIMARY CANCERS

The evidence of monoclonal evolution of a cell population containing a specific TP53 mutation is also relevant in determining whether multiple primary tumours, which are frequently observed in the oesophagus and upper aerodigestive tract, originate and develop as independent primary lesions or are the result of the spreading and invasiveness of a tumour into the surrounding mucosa. Various studies (Chung *et al*, 1993; Nees *et al*, 1993; Shin *et al*, 1994; Hayashi *et al*, 1996) have shown that the multiple primary tumours as well as the corresponding second primary cancers contain different TP53 mutations, indicating that the various cancers and related precursor lesions behave as independent monoclonal biological entities. These molecular fingerprints provide support for the proposal derived from histopathological observations by Slaughter *et al* (1953) that these multifocal monoclonal primary tumours are probably the result of prolonged exposure of the upper aerodigestive tract to the same carcinogen(s)—for example, tobacco smoke and alcohol—a phenomenon that he called "field cancerization".

A recent study of TP53 alterations in tumours of the upper areodigestive tract gives further molecular support to this hypothesis (Waridel *et al*, 1997). This study is based on the use of a highly sensitive functional assay in yeast that tests the transcriptional competence of human TP53 cDNA isolated from tumour samples. Multiple biopsy specimens of histologically normal tissues of the upper aerodigestive tract were taken and clonal TP53 mutations were identified in 76% of biopsy samples from patients with multiple tumours, compared with only 12% of biopsy samples from patients with single tumours. The presence of TP53 mutation in normal tissue is thus predictive of a multifocal pattern of disease. These results suggest that expansion of multiple independent clones of mutant TP53 containing cells is an important mechanism of field cancerization.

MOLECULAR EPIDEMIOLOGY

Epidemiological studies have clearly shown that smoking and alcohol as well as some nutritional and cultural habits are associated with SCC of the oesophagus (Muñoz and Day, 1997). A recent epidemiological study (Gammon *et al*, 1997) has shown that smoking is also linked to the risk of developing ADC of the oesophagus (and of gastric cardia). However, this study revealed certain epi-

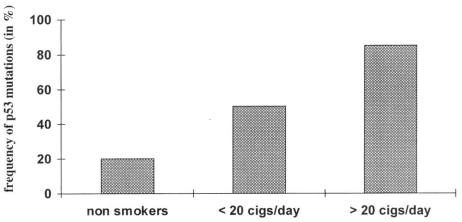

Fig. 2. Frequency of TP53 mutations in squamous cell carcinomas of smokers and non-smokers. From: Montesano et al (1996)

demiological features that differentiate this cancer type from SCC, namely that the association with smoking is much weaker, that no interaction is detected between smoking and alcohol and in fact a reduced cancer risk is attributed to wine drinking, while cessation of smoking does not result in a reduction of cancer risk. No information is given in this study on the intake of fresh fruits and vegetables, which in the case of SCC would be expected to reduce the cancer risk. These findings indicate that different risk factors are involved in the pathogenesis of two types of oesophageal cancer (Zhang *et al*, 1997).

Increased Prevalence of TP53 Mutations in Smokers

In many areas of the world, tobacco and alcohol have been identified as major risk factors in the aetiopathogenesis of SCC of the oesophagus. Among 91 SCC patients for whom reliable data on exposure to tobacco and/or alcohol are available (Montesano *et al*, 1996) the frequency of TP53 mutations reveals a strong relationship with tobacco smoking (Fig. 2). Only 20% of non-smoking SCC patients have TP53 mutations, in contrast to 80% of patients who smoked more than 20 cigarettes per day. Individuals smoking less than 20 cigarettes per day have a TP53 mutation frequency of about 50%. The relationship with alcohol consumption is less clear, since TP53 mutations are found in 32% of nondrinkers, in 51% of patients reporting a consumption equivalent to less than 1 litre of wine per day and in 58% of heavy drinkers. However, the independent impact of each of these major risk factors is difficult to assess, since most of the patients with TP53 mutations were exposed to both tobacco and alcohol and the contribution of other less well defined risk factors is unknown. Similar findings have been reported for SCC of the head and neck (Field *et al*, 1991; Brennan *et al*, 1995a).

Distinct TP53 Mutation Spectra in Squamous Cell Carcinoma and Adenocarcinoma

Mutations of the *TP53* tumour suppressor gene can be the result of DNA damage resulting from altered endogenous cellular processes or from exposure to exogenous environmental carcinogens (Jones *et al*, 1991; Greenblatt *et al*, 1994). It is reasonable to postulate that a specific type of TP53 mutation is indicative of a DNA lesion that occurred in the early stages of the natural history of a given cancer. Thus the spectrum of TP53 mutations in the monoclonal population of a tumour could reflect past exposure to specific risk factors. Various examples of specific mutation patterns have been reported in association with aflatoxin B1 and hepatocellular carcinoma, vinyl chloride and hemangiosarcoma of the liver, ultraviolet/psoralens and ultraviolet A exposure and skin cancer and tobacco and lung cancer (Harris, 1996; Hollstein *et al*, 1996; Hainaut *et al*, 1997; Montesano *et al*, 1997). This could be particularly relevant in the case of oesophageal carcinogenesis, in which, as discussed above, TP53 mutations have been shown to occur at an early stage. Thus the TP53 mutation spectra could provide valuable insights for identification of risk factors and their interaction.

SCC and ADC of the oesophagus differ significantly in their patterns of mutations in the *TP53* tumour suppressor gene (Fig. 3). In SCC the predominant type of mutation is transitional A:T base pairs, which represent more than 30% of all mutations. Together, these mutations account for less than 14% of the mutants in all other types of cancer. The spectrum of TP53 mutations in SCC is thus indicative of the involvement of exogenous carcinogens, in agreement with epidemiological data supporting the role of exogenous agents, such as tobacco, alcohol and nutritional components. The high frequency of mutations at A:T base pairs may reflect enhanced depurination of DNA upon reaction of carcinogens with adenine and/or exposure to DNA reactive agents such as acetaldehyde, a metabolite of ethanol.

In agreement with the notion that different risk factors are involved as causative events in different geographical areas, the spectrum of TP53 mutations in SCC from a high risk area in China significantly differs from that of SCC in Western Europe. In China, a high prevalence of G to T transversion is observed (35% compared with 12% in Europe), whereas mutations at A or T base pairs are less frequent (15% compared with 33% in Europe). In a recent analysis of 50 SCC from a high risk area in South Thailand (Chanvitan *et al*, 1995) we have found a mutation spectrum closely similar to that of China (Tanière P, Martel-Planche G, Lombard-Bohas C, Berger F, Takahashi S, Montesano R and Hainaut P, unpublished).

In ADC, TP53 mutations show a very high frequency of G:C to A:T transitions at CpG dinucleotides (~60%). To date, this is the highest level of CpG transition found in any cancer type (other cancer types with frequent CpG transitions are brain tumours and colon carcinoma, with, respectively, ~38% and

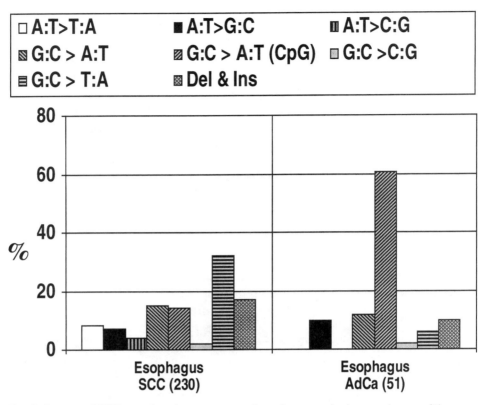

Fig. 3. Spectra of TP53 mutations in squamous cell carcinoma and adenocarcinoma of the oesophagus. Data are expressed as percentages of the total number of mutations found in these cancers as reported in the IARC TP53 mutation database. From: Hainaut et al (1998)

~47% G:C to T:A transversions). In contrast, mutations at A:T base pairs are rare compared with SCC.

Transitions at CpG dinucleotides are generally considered as the hallmark of mutations occurring spontaneously through hydrolytic deamination of 5-methylcytosine. Recent evidence (Shen *et al*, 1995; Yang *et al*, 1995) indicates that the mutability of CpG dinucleotides might also result from enzymatic deamination and methylation by methyltransferases, which bind with high affinity to the premutagenic DNA mismatches G:U and G:T, thereby preventing their efficient repair by mismatch repair proteins. In this respect, the studies on the role of altered methylation patterns of endogenous gene CpG islands in cell cycle control and carcinogenesis are of interest (Baylin, 1997; Chuang *et al*, 1997). The observation of a low frequency of microsatellite instability (Gleeson *et al*, 1996; Muzeau *et al*, 1997a) and the absence of oesophageal cancer in Lynch syndrome patients suggest that inherited defects in mismatch repair processes are not critical determinants in the development of this cancer.

PERSPECTIVES

Epidemiological studies have clearly shown that tobacco smoking, alcohol and some nutritional factors are associated with SCC of the oesophagus and that prevention of exposure to these risk factors could decrease the mortality due to this cancer. The role of human papillomavirus (HPV) infection in oesophageal cancer is not as evident as in anogenital cancers (Howley, 1994), although recent data suggest a role for HPV infection (He *et al*, 1997). A multicentre randomized trial in Europe showed that the survival of oesophageal cancer patients after surgery is ~20% at 5 years and that preoperative chemoradiotherapy did not improve survival (Bosset *et al*, 1997) and it is expected that in other regions of the world the situation is even worse. A similarly pessimistic picture is provided by the limitations of the pathology as a reliable tool for screening of precursor lesions or early cancer (Fennerty, 1997).

A more promising approach may be provided by the use of mutant genes and other genetic markers in combination with histopathology in the early diagnosis and staging as well as in the prognosis of oesophageal cancer. Analysis of TP53 has demonstrated its usefulness to generate hypotheses on the molecular mechanisms that are causing oesophageal cancers. Moreover, the identification of TP53 mutation as an early, clonal event provides us with a potential molecular marker for the identification of precursor lesions and the follow-up of tumour progression. The results recently obtained in the staging of cancer of the head and neck and some other cancers are promising (Brennan *et al*, 1995b; Caldas and Ponder, 1997; Waridel *et al*, 1997), although large prospective, multicentre studies are required for their validation. A better understanding of the natural history of oesophageal cancer is required for a proper interpretation of the significance of TP53 mutations in the screening, diagnosis and prognosis of this cancer. There is very little knowledge of the nature of the target cell in the origin of either SCC or ADC of the oesophagus or on the possible alterations in differentiation from the columnar to the epidermoid epithelium occurring during embryonal development (Johns, 1952) and the development of oesophageal cancer in adult life.

A more precise identification of the biological relevance of the precursor lesions may improve the clinical management of oesophageal cancers. This, in turn, may help to design and select adequate therapeutic strategies taking into account the specific nature of the genetic alterations observed in the tumour. In light of the poor achievements of current therapy protocols, the use of molecular markers as important criteria in the pathological and clinical evaluation appear to be our best hope for the significant reduction of mortality from oesophageal cancer in the future, in addition to primary prevention through control of tobacco and alcohol consumption.

SUMMARY

Oesophageal cancer is the fifth most frequent cause of cancer death world wide and most of these cancers occur in developing countries. The survival rate for

SCC or ADCs of the oesophagus is equally poor, mainly due to their late detection and the poor efficacy of the therapy. A short review of the natural history of these cancers, and in particular the occurrence of genetic and cellular alterations associated with cancer progression, is presented and discussed in the context of the relevance to aetiology and pathogenesis. SCCs and ADCs show a distinct pattern of TP53 mutations, namely a high prevalence of G>A transitions at CpG sites in ADCs whereas in SCCs a higher prevalence of G to T transversions and mutations at A:T base pairs is present. In both types of cancers TP53 mutations occur very early and are followed by the accumulation of other genetic alterations during the process of oesophageal carcinogenesis. The value of these genetic alterations in assessing the multifocal monoclonal origin of oesophageal cancer is also addressed.

Acknowledgements

We thank Dr Barnas, Dr Muñoz and Dr Tanière for comments and for communication of unpublished data, and Miss Hernandez for assistance in analysis of the IARC *TP53* mutation database. The secretarial help of Mrs Wrisez is also acknowledged.

References

Aas T, Borresen AL, Geisler S *et al* (1996) Specific P53 mutations are associated with de novo resistance to doxorubicin in breast cancer patients. *Nature Medicine* **2** 811–814

Aoki T, Mori T, Du X, Nisihira T, Matsubara T and Nakamura Y (1994) Allelotype study of esophageal carcinoma. *Genes, Chromosomes and Cancer* **10** 177–182

Barnas C, Martel-Planche G, Furukawa Y, Hollstein M, Montesano R and Hainaut P (1997) Inactivation of the p53 protein in cell lines derived from human esophageal cancers. *International Journal of Cancer* **71** 79–87

Barrett MT, Galipeau PC, Sanchez CA, Emond MJ and Reid BJ (1996a) Determination of the frequency of loss of heterozygosity in esophageal adenocarcinoma by cell sorting, whole genome amplification and microsatellite polymorphisms. *Oncogene* **12** 1873–1878

Barrett MT, Sanchez CA, Galipeau PC, Neshat K, Emond M and Reid BJ (1996b) Allelic loss of 9p21 and mutation of the CDKN2/p16 gene develop as early lesions during neoplastic progression in Barrett's esophagus. *Oncogene* **13** 1867–1873

Barrett MT, Schutte M, Kern SE and Reid BJ (1996c) Allelic loss and mutational analysis of the DPC4 gene in esophageal adenocarcinoma. *Cancer Research* **56** 4351–4353

Baylin SB (1997) Tying it all together: epigenetics, genetics, cell cycle, and cancer. *Science* **277** 1948–1949

Bennett WP, Hollstein MC, Metcalf RA *et al* (1992) p53 mutation and protein accumulation during multistage human esophageal carcinogenesis. *Cancer Research* **52** 6092–6097

Berrino F, Sant M, Verdecchia A, Capacaccia R, Hakulinen T and Esteve J (1995) *Survival of Cancer Patients in Europe—The Eurocare Study*, pp 1–463, IARC, Lyon

Borresen-Dale A-L, Lothe RA, Meling GI, Hainaut P, Rognum TO and Skovlund E (1997) *TP53* and long term prognosis in colorectal cancer; mutations in the L3 Zn-binding domain predict poor survival. *Clinical Cancer Research* **4** 203–210

Bosset JF, Gignoux M, Triboulet JP *et al* (1997) Chemoradiotherapy followed by surgery compared with surgery alone in squamous-cell cancer of the esophagus. *New England Journal of*

Medicine **337** 161–167

Brennan JA, Boyle JO, Koch WM *et al* (1995a) Association between cigarette smoking and mutation of the p53 gene in squamous-cell carcinoma of the head and neck. *New England Journal of Medicine* **332** 712–717

Brennan JA, Mao L, Hruban RH *et al* (1995b) Molecular assessment of histopathological staging in squamous-cell carcinoma of the head and neck. *New England Journal of Medicine* **332** 429–435

Caldas C and Ponder BA (1997) Cancer genes and molecular oncology in the clinic. *Lancet* **349 (Supplement 2)** SII16–SII18

Casson AG, Mukhopadhyay T, Cleary KR, Ro JY, Levin B and Roth JA (1991) p53 gene mutations in Barrett's epithelium and esophageal cancer. *Cancer Research* **51** 4495–4499

Chanvitan A, Nekarda H and Casson AG (1995) Prognostic value of DNA index, S-phase fraction and p53 protein accumulation after surgical resection of esophageal squamous-cell carcinomas in Thailand. *International Journal of Cancer* **63** 381–386

Chuang LS-H, Ian HI, Koh TW, Ng H-H, Xu G and Li BFL (1997) Human DNA-(cytosine-5) methyltransferase-PCNA complex as a target for p21WAF1. *Science* **277** 1996–2000

Chung KY, Mukhopadhyay T, Kim J *et al* (1993) Discordant p53 gene mutations in primary head and neck cancers and corresponding second primary cancers of the upper aerodigestive tract. *Cancer Research* **53** 1676–1683

Correa P (1982) Precursors of gastric and esophageal cancer. *Cancer* **50** 2554–2565

Correa P (1996) Morphology and natural history of cancer precursors, In: Schottenfeld D and Fraumeni JF (eds). *Cancer Epidemiology and Prevention*, 2nd ed, pp 45–64, Oxford University Press, Oxford

Day NE and Varghese C (1994) Oesophageal cancer. *Cancer Surveys* **19/20** 43–54

Esteve A, Martel Planche G, Sylla BS, Hollstein M, Hainaut P and Montesano R (1996) Low frequency of p16/CDKN2 gene mutations in esophageal carcinomas. *International Journal of Cancer* **66** 301–304

Fennerty MB (1997) Barrett's esophagus: what do we really know about this disease? *American Journal of Gastroenterology* **92** 1–3

Field JK, Spandidos DA, Malliri A, Gosney JR, Yiagnisis M and Stell PM (1991) Elevated P53 expression correlates with a history of heavy smoking in squamous cell carcinoma of the head and neck. *British Journal of Cancer* **64** 573–577

Foulds L (1975) *Neoplastic Development*, Academic Press, New York

Galipeau PC, Cowan DS, Sanchez CA *et al* (1996) 17p (p53) allelic losses, 4N (G(2)/tetraploid) populations, and progression to aneuploidy in Barrett's esophagus. *Proceedings of the National Academy of Sciences of the USA* **93** 7081–7084

Gammon MD, Schoenberg JB, Ahsan H *et al* (1997) Tobacco, alcohol, and socioeconomic status and adenocarcinomas of the esophagus and gastric cardia. *Journal of the National Cancer Institute* **89** 1277–1284

Gao H, Wang LD, Zhou Q, Hong JY, Huang TY and Yang CS (1994) p53 tumor suppressor gene mutation in early esophageal precancerous lesions and carcinoma among high-risk populations in Henan, China. *Cancer Research* **54** 4342–4346

Gleeson CM, Sloan JM, McGuigan JA, Ritchie AJ, Weber JL and Russell SE (1996) Ubiquitous somatic alterations at microsatellite alleles occur infrequently in Barrett's-associated esophageal adenocarcinoma. *Cancer Research* **56** 259–263

Goh HS, Yao J and Smith DR (1995) p53 point mutation and survival in colorectal cancer patients. *Cancer Research* **55** 5217–5221

Greenblatt MS, Bennett WP, Hollstein M and Harris CC (1994) Mutations in the p53 tumor suppressor gene: clues to cancer etiology and molecular pathogenesis. *Cancer Research* **54** 4855–4878

Hainaut P, Soussi T, Shomer B *et al* (1997) Database of p53 gene somatic mutations in human tumors and cell lines: updated compilation and future prospects. *Nucleic Acids Research* **25** 151–157

Hainaut P, Hernandez T, Robinson A *et al* (1998) IARC database of p53 gene mutations in human tumors and cell lines: updated compilation, revised formats and new visualisation tools. *Nucleic Acids Research* **26** 205–213

Hammoud ZT, Kaleem Z, Cooper JD, Sundaresan RS, Patterson GA and Goodfellow PJ (1996) Allelotype analysis of esophageal adenocarcinomas: evidence for the involvement of sequences on the long arm of chromosome 4. *Cancer Research* **56** 4499–4502

Harris CC (1996) The 1995 Walter Hubert Lecture—molecular epidemiology of human cancer: insights from the mutational analysis of the p53 tumour suppressor gene. *British Journal of Cancer* **73** 261–269

Hayashi K, Metzger R, Salonga D *et al* (1997) High frequency of simultaneous loss of p16 and p16beta gene expression in squamous cell carcinoma of the esophagus but not in adenocarcinoma of the esophagus or stomach. *Oncogene* **15** 1481–1488

Hayashi T, Sagawa H, Kobuke K, Fujii K, Yokozaki H and Tahara E (1996) Molecular-pathological analysis of a patient with three synchronous squamous cell carcinomas in the aerodigestive tract. *Japanese Journal of Clinical Oncology* **26** 368–373

He D, Zhang D-E, Lam K-Y *et al* (1997) Prevalence of HPV infection in esophageal squamous cell carcinoma in Chinese patients and its relationship to the *p53* gene mutation. *International Journal of Cancer* **72** 959–964

Hollstein MC, Metcalf RA, Welsh JA, Montesano R and Harris CC (1990) Frequent mutation of the p53 gene in human esophageal cancer. *Proceedings of the National Academy of Sciences of the USA* **87** 9958–9961

Hollstein M, Shomer B, Greenblatt M *et al* (1996) Somatic point mutations in the p53 gene of human tumors and cell lines: update compilation. *Nucleic Acids Research* **24** 141–146

Howley PM (1994) Viral carcinogenesis, In: Mendelsohn J and Howley PM (eds). *Molecular Biology of Cancer*, pp 38–58, WB Saunders, Philadelphia, Pennsylvania

Igaki H, Sasaki H, Kishi T *et al* (1994) Highly frequent homozygous deletion of the p16 gene in esophageal cancer cell lines. *Biochemical and Biophysical Research Communications* **203** 1090–1095

Jiang W, Zhang Y-J, Kahn SM *et al* (1993) Altered expression of the cyclin D1 and retinoblastoma genes in human esophageal cancer. *Proceedings of the National Academy of Sciences of the USA* **90** 9026–9030

Johns BAE (1952) Developmental changes in the oesophageal epithelium in man. *Journal of Anatomy* **86** 431–442

Jones PA, Buckley JD, Henderson BE, Ross RK and Pike MC (1991) From gene to carcinogen: a rapidly evolving field in molecular epidemiology. *Cancer Research* **51** 3617–3620

Kim R, Weissfeld JL, Reynolds JC and Kuller LH (1997) Etiology of Barrett's metaplasia and esophageal adenocarcinoma. *Cancer Epidemiology Biomarkers and Prevention* **6** 369–377

Kitahara K, Yasui W, Yokozaki H *et al* (1997) Expression of cyclin D1, CDK4 and p27KIP1 is associated with the p16MTS1 gene status in human esophageal carcinoma lines. *Journal of Experimental Therapeutics and Oncology* **1** 7–12

Levine AJ (1997) p53, the cellular gatekeeper for growth and division. *Cell* **88** 323–331

Maesawa C, Tamura G, Nishizuka S *et al* (1997) MAD-related genes on 18q21.1, Smad2 and Smad4, are altered infrequently in esophageal squamous cell carcinoma. *Japanese Journal of Cancer Research* **88** 340–343

Mandard AM, Marnay J, Lebeau C, Benard S and Mandard JC (1997) Expression of p53 in oesophageal squamous epithelium from surgical specimens resected for squamous cell carcinoma of the oesophagus, with special reference to uninvolved mucosa. *Journal of Pathology* **181** 153–157

Miura K, Okita K, Furukawa Y, Matsuno S and Nakamura Y (1995) Deletion mapping in squamous cell carcinomas of the esophagus defines a region containing a tumor suppressor gene within a 4-centimorgan interval of the distal long arm of chromosome 9. *Cancer Research* **55** 1828–1830

Montesano R, Hollstein M and Hainaut P (1996) Genetic alterations in esophageal cancer and their relevance to etiology and pathogenesis: a review. *International Journal of Cancer* **69** 225–235

Montesano R, Hainaut P and Wild CP (1997) Hepatocellular carcinoma: from gene to public health. *Journal of the National Cancer Institute* **89** 1844–1851

Mori T, Yanagisawa A, Kato Y *et al* (1994) Accumulation of genetic alterations during esophageal carcinogenesis. *Human Molecular Genetics* **3** 1969–1971

Muñoz N (1997) Le dépistage du cancer de l'oesophage est-il réalisable? *Semaines des Hôpitaux de Paris* **73** 633–635

Muñoz N and Day NE (1997) Esophageal cancer, In: Schottenfeld D and Fraumeni JF (eds). *Cancer Epidemiology and Prevention*, 2nd ed, pp 681–706, Oxford University Press, Oxford

Muzeau F, Flejou JF, Belghiti J, Thomas G and Hamelin R (1997a) Infrequent microsatellite instability in oesophageal cancers. *British Journal of Cancer* **75** 1336–1339

Muzeau F, Flejou JF, Thomas G and Hamelin R (1997b) Loss of heterozygosity on chromosome 9 and p16 (MTS1, CDKN2) gene mutations in esophageal cancers. *International Journal of Cancer* **72** 27–30

Nees M, Homann N, Discher H *et al* (1993) Expression of mutated p53 occurs in tumor-distant epithelia of head and neck cancer patients: a possible molecular basis for the development of multiple tumors. *Cancer Research* **53** 4189–4196

Neshat K, Sanchez CA, Galipeau PC, Levine DS and Reid BJ (1994) Barrett's esophagus: the biology of neoplastic progression. *Gastroenterology and Clinical Biology* **18** D71–76

Nowell PC (1976) The clonal evolution of tumor cell populations. *Science* **194** 23–28

Ory K, Legros Y, Auguin C and Soussi T (1994) Analysis of the most representative tumour-derived p53 mutants reveals that changes in protein conformation are not correlated with loss of transactivation or inhibition of cell proliferation. *EMBO Journal* **13** 3496–3504

Sarbia M, Porschen R, Borchard F, Horstmann O, Willers R and Gabbert HE (1994) p53 protein expression and prognosis in squamous cell carcinoma of the esophagus. *Cancer* **74** 2218–2223

Shen JC, Zingg JM, Yang AS, Schmutte C and Jones PA (1995) A mutant HpaII methyltransferase functions as a mutator enzyme. *Nucleic Acids Research* **23** 4275–4282

Shin DM, Kim J, Ro JY *et al* (1994) Activation of p53 gene expression in premalignant lesions during head and neck tumorigenesis. *Cancer Research* **54** 321–326

Slaughter DP, Southwick HW and Smejkal W (1953) Field cancerization in oral stratified squamous epithelium. *Cancer* **6** 963–968

Spechler SJ (1997) Esophageal columnar metaplasia (Barrett's esophagus). *Gastrointestinal Endoscopy Clinics of North America* **7** 1–18

Stone S, Jiang P, Dayananth P *et al* (1995) Complex structure and regulation of the P16 (MTS1) locus. *Cancer Research* **55** 2988–2994

Tanaka H, Shimada Y, Imamura M, Shibagaki I and Ishizaki K (1997) Multiple types of aberrations in the p16 (INK4a) and the p15 (INK4b) genes in 30 esophageal squamous-cell-carcinoma cell lines. *International Journal of Cancer* **70** 437–442

Wang DY, Xiang YY, Tanaka M *et al* (1994) High prevalence of p53 protein overexpression in patients with esophageal cancer in Linxian, China and its relationship to progression and prognosis. *Cancer* **74** 3089–3096

Wang LD, Shi ST, Zhou Q *et al* (1994) Changes in p53 and cyclin D1 protein levels and cell proliferation in different stages of human esophageal and gastric-cardia carcinogenesis. *International Journal of Cancer* **59** 514–519

Wang L, Li W, Wang X *et al* (1996) Genetic alterations on chromosomes 3 and 9 of esophageal cancer tissues from China. *Oncogene* **12** 699–703

Waridel F, Estreicher A, Bron L *et al* (1997) Field cancerisation and polyclonal p53 mutation in the upper aerodigestive tract. *Oncogene* **14** 163–169

World Health Organization (1997) *The World Health Report 1997, Conquering Suffering, Enriching Humanity*, World Health Organization, Geneva

Yang AS, Shen JC, Zingg JM, Mi S and Jones PA (1995) HhaI and HpaII DNA methyltransferases bind DNA mismatches, methylate uracil and block DNA repair. *Nucleic Acids Research* **23** 1380–1387

Zhang ZF, Kurtz RC and Marshall JR (1997) Cigarette smoking and esophageal and gastric cardia adenocarcinoma. *Journal of the National Cancer Institute* **89** 1247–1249

Zhuang Z, Vortmeyer AO, Mark EJ *et al* (1996) Barrett's esophagus: metaplastic cells with loss of heterozygosity at the APC gene locus are clonal precursors to invasive adenocarcinoma. *Cancer Research* **56** 1961–1964

The authors are responsible for the accuracy of the references.

Skin Precancer

D E BRASH[1] • J PONTÉN[2]

[1]*Departments of Therapeutic Radiology and Genetics and Yale Comprehensive Cancer Center, Yale School of Medicine, New Haven, Connecticut 06520;*[2]*Department of Pathology, University Hospital, S-751 85 Uppsala*

Introduction
Pathology
    Precursors of squamous cell carcinoma (SCC) of the skin
    Precursors of basal cell carcinoma (BCC)
    Precursors of melanoma
Epidemiology
    SCC precursors
    BCC precursors
    Melanoma precursors
Regression
    SCC precursors
    BCC precursors
    Melanoma precursors
Progression
    SCC
    BCC
    Melanoma
Stem cells
Genes
    PTCH and the hedgehog pathway
    TP53
    Melanoma
Carcinogen
    The molecular signature of UV radiation
    Mutations in precancers
    UV mutations in normal skin
    Mutations in tumours
Cellular events
    Acute UV exposure
    Apoptosis
Clonal expansion
Clonal lineages
Drugs
Animal models for skin precancer
Summary

INTRODUCTION

Skin precancers are perhaps the best studied precursors of cancer in humans or mice. The first clinical observation of squamous cell cancer (SCC) in people dates back to 1775, when Pott described scrotal cancer in chimney sweeps (Pott, 1771–75). Experiments began in 1914, when tar applied to rabbit skin resulted in malignant tumours (Yamagiwa and Ichikawa, 1914, 1918). In spite of meticulous descriptions, two major stumbling blocks in understanding natural or experimental precancers of the epidermis were a) how to distinguish pre-cancers from toxic and reactive responses and b) how to show that putative pre-cancers were indeed on a cell lineage leading to cancer. The outlines of a coherent picture have begun to emerge.

Fig. 1 assesses our understanding of various facets of skin precancer. Comparing such assessments between precancer types will spotlight needed experiments as well as organs in which crucial experiments can be done best. We will trace our current understanding of skin precancer down from the pathology and epidemiology to findings at the molecular level. Along the way, we will do our best to erase common misconceptions. Then, we will trace the effects of molecular changes back up to changes in cell behaviour. Two themes will recur at every step: mutation and clonal expansion.

PATHOLOGY

Morphological observation of human skin reveals a long series of events leading to in situ and invasive cancer. As with all neoplasias, the process is extended in time, so that decades can elapse between early dysplasia and invasive cancer. The rate at which precancer and cancer develop is consonant with a species' lifespan; indeed, it would be appropriate to use for example "mouse-years", "rabbit-years" and "human-years" rather than chronological time to describe a biological rate for carcinogenesis. Since cell doubling rates are comparable between mammals, this fact remains totally unexplained. Our description of the series of events will, in conformity with the definitions of the chapter by Pontén, use the terms of Table 1. The morphological intricacies of adnexal precancers have already been described (Kao, 1990).

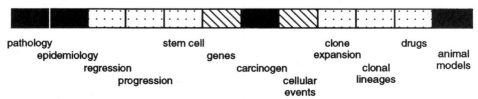

Fig. 1. A subjective assessment of our current understanding of skin precancer. Dotted squares, some facts are known and plausible hypotheses exist; hatched, important elements are known; solid, well understood

TABLE 1. Terminology for skin precancers

Preferred term	Synonyms	Comments
Keratinocyte stages		
Dysplasia	Actinic keratosis; solar keratosis; Bowenoid lesion	Actinic or solar keratosis denotes a combination of dysplasia with solar damage to the dermis
	Arsenical keratosis	Dysplasia in palms/sole after exposure to arsenic
Squamous cell carcinoma in situ	Bowen's disease	Distinguished from dysplasia by focal or total loss of ordered differentiation
Invasive squamous cell cancer		Penetration through basal membrane
Basal cell cancer	Basalioma, rodent ulcer	
Melanocyte stages		
Dysplastic naevus		
Melanoma in situ	Superficially spreading melanoma without dermal invasion; Lentigo maligna in radial growth phase without dermal invasion; Hutchinson's melanotic freckle	
Malignant melanoma		All forms show dermal invasion

Precursors of Squamous Cell Carcinoma (SCC) of the Skin

Epidermal dysplasias are defined by clinical characteristics and by a loss of cell uniformity and architectural orientation (Brownstein and Rabinowitz, 1979; MacKie, 1992; Schwartz and Stoll, 1993). Clinically, the visible lesion is a circumscribed, raised, reddish lesion, often rough because of hyperkeratosis. It typically appears on sun exposed parts of the body and is usually associated with solar damage to the elastin of the underlying dermis. Multiple lesions may accumulate over the course of years or may occur simultaneously. The age of onset is typically 40 years or later, but dysplasia is now being seen in 20 year olds heavily exposed to the sun.

Keratinocytes in dysplasias vary in size, shape and orientation. Some may be prematurely keratinized (termed "dyskeratosis"). Basal cells may crowd together, even forming budlike extensions toward the dermis without penetrating the basement membrane. Individual nuclei show "atypia", that is an increased affinity for basic dyes, a coarse chromatin structure and departure from the normal smooth and rounded contour. Some nuclei may persist into the stratum corneum ("parakeratosis"). The number of cells replicating their DNA is three times higher than normal, and many such cells are not restricted to basal or suprabasal levels (Pearse and Marks, 1977). A sharp, slanted border is seen under the microscope, with the basal region broader than the surface. Close inspection sometimes reveals horizontal extension of dysplastic cells into neighbouring epidermal territory. These microscopic features are quite similar to those of carcinoma in situ and SCC, except in being confined to a fraction of the epidermis. Lateral growth of the dysplasia spares the apertures of hair follicles. The dysplasia's sharp border against surrounding normal epidermis strongly suggests proliferation of a group of abnormal cells rather than a reaction to a toxic agent.

Skin dysplasias have been classified in various ways. Typical categories of actinic keratoses are: hypertrophic (marked hyperkeratosis with parakeratosis and premature keratinization, as well as a thickened epidermis with downward proliferations); atrophic (minimal hyperkeratosis, thin epidermis with downward proliferations, and rete ridges absent); acantholytic (cleft between atypical basal cells and suprabasal cells, loss of intercellular bridges); and lichenoid (vacuolar degeneration of the basal layer, with a subepidermal immune infiltrate) (Lever and Schaumburg-Lever, 1990). Carcinoma in situ cannot always be sharply distinguished from dysplasia and can be considered a continuation of dysplasia. It should display cellular atypia in all layers and show thickening because of net downward growth without penetration of the dermis. It does not spare hair follicle openings. Dysplasias seem to arise in skin that is already abnormal. The epidermis adjacent to actinic keratoses has twice the normal number of replicating cells and occasional multinucleate cells (Pearse and Marks, 1977).

Microscopic features of dysplasia may provide clues to mechanistic understanding. Taken together, they suggest a clonal proliferation of cells that have undergone genetic alterations of sufficient extent to disturb DNA synthesis, DNA packing and combination with nuclear proteins, and also parts of the differentiation program. Dysplasias differ from each other in their fine features, such as degree of atypia and disturbance of differentiation, suggesting that the set of genes mutated, or the site mutated within a gene, may differ from lesion to lesion. Moreover, the usual subdivision into slight, moderate and strong dysplasia is a simplification imposed on a continuum of departures from normal. Thus even early lesions may contain both essential and ancillary mutations.

Pterygia are keratinocyte growths over the cornea. They arise where the eye's conjunctival and corneal epithelium meet. The dermis underlying a pterygium shows solar degeneration. The epidermis can be thin owing to atrophy or thickened through proliferation, but cellular atypia is rare (Spencer, 1996). Less often, the epithelium exhibits dysplasia or SCC.

Precancers may have precursors. When dermatologists treat dysplasias with 5-fluorouracil, the lesions redden and encrust. In addition, new red spots 2–10 mm in diameter appear at sites not previously judged to be abnormal. These "latent actinic keratoses" are assumed to arise from subclinical precursors (Schwartz and Stoll, 1993). Going back even further, it has recently been found that normal sun exposed skin contains many clones of apparently normal keratinocytes that are mutated in the *TP53* tumour suppressor gene (Jonason *et al*, 1996; Ren *et al*, 1996a, 1996b, 1997b). The *TP53* gene will be discussed in more detail later. It has the convenient property that most *TP53* mutations lead to overly stable TP53 protein. Therefore, staining the epidermis with antibody to TP53 protein reveals cells that probably have mutations. Using this technique on whole mounts of epidermis, or on serial paraffin sections, reveals a three dimensional arrangement of mutated cells. Instead of being scattered throughout the epidermis, *TP53* mutated cells are present as tiny clones 60–3000 cells in size (Fig. 2). Mutations in the *TP53* gene have been confirmed by microdissection and sequencing. Often, the clones encase a hair follicle or form a cone having its apex at the dermal–epidermal junction. The degree of TP53 immunopositivity decreases in the differentiated cells of the upper part of the clones (as it does in dysplasias and SCCs). Because the antibody method detects most *TP53* mutations, it reveals the actual mutation frequency in skin. Surprisingly, the frequency on sun exposed skin averages 30 clones/cm^2. Face and hands contain thousands, with almost one epidermal cell in 20 having a *TP53* mutation. The clonal arrangement reveals that these cancer prone cells are not sitting still while waiting for additional genetic hits—they are proliferating.

Precursors of Basal Cell Carcinoma (BCC)

Sporadic BCCs apparently arise without precursors. Even small tumours appear to have all the characteristics of BCC. It should perhaps be mentioned, because of a controversial history, that BCCs are now known to originate from a single focus even when they appear multifocal in sections (Madsen, 1965;

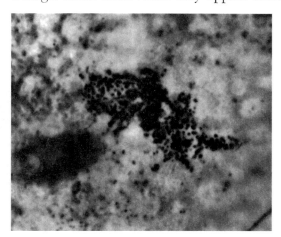

Fig. 2. A clone of TP53 mutated cells in normal human skin. Sun exposed skin contains over 30 clones/cm^2

Pontén *et al*, 1997). The *TP53* mutated clones are candidates for a BCC precursor, since many are found in hair follicles (see Stem Cells, below), but no definite evidence exists for this possibility. In contrast, a precursor of sorts exists in Gorlin syndrome (also called "naevoid basal cell carcinoma syndrome"). This autosomal dominant disorder is characterized by multiple BCCs (Springate, 1986; Gorlin, 1995). It is also associated with non-cutaneous tumours. More to the point here, the syndrome includes striking congenital malformations such as pits of the palms and soles, keratocysts of the jaw, midline brain malformations, spine and rib abnormalities, ectopic calcification, macrocephaly with coarse facies and generalized overgrowth. The pits, about 2 mm wide and about 2 mm deep, result from an absence of the thick keratinized layer typical of the palm and sole. Microscopically, the pits have irregular rete ridges with small and crowded basal cells. They occasionally show basaloid budding into the dermis and have been said to resemble tiny BCCs (Howell and Mehregan, 1970). Studies of the pits seen in Gorlin syndrome may thus shed some light on sporadic BCC.

Precursors of Melanoma

Human melanocytes normally remain at the dermal–epidermal junction and rarely proliferate. A freckle ("lentigo") results from an accumulation of apparently normal melanocytes at the dermal–epidermal junction (Clark *et al*, 1990). A mole (or "common acquired melanocytic naevus") consists of melanocytes that may extend suprabasally and dermally but are normal in appearance and are not accompanied by an inflammatory infiltrate (Clark and Mihm, 1969). Moles begin to appear between ages 1 and 5 years. The number of moles then increases until age 15 in males and age 25 in females, with the most sun exposed sites reaching peak values first (Nicholls, 1973). They then slowly disappear, as described under Regression, below.

Dysplastic naevi differ from ordinary moles. They are multiple pigmented lesions that vary markedly in size, shape, colour and texture, both within a lesion and across a patient's skin (Clark *et al*, 1990; Kopf *et al*, 1991). The histological structure of dysplastic naevi is a subject of some debate. Occasional melanocytes are pleomorphic, with dark staining nuclei, and may be accompanied by inflammatory cells (Kopf *et al*, 1991). Clark has insisted that only lesions with nuclear atypia should be termed "dysplastic naevi", even if the patient has multiple lesions that are similar at the clinical level (Clark *et al*, 1990). The dysplastic naevi begin as small, uniformly pigmented lesions that appear in large numbers about age 5 to 6 years (Kopf *et al*, 1991). Around puberty some of the smaller lesions take on the appearance of dysplastic naevi. Individuals who have dysplastic naevi have a risk of melanoma 6 to 150 times higher than normal, depending on the study (Kopf *et al*, 1991). An apparent familial syndrome of dysplastic naevi is termed dysplastic naevus syndrome. The possibility that freckles, moles and dysplastic naevi constitute a continuum of lesions able to progress to melanoma will be discussed below under Progression.

Lentigo maligna ("Hutchinson's melanotic freckle") is a freckle like pigmented flat patch. It appears on sun exposed skin about age 60, grows slowly, and with time changes from tan coloured to black (Clark and Mihm, 1969). Histologically, lentigo maligna is composed of almost contiguous intraepidermal melanocytes, many of which are pleomorphic to varying extents. The underlying dermis exhibits degenerative changes typical of sun damaged skin. Lentigo maligna differs from malignant melanoma of lentigo maligna origin only in remaining intraepidermal.

EPIDEMIOLOGY

SCC Precursors

Epidemiology tells us that most skin dysplasias are caused by sunlight. These actinic keratoses are most frequent on sun exposed body sites of fair skinned individuals who have a tendency to burn rather than tan. Anecdotally, red or blonde hair is also a predisposing factor. In addition, dysplasias are most common in those who live at lower latitudes, have outdoor occupations and have a high cumulative exposure (Green *et al*, 1988; Marks, 1988; Vitasa *et al*, 1990). The relative risk contributed by each of these factors is on the order of 2. Skin dysplasias are rare in blacks, except for albinos or patients with xeroderma pigmentosum (Brownstein and Rabinowitz, 1979; Brauner, 1985). These factors are the same ones important for SCC and BCC (Urbach, 1984). Patients with actinic keratosis show a 30–50% deficit in repair of DNA photoproducts (Lambert *et al*, 1976; Abo-Darub *et al*, 1978; Sbano *et al*, 1978). This deficit is consistent in several studies, and its magnitude overlaps that of the less severe subgroups of xeroderma pigmentosum. The defect probably does not just reflect an overloading of DNA repair in individuals with light skin, since the defect is seen in lymphocytes as well as fibroblasts, and since the patients' sun exposed skin actually showed greater repair than sun shielded skin. Overall, it appears that susceptibility to skin precancer is a multi-genic trait.

In areas of the world with high sun exposure, such as Australia, more than half of people over age 40 have at least one dysplasia, and the average is 6 or 7 (Marks *et al*, 1989). In men over 70, the figure is 85%. Similarly, the clones of *TP53* mutant cells in normal skin are most frequent on areas that are chronically sun exposed (Jonason *et al*, 1996; Ren *et al*, 1996b). They also become more numerous with age and are associated with elastotic dermis, a classic indication of chronic sun damage (Ren *et al*, 1996b).

Epidemiology also reveals the stage in life at which sunlight is important. People who move from England to Australia before age 20 acquire the higher Australian dysplasia incidence, but the risk is much less if they move as adults (Marks *et al*, 1990). Similar timing is seen for SCC and BCC (Kricker *et al*, 1991). Some important sunlight exposure does occur in adulthood because, with sunscreens, adults can reduce the number of dysplasias by half (Thompson *et al*, 1993; Naylor *et al*, 1995).

Arsenic can cause the same lesions—dysplasias, carcinoma in situ (CIS; Bowen's disease) and SCC. Ingestion is typically through medicinals or in the drinking water in particular regions of the world such as parts of Taiwan and Argentina (Brownstein and Rabinowitz, 1979; Schwartz and Stoll, 1993; Braverman, 1998). In addition, use of arsenic in herbicides and insecticides up to the 1930s led to high levels in cigarettes. Arsenical keratoses are more nodular than actinic keratoses and often appear on sites of friction, such as palms and soles. They are not regularly accompanied by any dermal changes. The mechanism is unknown. Arsenical keratoses are associated with elevated frequencies of internal cancers (Braverman, 1998). CIS was once thought to be associated with internal cancers, but the strength of this correlation is unclear (Braverman, 1998).

Pterygia of the eye behave quite distinctly from epidermal dysplasias. The lesions are not rarer in blacks than whites, nor is the lesion correlated with eye colour or tendency to burn rather than tan (Moran and Hollows, 1984; Taylor et al, 1989). Yet pterygia are most frequent in parts of the world closest to the equator and are present in over 10% of the elderly population of northern Australia (Moran and Hollows, 1984). In fishermen wearing dosimeters, a direct dose–response relation has been found between pterygia and both ultraviolet B and A (Taylor et al, 1989). The cause is thus presumed to be ultraviolet radiation. The different behaviour compared with other sunlight related lesions is apparently due to the lack of melanin protection in the conjunctiva and cornea. There may also be a hereditary component to pterygium susceptibility (Hilgers, 1960).

BCC Precursors

The pits in the palms and soles of Gorlin patients are not congenital; they appear in the second decade of life. Because the soles are a major site, pits do not seem to be sunlight related. If pits are clonal defects resulting from a second genetic hit in the *PTCH* gene (see Genes, below), then this second event is probably not caused by sunlight. This fact is striking because sunlight does have a role in the BCCs of patients with Gorlin syndrome. The tumours are more frequent on sun exposed sites, though not limited to such sites. Also, BCCs are rare in black Gorlin patients even if the developmental anomalies or internal cancers are present (Howell, 1984).

Melanoma Precursors

Moles ("common acquired melanocytic naevi") begin to appear between ages 1 and 5 years. Their number is proportional to sunlight exposure during the first 10 years of life (Holman and Armstrong, 1984a; Cooke and Fraser, 1985). An abundance of moles confers a 10-fold increased risk for melanoma (Holman and Armstrong, 1984b; Holley et al, 1987). In addition to a dependence on sunlight, frequent moles are more likely in children who also have birthmarks, freckles and red hair (Nicholls, 1968). Individuals with many moles also have an elevated frequency of dysplastic naevi. Dysplastic naevi can arise sporadically or in families as an autosomal dominant trait (Clark *et al*, 1990). The presence of multiple sporadic dysplastic naevi increases the risk of melanoma 4–10-fold. Families who inherit a predisposition to dysplastic naevi also inherit a predisposition to melanoma, with an almost 100% lifetime risk. Lentigo maligna (Huchinson's freckle) most often occurs on exposed body sites of light skinned individuals (Clark and Mihm, 1969). It is strongly correlated with a tendency to burn rather than tan, with high sunlight exposure and with migration to Australia as a child, but it has no correlation with naevi (Holman and Armstrong, 1984a,b). Preinvasive melanomas are most common on the face and, in men, the ears (Green *et al*, 1993). In a 7 year period between 1980 and 1987, these preinvasive lesions increased by 50%; the greatest increases were for intermittently sun exposed sites such as the back and legs (Green *et al*, 1993).

Much more is known about melanomas themselves (reviewed in Koh *et al*, 1990; Lee, 1991). These studies may be instructive in designing or interpreting studies of the precursor lesions. It is surprisingly clear that most melanomas depend on sunlight. The tumours are most frequent in light skinned individuals who burn rather than tan, especially those living near the equator (Holman and Armstrong, 1984b). Melanomas are rare on the buttocks and the soles of the feet (Koh *et al*, 1990; Green *et al*, 1993). When expressed as lesions per unit area, melanomas in Australia are most frequent on the face, shoulders, back and, in men, the ears and neck (Green *et al*, 1993). The frequency of melanoma on the leg is nine times higher in women than in men, whereas the frequency on the breast is lower in women (Clark *et al*, 1990). The clinical cliché that most melanomas occur on the back in men and the lower legs in women, though true, reflects the greater surface area of these sites, as well as the elimination of two high frequency sites by long hairstyles in women. Thus there is no need to invoke systemic effects, such as UV induced suppression of circulating immune cells, to explain an oft recited concentration of melanomas on sun shielded sites. Indeed, though systemic effects could explain a supposed lack of concentration on the face and arms, they offer no explanation of the concentration on intermittently exposed sites.

That the back and leg are sites for melanoma at all suggests that intermittent sun exposure is important. Its effect is pronounced when these intermittent occasions expose large areas of skin. For example the additional melanomas seen in populations living near the equator occur precisely on those body sites usually partially protected (Nicholls, 1973). In less sunny areas, such as Norway and Denmark, the intermittently exposed sites predominate somewhat, even when normalized to surface area (Green *et al*, 1993). The presumption has been that these sites reflect recreational exposure, which is particularly likely to lead to sunburn. Intermittent exposure has also been proposed as an explanation of the observation that melanomas are twice as common in office workers as in outdoor workers (Holman *et al*, 1980; Lee, 1991). Several observations support the hypothesis: the increase in melanoma since the 1930s is greatest for intermittently sun exposed sites (Koh *et al*, 1990; Green *et al*, 1993); melanomas are not associated with solar elastosis at the same site (Schreiber *et al*, 1984); and a history of severe sunburn doubles the risk of melanoma (except for lentigo maligna melanoma) (Elwood *et al*, 1985; Green *et al*, 1985). A cautionary note is that this last correlation can be attributed completely to the tendency of certain skin types to burn rather than tan; that is, the actual sunburns could be just an assay for skin type (Elwood *et al*, 1985).

Much melanoma inducing sun exposure happens in childhood. Melanomas are more frequent in adults who moved to Australia as children rather than as adults (Holman and Armstrong, 1984a,b). After age 15, migrating to Australia does not affect the melanoma rate. Melanoma cases increase in the summer months; this fact suggests a short latency promotional effect of sunlight, but it might also reflect an ascertainment bias (Scotto and Nam, 1980). Similarly, melanoma cases rise at 9–12 year intervals that come 2 years after peaks of sunspot activity; internal cancers do not follow this pattern (Houghton and Viola, 1981). The short latency suggests that sunlight is acting as a tumour promoter rather than a mutagen. Since sunspots make very little change to the UVB reaching the Earth's surface (Houghton and Viola, 1981; Koh *et al*, 1990), other effects of sunspots may be responsible—such as increasing the ionized particles of the solar wind. Many investigators have noted a doubling of melanoma each decade since the 1930s (Glass and Hoover, 1989; Koh *et al*, 1990). The dependence of melanoma on sunlight does not neccessarily mean that an increase in melanoma must be caused by an increase in sun exposure. Yet, increased recreational exposure is usually blamed for the "melanoma epidemic". The chief direct evidence for this supposition appears to be the observation that increases have been greatest for intermittently sun exposed sites such as the trunk and limbs, with some investigators seeing no change in melanomas of the head and neck (Koh *et al*, 1990).

Some melanomas are clearly independent of sunlight. Melanomas of the mucosa, palms, soles and nailbeds are equally frequent in whites and blacks, are not associated with precursor naevi and have remained relatively constant in frequency during the same decades that melanomas of the skin have become epidemic (Elder and Clark, 1986). Eye melanomas are more frequent in whites than blacks, but they do not depend on latitude and have not increased over the past several decades (Strickland and Lee, 1981).

REGRESSION

SCC Precursors

The hallmark of precancers is their tendency to regress. Observing Australian patients over the course of a year revealed that 26% of skin dysplasias (actinic keratoses) initially present regressed (Marks *et al*, 1986). Anecdotally, actinic keratoses tend to regress when the patient moves to a less sunny climate

(MacKie, 1992). Pterygia have been reported to regress in late life or when the patient moves away from the sunny environment (Hilgers, 1960; Youngson, 1972). *TP53* mutated clones can be generated in mice by irradiating them with UVB for several weeks (Berg *et al*, 1996). After irradiation ends, the clones begin to disappear.

The mechanism of regression is unknown. Several observations have been interpreted as supporting an immune involvement. Histologically, about 20% of dysplasias contain vacuolated basal cells and 7% a subepidermal mononuclear infiltrate, suggesting an immune response (Tan and Marks, 1982). A second line of evidence often cited is that skin cancers develop in patients who are immunodeficient due to leukaemia or lymphoma. In most such reports, controls or patient data are absent, but an 8-fold elevation does seem to be the case in chronic lymphocytic leukaemia (Gunz and Angus, 1965; Manusow and Weinerman, 1975). An important caveat is that most of these patients had received radiation or immunosuppressive drugs. Another frequently cited fact is that dysplasias (and SCCs) are at least ten times more frequent in transplant patients receiving immunosuppressive drugs than in the general population (Boyle *et al*, 1984). The dysplasias arise quickly, 2–6 months after treatment begins, particularly on sun exposed sites of fair skinned individuals; these dysplasias apparently convert more readily than usual to SCCs (Walder *et al*, 1971; Marshall, 1974; McLelland *et al*, 1988). The resulting SCCs, in turn, are unusually aggressive, resistant to radiation therapy and prone to metastasis (Walder *et al*, 1971; Maize, 1977). But non-immune explanations are readily available. Azathioprine and cyclophosphamide are DNA damaging agents and potentially mutagenic (Penn, 1978). Cyclosporin inhibits keratinocyte proliferation (Urabe *et al*, 1989). These drugs may thus induce apoptosis, acting as tumour promoters by favouring the clonal expansion of the death resistant cells created by sunlight induced mutations (see Clonal Expansion, below).

Other facts speak against an immune role in regression. In contrast to immunosuppressed patients, genetically immunodeficient individuals do not have more skin cancers (Gatti and Good, 1971; Waldmann *et al*, 1972; German, 1983). Moreover, when dysplasias are transplanted to nude mice, the lesions remain unchanged for up to 9 months (Thomas *et al*, 1985). This result implies that immune surveillance is not responsible for preventing progression, although regression might require immune mechanisms. An alternative mechanism for regression is a shift in the balance between cell renewal and apoptosis, towards net negative growth. In several circumstances cells with abnormal cell cycles are known to be removed by apoptosis (White, 1994). Apoptotic regression may prevail once exposure to causative agents ceases, as discussed below under Clonal Expansion.

SCC does not spontaneously regress. A barrier seems to be passed once invasiveness has developed. This issue has been somewhat difficult to settle because of confusion with self healing keratoacanthoma, which can be virtually indistinguishable from highly differentiated SCC.

BCC Precursors

The palmar and plantar pits seen in Gorlin patients do not regress (Howell and Mehregan, 1970). BCCs also do not regress in clinical practice. But in human autotransplant experiments BCCs transferred from their original site regressed, suggesting that an abnormal underlying dermis is required for maintenance of the tumour (van Scott and Reinertson, 1961).

Melanoma Precursors

Moles routinely regress after reaching a peak incidence about age 15 in males or age 25 in females. They first acquire a light halo and eventually become depigmented spots (Nicholls, 1973). By age 80 moles are absent. Lentigo malignas often regress partially, leaving a hypopigmented spot, and then continue growing in other directions. They can even regress completely (Clark and Mihm, 1969).

Melanomas themselves are one of four human tumours that undergo spontaneous remission at an appreciable rate (Everson and Cole, 1966). (The others are renal cell carcinoma, neuroblastoma and choriocarcinoma.) About 5% of melanomas regress completely, five times the rate for tumours in general (Everson and Cole, 1966; Nathanson, 1976). Partial regression is more common, occurring in approximately 50% of thin melanomas and 10% of lesions >3 mm thick (Clark et al, 1990; Blessing and McLaren, 1992). Nearly all regressing lesions are superficial spreading melanomas and few are nodular, either because the radial, preinvasive phase is more susceptible to regression or because thicker lesions obscure any partial regression. Regression is also most common in lesions of the trunk and lower limb. These are, of course, the same intermittently exposed sites showing the dramatic recent rise in tumour incidence. This may seem a contradiction, but partial regression is actually associated with a poor prognosis, particularly if a vertical growth phase is present. Regression of melanomas is typically associated with an immune infiltrate and apoptosis, suggesting an immune role. Melanomas are more frequent in immunosuppressed patients (Green et al, 1981), but interpretation of this fact may be subject to the caveat raised above in connection with carcinomas. However, if UV induced immunosuppression is involved in human melanoma—presumably by suppressing immune regression—the site distributions imply that the culprit would need to be intermittent high UVB exposures.

PROGRESSION

Demonstrating progression unequivocally would require the same genetic marker to be present in lesions of different morphology believed to belong to the same clone (see Clonal Lineages, below). In addition, the putative more advanced stage should have acquired additional mutations beyond those present in the founder lesion. Such an approach is now feasible and is beginning to be employed on a scale that will permit solid conclusions. However, it currently remains formally unproven that dysplasia, CIS and SCC are indeed manifestations of progression within one neoplastic clone. The alternative explanation that the lesions arise independently and have their own typical natural histories is not excluded. Similar reservations apply to the development of melanoma.

SCC

Many textbooks assert a progression from dysplasia to CIS and SCC, with the transitional state being hyperplasia of the suprabasal layer ("acanthosis"). Somewhat anecdotally, it is reported that SCCs arising from a dysplasia are much less likely to metastasize than those that arise from a scar or arise without an obvious precursor (Graham and Helwig, 1964; Lund, 1965). Longitudinal observation of patients showed that about 60% of SCCs in Australia arose at the site of a dysplasia (actinic keratosis) that had been clinically diagnosed the previous year (Marks *et al*, 1988). The remaining 40% arose on what had been clinically normal skin a year earlier. The risk of a dysplasia transforming to SCC was less than 1 in 1000 per year. Dysplasias are often found in the company of SCCs but not with BCCs (Marks, 1988).

Histological documentation for progression is less convincing, however. One study states that 20% of skin dysplasias (actinic keratoses) contain regions of SCC (Montgomery, 1939). Texts often cite this paper (or cite other texts that cite it), but the original contains little supporting data. In clinical pathology practice it is certainly rare to observe transitions between dysplasia, CIS and SCC. The common morphological impression of SCC is that it has arisen de novo. When lesions do adjoin, it is inherently uncertain whether an apparently non-invasive dysplasia or CIS actually represents an extension of the invasive cancer into adjacent epidermis.

Of the thousands of *TP53* mutated clones on sun exposed skin, it is clear that most never progress to dysplasia, let alone carcinoma. Using the observed figure of 30 clones/cm^2 in chronically sun exposed skin (Jonason *et al*, 1996; Ren *et al*, 1997b) and 0.2 m^2 of such skin (10% of total skin) gives a total of 60 000 clones per person. In comparison, the average number of actinic keratoses, even in Australia, is six to seven; one person in five gets a skin tumour in his lifetime in the USA. In Scandinavia, where one person in five contracts dysplasia, the likelihood that a *TP53* mutant clone will progress to dysplasia is about 1 in 300 000 (Ren *et al*, 1997a). This failure to progress could be due to regression, squamous differentiation, or failure to sustain a mutation in an additional gene.

Pterygia are said not to be precancerous, but it is unclear to what extent this fact is due to renaming of the lesions as "solar keratoses" or SCC once atypia is present (Spencer, 1996). If corneal SCCs in fact do not arise from pterygia, they would be a precancerless SCC. Pterygia would constitute a negative control for thinking about precancers—an apparently clonal lesion that can regress, but does not progress to cancer.

BCC

Most of the many BCCs in patients with Gorlin syndrome do not arise on the palms and soles, so they did not arise from the BCC like pits. Pits do occasionally progress to BCC, however (Howell and Mehregan, 1970). These BCCs are much less aggressive than those on the head and neck of the same patient (Howell, 1984).

Melanoma

Most naevi never progress to melanoma. Each year one melanoma develops per 7000 common naevi or 80 dysplastic naevi (Kraemer *et al*, 1983). On the other hand, about one third of malignant melanomas adjoin a dysplastic naevus (Kopf *et al*, 1991); the figure rises to over 70% in families with dysplastic naevus syndrome (Clark *et al*, 1990). Melanomas appearing after immunosuppression also appear to arise from a precursor naevus located at the tumour margin (Green *et al*, 1981). Histological observations have led to the proposal that the early sequence of melanoma development is (Clark *et al*, 1984, 1990): lentigo (a freckle), consisting of an increased number of basal melanocytes; common acquired melanocytic naevus (a mole), with a dermal component that may begin when a clone of melanocytes migrates to the crest of a rete ridge and forms a cord; and a naevus with an aberrant cell pattern (abnormal "architecture"). Many clinicians call the latter lesion a dysplastic naevus, but Clark reserves this term for the next stage. Melanoma begins when the naevus with aberrant architecture develops a localized subpopulation of cells that show nuclear atypia. This stage begins to be reached in the thirties. Succeeding stages can include: a radial growth phase; a vertical growth phase, which begins with a new subpopulation of cells in the radial lesion; and metastasis. Metastatic potential is a feature of the vertical growth phase. Lentigo maligna can progress to lentigo maligna melanoma, which invades locally but metastasizes somewhat less often than superficial spreading melanoma (Clark and Mihm, 1969).

The invasive proclivity of a melanoma precursor may vary from body site to body site. First, the site to site variation in the proportion of melanomas having an adjacent naevus cannot be explained by the variation in naevus density (Green, 1992). Second, the density of preinvasive melanomas varies as face >> ears >> neck > shoulders and back but for invasive melanomas the order is ears > shoulders > face and back (Green *et al*, 1993). It may also be relevant that melanomas begin to occur before age 40 on the shoulders and back, but after age 40 on the face, ears and neck (Green *et al*, 1993).

There may be a new kind of melanoma that, while locally invasive, has no tendency to become thicker, grow vertically or metastasize (Burton *et al*, 1993). The evidence is still indirect. In the late 1980s, widely separated regions of the world saw a sudden and striking increase in thin melanomas. These were correctly ascribed to increased attentiveness to early lesions. The surprise is that excising these lesions did not lead to a decrease in late stage or metastatic lesions. As a result, it was proposed that clinicians were seeing a previously overlooked lesion that has a different prognosis. Learning to distinguish these melanomas from lethal ones is thus a high priority.

STEM CELLS

A stem cell's job is to resist differentiation, allowing it to send new cells down the differentiation pathway. Two properties often ascribed to stem cells, frequent replication and immortality, are not essential to this definition. In some systems, apparently including skin, the stem cells generate "transit amplifying cells" that undergo several cell divisions and then differentiate. Stem cells are the most likely cell of origin for human skin cancer, since sunlight exposure in childhood contributes to a tumour six decades later. Similarly, the tumour promoters with which mice must be treated in order to yield a tumour (see Animal Models, below) can be given a year after carcinogen treatment (Potten and Morris, 1988). It is formally possible that a transit amplifying cell could also lead to a tumour if a mutation blocks the cell's commitment to differentiation. The mutation would have created a stem cell.

In the bone marrow, stem cells constitute about 0.05% of the population (Miller *et al*, 1993a). When mouse skin is X-irradiated so that it must be repopulated, about 10% of the basal keratinocytes are clonogenic (Potten and Hendry, 1973). It is not clear whether the 10% figure represents stem cells only or also includes transit amplifying cells. Indeed, a radiobiological subpopulation could in principle simply represent a fraction of cells in a radiation resistant phase of the cell cycle. Yet, the 10% figure is commonly cited as being the fraction of basal cells that are stem cells. This number is 200 times higher than that in the haemopoietic system, though perhaps because only one level of transit amplification is used.

Murine dorsal skin is relatively flat and free of dermal papillae and rete ridges. It appears to consist of hexagonal columns of about 15 cells: a basal layer consisting of a single putative stem cell surrounded by approximately 10 transit amplifying cells, all overlain by a column of about three large, flattened, hexagonal keratinocytes undergoing squamous differentiation (reviewed in Potten and Morris, 1988). Mitotic figures tend to be seen in the basal layer at the periphery of the column. This arrangement has been called an epidermal proliferating unit. Retroviral labelling of proliferating murine keratinocytes reveals columns of cells in roughly this pattern (Mackenzie, 1997). However, these columns do not seem to be monoclonal (Miller *et al*, 1993a). Columns are not seen in skin of the palm or sole (Miller *et al*, 1993a).

Stem cells in skin cannot yet be identified directly, because no markers exist for differentiation resistant keratinocytes. However, plating primary human epidermal cultures at low density yields three clone sizes, reflecting three classes of proliferation potential (Barrandon and Green, 1987). The largest, termed "holoclones", are presumed to arise from stem cells; in contrast, smaller "para-clones" result from cells that divide several times and then differentiate, as expected of a transit amplifying cell. In intact epidermis, basal cells adhere to the dermal–epidermal junction via receptors for extracellular matrix proteins such as collagen, fibronectin, and laminin. At the time basal keratinocytes commit to upward migration and squamous differentation the activity of these receptors, which are heterodimers containing β1 integrin, is downregulated. Somewhat correspondingly, keratinocytes isolated from cultured human epidermis on the basis of having high β1 integrin gene expression have the greatest proliferative capacity. Cells expressing less β1 integrin proliferate several times, and their daughters undergo differentiation, akin to transit amplifying cells (Jones and Watt, 1993). In tissue sections, cells with two-fold elevated β1 integrin expression lie at tips of dermal papillae or rete ridges (Jones *et al*, 1995). They also are less often in S phase. However, these cells constitute about 40% of the basal layer, so it would appear that β1 integrin also marks non-stem cells. These could be transit amplifying cells, but then the rarity of S phase is perplexing.

An alternative strategy has been to seek cells that replicate their DNA infrequently. When mouse dorsal skin is radiolabelled by injection every 6 hours for a week, over 90% of the basal cells incorporate radiolabelled nucleotide (Morris *et al*, 1985). A month later, only 2% of the cells remain labelled; these label retaining cells are at or near the central cell of a column. These could well be stem cells, since they lose their label over a time scale of months; only about 10% of the columns had their central cell labelled at the end of the 1 week procedure. The same cells retain radiolabelled chemical carcinogens, again indicating infrequent replication (Potten and Morris, 1988). The tumour promoter 12-*O*-tetradecanoylphorbol-13-acetate (TPA) increases the proliferation of these putative stem cells, but not the surrounding cells (Morris *et al*, 1985). In monkey palm skin, the label retaining stem cells lie at the bottom of the deepest rete ridges (Miller *et al*, 1993a). Hair follicles also contain label retaining cells; here, they are in the bulge region at the base of the erector pili muscle (Miller *et al*, 1993a). Both follicular and rete ridge label retaining cells are undifferentiated (Akiyama *et al*, 1995). The proliferative potential of cells microdissected from hair follicles is greatest for cells at the level of the bulge (Moll, 1995). Several researchers have suggested that the epidermal proliferating units are responsible for day to day epidermal maintenance, whereas the bulge region cells serve as a reserve of "ultimate" stem cells.

Which stem cells give rise to skin precancers and cancers? On the basis of morphology, SCCs have been thought to arise from the interfollicular basal cells that give rise to squamously differentiating progeny. Though a transformed cell could have an arbitrary morphological relationship to its precursor, early SCCs do appear to arise from epidermis between hair follicles (Miller *et al*, 1993b). BCCs, whose cells resemble basal cells in failing to keratinize, have received more scrutiny. Two schools of thought have maintained either that they arise from interfollicular basal cells that retain their basal morphology or that they arise from keratinocytes in hair follicles or sebaceous glands. Histological observations of early lesions tend to support the hair follicle origin, although some BCCs arise at interfollicular sites (Madsen, 1955; Miller, 1991, 1993b). The hedgehog signalling pathway (discussed in Genes, below) is mutated in most basal cell carcinoma and does have a normal expression pattern restricted to hair follicles (Dahmane et al, 1997; Oro et al, 1997). Because clones of TP53 mutated cells occur in hair follicles as well as interfollicular skin, they could in principle be precursors to BCC as well as SCC.

In mice the hair follicle keratinocytes appear to be the source of cancers. The yield of skin tumours (papillomas) after treating with a chemical carcinogen varies with the hair cycle. Two to five times more tumours are generated when the carcinogen is applied during the growth phase of the follicle (anagen) than in the resting phase (telogen) (Miller et al, 1993c). Anagen is the time when the label retaining cells of the bulge region undergo transient proliferation. Additional clues come from experiments with transgenic mice. When mice are constructed with a RAS oncogene driven by a promoter expressed only in the suprabasal cells, painting their skin with carcinogenic chemicals gives only papillomas. (This last fact does suggest that suprabasal cells can lose their commitment to differentiation and travel part way down the path to tumorigenesis.) However, if the RAS oncogene is driven by a keratin 5 promoter, which is expressed only in the follicle, chemical carcinogens generate invasive tumours (Brown and Balmain, 1995).

For the TP53 mutant clones in human skin, it is possible to calculate how many cells are potential targets of sunlight. Mutations after low UV doses occur in mammalian genes at a frequency of 10^{-5} per cell generation or less (McGregor et al, 1991). Because the number of nucleated keratinocytes in human skin is about $5 \times 10^6/cm^2$ (Bergstresser et al, 1978), about 50 cells/cm^2 would receive a TP53 mutation each generation. This figure roughly equals the number of mutated clones actually observed, 30/cm^2. Thus, if the clones reflect a single cell generation's production of mutations, this correspondence suggests that they arise from transit amplifying cells as well as stem cells. If clones persist for ten generations, however, they could arise solely from stem cells. The tendency of TP53 mutated clones in mice to regress on a scale of weeks (Berg et al, 1996) suggests that the former case applies.

Stem cells are rather dangerous. Their ability to replicate means that a mutation that confers a growth advantage may allow the mutant cell to overrun a tissue (Cairns, 1975). Several lines of defence have been proposed, including compartmentalizing stem cells and minimizing their numbers. The latter is achieved by using stem cells to make transit amplifying cells, which do most of the dividing. Stem cells would then spend most of their lives in resting phase. If stem cells are usually held in resting phase, there is a potentially important implication for cancer. Any cell that can escape resting phase has a selective advantage over its neighbours (Cairns J, personal communication). Such escape would be mediated by a mutation in exactly those genes that are now called "tumour suppressor" genes. The analogue of these events has been seen in bacteria escaping from nutritionally imposed stationary phase. The conclusion is that mutations and tumours should not be thought of as events limited to dividing cells. In this regard, it is probably important—in a way not yet understood—that the *TP53* tumour suppressor gene appears able to switch a cell from dividing like a differentiating cell to dividing like a stem cell (Sherley *et al*, 1995).

GENES

Two genes have been identified that normally prevent cancers but are inactivated in SCC or BCC. *PTCH*, a component of a cellular signalling pathway, is mutated in perhaps 90% of BCCs. Inherited mutations in the gene cause Gorlin syndrome, which predisposes the carrier to multiple BCCs. *TP53*, which encodes a transcription factor that regulates the cell cycle and cell death, is mutated in the majority of BCC, SCC, CIS, skin dysplasias and *TP53* immunopositive patches. The locations of undiscovered tumour suppressor genes are often indicated by regions of DNA that are frequently lost in sporadic tumours. Dysplasias show allelic loss at several different loci (Rehman *et al*, 1994), so even precancers may have multiple abnormal genes. For example, telomerase is normally present only in the skin's basal layer (Harle-Bachor and Boukamp, 1996), but it is elevated in half of sun-exposed skin samples and over 80% of dysplasias, SCC's, BCC's and melanomas (Ueda et al, 1997).

PTCH and the Hedgehog Pathway

When the Gorlin syndrome gene was mapped, to chromosome 9q22.3, it became clear that most sporadic BCCs are mutated in the same region. Minute BCCs are as likely as large tumours to have chromosome 9 allelic loss (Shanley *et al*, 1995), so this loss appears to be an early event. These insights may provide models for precancerous events in BCC. For example 9q22.3 is also lost in the jaw cysts of Gorlin patients (Levanat *et al*, 1996). Gorlin syndrome patients inherit a point mutation, and loss of the second allele in a single cell leads to either a tumour or a clonal developmental defect such as a jaw cyst.

Once cloned, the Gorlin gene was found to be the human homologue *PTCH* of the *Drosophila* gene *ptc* ("patched") (Hahn *et al*, 1996a; Johnson *et al*, 1996; Gailani and Bale, 1997). Forty-two mutations have been identified in Gorlin patients, distributed across the 24 exons of the gene (Chidambaram *et al*, 1996; Hahn *et al*, 1996a; Johnson *et al*, 1996; Unden *et al*, 1996; Wicking *et al*, 1997). One-third of the mutations are base substitutions, nearly all leading to premature stop codons or splice-site mutations. One-third are 1 or 2 basepair deletions or insertions, resulting in frameshifts, and another third are 4 to 76 base deletions or insertions. Each kind of mutation would inactivate the protein, as expected for a tumour suppressor gene. The unusually high frequency of deletions and insertions may simply reflect the fact that mutations were obtained by first screening for single strand conformation polymorphisms. Since *PTCH* mutations have been found in only 15% of Gorlin families, any skewing of mutation types may be appreciable. It is not yet known whether the gene has mutation hotspots or functionally important protein domains, since deletions, insertions and stop codon mutations will be effective anywhere in the gene.

Sporadic BCCs have also been sequenced. One-third had *PTCH* alterations detectable by screening for single strand conformation polymorphisms (Gailani *et al*, 1996b; Hahn *et al*, 1996a; Johnson *et al*, 1996; Unden *et al*, 1996). Direct sequencing of two BCCs that did not have allelic loss or conformation poly-morphisms showed point mutations in both, suggesting that nearly all BCCs contain *PTCH* mutations (Gailani *et al*, 1996b). However, this result also shows that screening can miss two-thirds of the mutations in *PTCH*. The mutations in sporadic tumours were somewhat different from those in the germline. Over half were base substitutions, and these often led to aminoacid changes. Only a third were small or large deletions or insertions. One missense mutation near the 3′ end of the coding sequence was recently identified in a family with BCCs but no other signs of the Gorlin syndrome. Thus it is possible that some patients with multiple BCCs, but no family history, are actually new cases of a milder form of Gorlin syndrome.

What does the PTCH protein do? Its cDNA sequence predicts that *PTCH* encodes a large glycoprotein with 12 membrane spanning domains and two large extracellular loops (Hooper and Scott, 1989; Nakano *et al*, 1989). From previous studies of *Drosophila*, Ptc is known to be part of the hedgehog sig-nalling pathway, which is important in determining early embryonic patterning and cell fate (reviewed in Perrimon, 1995; Dean, 1996). The current model envisions patched in a complex with smoothened, a membrane protein having seven membrane spanning domains and characteristics of a G protein coupled receptor (Alcedo *et al*, 1996; Chen and Struhl, 1996; van den Heuvel and Ingham, 1996) (Fig. 3). Alone, smoothened appears to be constitutively active; acting through cubitus interruptus, it induces overexpression of target genes for proteins such as wingless, decapentaplegic and patched (Stone *et al*, 1996). However, the complex with patched inhibits smoothened's activity. The secret-ed signalling protein hedgehog binds to the patched side of the patched-smoothened complex (Marigo *et al*, 1996; Stone *et al*, 1996). This binding inhibits the inhibition of smoothened, thereby inducing transcription of smoothened's downstream target genes. Thus, if patched is in the active form it will turn off its own transcription; little protein will be present. If a hedgehog signal is present, switching patched to the inactive form, more patched will be made and promptly inactivated by hedgehog. Thus, patched is most visible in the part of the embryo where it is in the inactive form and the hedgehog path-way is on. Similarly, an inactivating mutation in patched would lead to an increase in its transcription.

BCC tumours support this model for PTCH. Expression of patched is bare-ly detectable in epidermis or cultured keratinocytes (even for Gorlin patients) but is readily detectable in tumours (Gailani *et al*, 1996b). This result suggests upregulation of the gene once both alleles of *PTCH* are mutated. Clonal devel-opmental abnormalities, such as jaw cysts, probably arise in a similar way. In

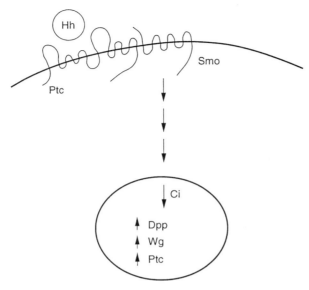

Fig. 3. Interactions between patched (Ptc), smoothened (Smo) and hedgehog (Hh) proteins in *Drosophila*. Patched represses transcription of hedgehog target genes by inactivating smoothened. Hedgehog binds to patched, thereby activating smoothened and causing increased transcription of wingless (Wg), decapentaplegic (Dpp) and patched (Ptc). In the absence of patched, smoothened may be constitutively activated resulting in the overexpression of these genes. Cubitus interruptus (Ci) is a transcription factor that is activated in the presence of hedgehog

other tissues, the gene dosage abnormality caused by losing just one functional copy of *PTCH* is evidently sufficient to perturb normal embryological development. This perturbation results in the non-clonal developmental anomalies of Gorlin syndrome, such as the spine and rib abnormalities or generalized overgrowth.

How does *PTCH* inactivation result in tumours? The answer may lie in the resulting upregulation of other hedgehog target genes. The vertebrate homologue of wingless, WNT1, is known to cause mammary tumours in mice when activated (reviewed in Nusse, 1994). Decapentaplegic is a member of the transforming growth factor-β (TGFB) superfamily, with closest homology to the vertebrate bone morphogenetic protein (BMP) subfamily. Members of the TGFB family have complex roles in cell growth and differentiation (reviewed in Hogan *et al*, 1994). A component of the decapentaplegic signal transduction pathway is mad (Sekelsky *et al*, 1995). One human homologue of the mad gene, *DPC4*, has been shown to act as a tumour suppressor in both pancreatic and colon cancer (Hahn *et al*, 1996b; Thiagalingam *et al*, 1996). Cubitus interruptus is a *Drosophila* transcription factor related to human GLI proteins (Motzny and Holmgren, 1995). Human *GLI1* is believed to act as an oncogene in brain tumours (Kinzler *et al*, 1987). The protein is expressed in human hair follicles and in BCCs, but not in SCCs. Overexpression in frog epidermis leads to nodular proliferations (Dahmane *et al*, 1997).

Human skin tumours may begin with upstream events in the same pathway. The most common vertebrate homologue of hedgehog is sonic hedgehog (SHH), required for correct patterning of the neural tube and somites and for anterior/posterior positioning of the limb bud (Riddle *et al*, 1993; Roelink *et al*, 1995). Its list of target tissues corresponds well with the clinical features of Gorlin syndrome, which include abnormalities of the brain, ribs, vertebrae and limbs. In addition, PTCH is expressed in all the target tissues of sonic hedge-hog. Transgenic mice overexpressing the *SHH* gene develop many features of Gorlin syndrome, and one *SHH* mutation has been identified in a BCC (Oro *et al*, 1997). Since, in *Drosophila*, *ptc* is one of at least 15 genes that have inter-acting roles in development, the mammalian homologues of these interactors may be important modifiers of BCC development.

TP53

TP53 is involved in both BCC and SCC. Indeed, the *TP53* gene is now known to be mutated in over half of all human cancers (Greenblatt *et al*, 1994). Every tumour may involve a defect in some part of the complete TP53 pathway (Agarwal *et al*, 1998). The TP53 protein is a transcription factor whose targets include genes regulating the cell cycle, such as *CDKN1A*, and genes regulating cell death, such as *BAX* (Levine, 1997).

TP53 mutations are present in carcinoma in situ (Campbell *et al*, 1993b). Going back further in time, over 60% of dysplasias contain *TP53* mutations (Nelson *et al*, 1994; Taguchi *et al*, 1994; Ziegler *et al*, 1994). This percentage may be underestimated for technical reasons, because dysplasias are not full thickness lesions; of the thickest biopsies, 75% contained mutations. The pres-ence of *TP53* mutations in dysplasia indicates that these precancers are clonal events rather than toxicity reactions. Different parts of the same dysplasia have identical mutations, confirming a clonal origin (Ziegler *et al*, 1994; Ren *et al*, 1996a). Patients with multiple dysplasias have different *TP53* mutations in each lesion (Ziegler *et al*, 1994). Therefore, each dysplasia is the record of a separate UV photon absorption event and subsequent mutation, followed by clonal expansion. The mutations in the DNA changed aminoacids in the TP53 protein, implying that the mutations had been selected for. They thus contributed to the development of the precancer. Had mutations often been found that did not change the protein, we would be forced to conclude that the mutations were an incidental side effect of dysplasia.

These precancer mutations are probably important in cancer development, because *TP53* mutations are present in skin carcinomas. Over 90% of the SCCs from the USA have a mutation somewhere in the *TP53* tumour suppressor gene (Brash *et al*, 1991, 1996). Although BCCs differ from SCCs in being diploid and rarely metastasizing, *TP53* mutations are present in nearly all of these tumours as well (Brash *et al*, 1996; Pontén *et al*, 1997). The *TP53* mutations are present even in small BCCs—presumably early lesions (Gailani *et al*, 1996a).

Are the *TP53* mutations found in dysplasias actually due to small SCCs arising within the dysplasia? This possibility was ruled out by microdissecting dysplasias before DNA sequencing; in all cases, the mutations were present throughout the lesion (Ziegler *et al*, 1994). Thus, the *TP53* mutations did not arise after the dysplasia emerged. Did they arise before the dysplasia, so that a dysplasia arises within a large *TP53* mutated clone of cells in sun damaged skin? This question was addressed by examining biopsy samples of normal skin flanking the dysplasia, to determine whether they contain the same mutation found in the lesion. Using the sensitive single-nucleotide primer extension (SNuPE) technique, able to detect one part in 10^4, it was found that the frequency of such mutations was orders of magnitude less than 100% (Ziegler *et al*, 1994). Evidently the *TP53* mutations arise at the same time as the clonal expansion of the dysplasia, suggesting that they are responsible for the dysplasia. The *TP53* mutations in dysplasias may also illuminate the process of clonal evolution of the tumour. Although mutations in SCC and BCC were clustered into hotspots, the aminoacid substitution mutations in dysplasias were spread nearly evenly across the *TP53* gene (Fig. 4). This result suggests that between the precancer and the cancer a selection occurs; some *TP53* alleles can lead to an SCC, whereas others are more likely to regress.

Going back still further, *TP53* mutations are present in most TP53 immunopositive clones (Jonason *et al*, 1996; Ren *et al*, 1996a). Unlike SCCs and dysplasias, however, allelic loss at the *TP53* locus was not seen (Ren *et al*, 1997a). The mutations again change an aminoacid, implying that the mutations were selected for and so had a causal role in clonally expanding the initial mutated cell.

Melanoma

Genes involved in hereditary and sporadic melanoma have been reviewed (Albino *et al*, 1997). The tumour suppressor gene *CDKN2A* is mutated in several familial melanoma kindreds (Hussussian *et al*, 1994). This gene encodes an inhibitor of CDK4, a cell cycle regulator. Most cell lines derived from sporadic melanomas or melanoma metastases have allelic loss or mutations in *CDKN2A* (Kamb *et al*, 1994; Liu *et al*, 1995; Pollock *et al*, 1995), but the mutations are rarer in primary melanomas (Gruis *et al*, 1995; Healy *et al*, 1996; Herbst *et al*, 1997). Allelic loss of *CDKN2A* or loss of an adjacent gene may be more important than point mutation. Similarly, in many tumour types *CDKN2A* expression is inactivated by methylation of an upstream regulatory region (Gonzalez-Zulueta *et al*, 1995; Herman *et al*, 1995). The latter avenues of investigation may be more fruitful relative to precancers.

In many melanomas, the level of TP53 protein is abnormally high. Unlike most tumour types, however, immunostaining is not uniform throughout the tumour but occurs in cell clusters or in scattered cells. Perhaps for this reason, the percentage of positive tumours reported ranges from 30% to 80% (Stretch *et al*, 1991; Sparrow *et al*, 1995; Weiss *et al*, 1995; Albino *et al*, 1997). Upon

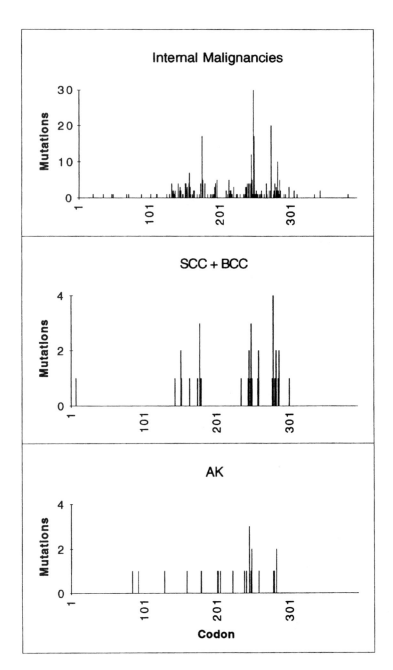

Fig. 4. Distribution of *TP53* mutations in skin precancers and cancers. The mutation hotspots in SCC and BCC compared to dysplasias suggest that only certain mutations able to cause dysplasia can progress to SCC. AK = actinic keratosis. Reproduced by permission of Blackwell Science, Inc. from Brash et al (1996)

DNA sequencing, however, only 2–25% of the tumours have *TP53* mutations (Florenes *et al*, 1994; Sparrow *et al*, 1995; Weiss *et al*, 1995; Albino *et al*, 1997). Pursuing the possibility of *TP53* mutations in naevi or in lentigo maligna may therefore not be rewarding. The gene encoding β-catenin, a signalling protein, is mutated in some melanoma cell lines (Rubinfeld *et al*, 1997).

CARCINOGEN

Skin cancers are the only human tumours for which it is possible to monitor, and even modify, an important naturally occurring carcinogen—ultraviolet light. Moreover, samples from precancer and cancer are easily obtained. This access has paved the way towards understanding some basic carcinogenetic mechanisms; these are most likely of general significance. The aetiological role of sunlight in skin cancer was noted early, at a time when other cancers were thought to be due to stray germinal tissue or parasites (Hyde, 1906). The epidemiological studies discussed previously implicate the UV portion of sunlight as the cause of most human skin cancers. Molecular studies of mutations have sealed this verdict.

The Molecular Signature of UV Radiation

The kinds of mutations made by UV have been studied for many years, in organisms from viruses to humans. In all cases the types of mutations are the same:

1. They occur at dipyrimidine sites, bases at which a C or T nucleotide is adjacent to another C or T. Two-thirds of the mutations are C→T substitutions.
2. In about 10% of cases, two adjacent cytosines mutate, leading to a CC→TT. These mutations are very distinctive and are caused by almost no other agents, and then only rarely (Hutchinson, 1994).

Finding both types of mutations in a collection of tumours eliminates all agents except UV. These unique properties of classic UV mutations give us a tool for deducing backwards, from the mutations found in the tumours to the original carcinogen. A third of UV-induced mutations include C→A and T→C substitutions. Because UV photoproducts join two adjacent bases, this third also includes deletions or insertions of one or two bases (Drobetsky *et al*, 1987). We treat these mutations as "non-informative", however, because they can also be made by other carcinogens. Although they are made by UV, and must be present when the classic UV mutations are present, their presence does not help us deduce backward.

These kinds of mutations occur because the most frequent UV photoproducts involve adjacent pyrimidines (reviewed in Brash, 1988). These are the "cyclobutane dimer" and the "pyrimidine-pyrimidone (6-4) photoproduct". The former are less quickly repaired than the latter (Mitchell and Nairn, 1989). Why the mutation is C→T is less clear, although several plausible models have been proposed. Both photoproducts lead to an abnormal DNA structure, bending the DNA or creating an imitation of an abasic site.

Mutations in Precancers

Nearly all *TP53* mutations in dysplasias (actinic keratoses) or CIS occur at adjacent pyrimidines, as expected for UV from sunlight (Brash *et al*, 1991, 1996; Ziegler *et al*, 1993). Moreover, about two-thirds of the mutations are C→T substitutions, and several of these are CC→TT. The mutations change an aminoacid of the TP53 protein, so the UV like mutations are not simply an indicator of lifetime sunlight exposure. If they were, mutations that do not change an aminoacid would often be seen—such as C→T substitutions at the third position of redundant codons. Although sunlight must initially make such mutations, the cells evidently never expand into a clone.

UV Mutations in Normal Skin

Sequencing *TP53* in the mutant clones of normal skin reveals a familiar pattern: sunlight induced C→T and CC→TT mutations at dipyrimidine sites (Jonason *et al*, 1996; Ren *et al*, 1996a). Because these mutations changed an aminoacid, the mutations were selected for and so had a causal role in the clonal expansion of the initial mutated cell. Supporting these observations are two experiments performed before the discovery of discrete clones of mutated cells. The pathognomic CC→TT mutations had been used as a measure of sunlight exposure in normal skin. The frequency was higher in sun exposed skin than in non-exposed skin, of the order of 10^{-6}, and was higher in sun exposed skin from skin cancer patients than from cancer free volunteers (Nakazawa *et al*, 1994). It was previously mentioned that normal skin flanking a dysplasia (actinic keratosis) had been examined for the same mutation found in the dysplasia. The mutation frequency was not 100%, but it was not zero, either. Frequencies were typically 10^{-3} to 10^{-2} (Ziegler *et al*, 1994).

Mutations in Tumours

Mutations in skin tumours support a continuity between precancer and cancer. The *TP53* mutations in SCC and BCC occur at adjacent pyrimidines; about two-thirds of the mutations are C→T substitutions, as expected, and several of these are CC→TT (Brash *et al*, 1991, 1996; Ziegler *et al*, 1993). This pattern differs from the mutations seen in *TP53* in internal cancers such as colon or breast (Brash *et al*, 1991; Greenblatt *et al*, 1994): whereas many of the same codons mutate, they do so by different base substitutions. The mutations again change an aminoacid of the TP53 protein. The role of UV in generating the *TP53* mutations in tumours has been directly confirmed in mice: UV induced skin tumours have UV like mutation patterns (Kress *et al*, 1992; Kanjilal *et al*, 1993). In addition, the numerous skin cancers in patients with the repair defective disorder xeroderma pigmentosum also have C→T mutations at dipyrimidine sites in the *TP53* gene (Dumaz *et al*, 1993; Sato *et al*, 1993).

When the locations of tumour mutations are plotted across the *TP53* gene, internal cancers show five hotspots. These are at CG sequences, which are known to be the sites of 5-methylcytosine in mammalian cells (Greenblatt *et al*, 1994). It appears that these sites are hotspots because body temperature leads to slow deamination of the cytosine which, because of the 5-methyl group, becomes a thymine. In the skin cancers there are nine hotspots (Ziegler *et al*, 1993). These fall into three categories. Some are important to the function of the TP53 protein. A second category of hotspots confirms the causality of sunlight. Codons 175 and 273 are frequent hotspots in internal cancers but were not recovered in the skin cancers. Those are the two internal cancer hotspots at which the mutating pyrimidine is flanked by two purines. In the absence of a dipyrimidine site there should be no UV photoproducts and no mutations in a cancer induced by sunlight. A third category comprises hotspots specific for skin cancers and not seen in internal cancers. These are codons 177, 196, 278, 294 and 342. A plausible explanation would be either greater induction of UV photoproducts at these sites or slower DNA repair; the level of UV photoproducts at these hotspots was not unusual, however (Ziegler *et al*, 1993). A method was devised to measure DNA repair at individual bases in the genome of *Escherichia coli* by end-labelling single genes. It revealed that, even if excision repair at a site is eventually complete, a slow rate of repair renders the site a mutation hotspot (Kunala and Brash, 1992). In UV irradiated cultured fibroblasts, the *TP53* mutation hotspots in skin cancer are repaired more slowly than many of the other sites in the gene (Tornaletti and Pfeifer, 1994). It remains to be checked, however, that sites that are not skin cancer hotspots, but which can contribute to tumours, are repaired rapidly.

In the *PTCH* gene, sunlight is still a major player. But up to one-third of the *PTCH* mutations in sporadic BCCs may have a non-UV origin. About 40% of the mutations in sporadic BCCs are classic UV mutations, and another 15% are the expected non-informative mutations at dipyrimidine sites (Gailani *et al*, 1996b; Hahn *et al*, 1996a; Johnson *et al*, 1996; Unden *et al*, 1996). A further 15% are one or two base insertions or deletions, often adjacent to a C→T at a dipyrimidine site. UV like mutations thus account for 70% of the total. In contrast, about 20% of the mutations in sporadic BCCs resemble those seen in the germline of Gorlin syndrome patients—deletions or insertions larger than two base pairs. This finding accords with the clinical observation that about one-third of BCCs occur on parts of the body that are not chronically exposed to the sun. The non-UV mutations could be due to DNA polymerase errors or to an unknown aetiological agent. For example patients with multiple BCCs of the trunk tend to have unusual alleles of glutathione S-transferase and cytochrome P450 (Lear *et al*, 1997). Because these enzymes are involved in detoxifying endogenous and exogenous compounds, including some chemical carcinogens, it is possible that such compounds contribute to BCC aetiology.

In melanoma cell lines, many mutations in *CDKN2A* are C→T at dipyrimidine sites or CC→TT (Liu *et al*, 1995; Maestro and Boiocchi, 1995; Pollock *et al*, 1995). The rare mutations in primary melanomas and metastases may also be

UV related (Gruis *et al*, 1995; Healy *et al*, 1996; Herbst *et al*, 1997). But fluorescent lights induce pyrimidine dimers in DNA, so one wonders whether long term passage of cell lines accounts for the higher frequency of UV related mutations in vitro. The mutations seen in the β-catenin gene may also be UV induced (Rubinfeld *et al*, 1997).

CELLULAR EVENTS

Acute UV Exposure

Exposing normal skin to artificial sunlight causes TP53 protein to accumulate rapidly in epidermal nuclei (Campbell *et al*, 1993a; Hall *et al*, 1993). With large individual variations, the protein disappears within about 24–48 hours (Pontén *et al*, 1995). Although never formally proved, this response is interpreted as a reaction to acute DNA damage.

When unselected biopsy samples from normal skin are reacted with antibody against TP53, sun exposed skin is seen to contain not only clones of *TP53* mutated cells but also individual antibody positive cells (Ren *et al*, 1996b). These "dispersed pattern" cells are particularly common during the sunny months and do not increase with age. In analogy with acutely irradiated skin, these cells are apparently responding to acute damage caused by recent ambient UV. Skin having a dispersed TP53 pattern was experimentally shielded from sun exposure for more than a month, to see if the TP53 positivity disappeared. Such disappearance could be due to repair of the underlying DNA damage or to removal of cells via normal differentiation or apoptosis. A proportion of the positive cells did disappear. Others remained positive, suggesting that they had *TP53* mutations but had not proliferated.

Apoptosis

A number of studies indicate two different functions for TP53 at the cellular level. In one function, termed "the guardian of the genome" pathway, DNA damage increases the stability of the TP53 protein. This induction leads to a cell cycle arrest at a G_1 phase checkpoint (reviewed in Fisher, 1994). The conventional wisdom is that TP53 induction then facilitates DNA repair, either directly or by retarding cells in G_1. However, there is little evidence for a role of G_1 arrest in DNA repair, or even in enhancing survival (Brachman *et al*, 1993; Slichenmyer *et al*, 1993). Another category of TP53 function has been termed "cellular proofreading" (Brash, 1996). In this pathway, stabilization of TP53 leads to apoptosis, a form of programmed cell death (Fisher, 1994; Levine, 1997). The signal for UV induction of TP53 and apoptosis originates in unrepaired UV photoproducts in actively transcribed genes (Ljungman and Zhang, 1996). TP53 is also required for apoptosis of cells that have cell cycle abnormalities (reviewed in White, 1994). Killing a damaged or aberrant cell would prevent it from becoming cancerous.

Skin cells are discarded in differentiation, by means of apoptosis (reviewed in Haake and Polakowska, 1993), so it is reasonable that skin would use cellular proofreading as a way of removing precancerous cells. It has long been known that skin overexposed to sunlight contains "sunburn cells", keratinocytes with dense, pycnotic nuclei and intensely eosinophilic cytoplasm (Danno and Horio, 1987; Young, 1987). This morphology is typical of apoptotic cells. Sunburn cells do in fact contain the DNA strand breaks known to be present in apoptotic cells (Ziegler *et al*, 1994; Brash, 1997). These sunburn cells require TP53. Irradiating the skin of normal mice with UVB generates sunburn cells, but in *TP53* knock-out mice the frequency of sunburn cells is an order of magnitude lower (Ziegler *et al*, 1994). The heterozygous knockout, in which only one *TP53* allele is inactivated, is intermediate. These results indicate that keratinocytes in skin have a cellular proofreading mechanism for UV damaged cells.

It is now possible to envision how failure of cellular proofreading, due to a *TP53* mutation, could lead to skin cancer. On the one hand, the *TP53* cell will mishandle regulatory events, such as cell cycle arrest; cell division events, such as the stem cell/proliferative cell decision; and some differentiation events not discussed here. On the other hand, these cancer prone cells will escape the apoptosis that would normally have removed them. It should be kept in mind, however, that some point mutations in *TP53* do not interfere with apoptosis or with formation of sunburn cells (Li *et al*, 1996; Rowan *et al*, 1996).

In the case of skin, the apoptosis related defects leave the cell susceptible to further assaults from sunlight. For example the number of mutant cells generated by each additional UV exposure increases. This is because, in a death defective clone, a greater proportion of cells survive UV irradiation to carry an additional mutation. Yet, because mutation frequency is defined as mutations/survivor, the mutation frequency has not increased at all. Finally, there is a more insidious way by which apoptosis resistance allows sunlight to foster cancer at the level of the tissue rather than the genome. This will now be described in some detail.

CLONAL EXPANSION

How do mutant cells expand into a clone? Normal skin exposed to sunlight will accumulate DNA photoproducts, and some of these cells will undergo apoptosis. If a cell received a *TP53* mutation during a previous trip to the beach, it will become apoptosis resistant. The straightforward consequence is that one cancer prone cell will survive cellular proofreading. The situation is reminiscent of the long-standing observation that precancerous liver nodules are resistant to cytotoxic drugs (Farber and Rubin, 1991).

Yet, the situation may actually be much worse than this. The cancer prone cell's neighbours will still undergo apoptosis when damaged, as they should, so they could leave space for the *TP53* mutated cell to clonally expand. For example the mutant clones seen in sun exposed skin are much larger than the column of cells derived from a single proliferating cell (Mackenzie, 1997). After the *TP53* mutation, each visit to the beach will provide an additional chance for the *TP53* mutated cells to expand further. Sunlight exposure should thus act as a selection pressure favouring the clonal expansion of *TP53* mutated cells (Fig. 5). Hypoxia, which also induces TP53 and apoptosis, does select out for *TP53* mutated cells (Graeber *et al*, 1996). Sunlight may thus act twice: once to mutate the *TP53* gene and afterwards to select for clonal expansion of the *TP53* mutated cell. This model is supported, but not yet proven, by the observation that *TP53* mutated clones in mice regress in the absence of UV exposure (Berg *et al*, 1996). Similarly, in humans the *TP53* mutated clones are largest in sun exposed areas (Jonason *et al*, 1996).

In addition to being a mutagen, UVB radiation is a tumour promoter in mouse skin (Epstein and Epstein, 1962; Blum, 1969). Tumour promoters are agents that increase cancer incidence only when used after the carcinogen treatment (Berenblum, 1975; Potter, 1984; Cerutti, 1985). Several mechanisms have been proposed, but promotion is generally viewed as a process of increasing the number of previously mutated cells. It is therefore important to recognize that the selective pressure of sunlight proposed above operates only after there has already been a *TP53* mutation. Therefore, this selection pressure qualifies as tumour promotion. A *TP53* mutation thus creates a cellular copying machine. A moment's thought reveals that, once a cell has divided, more precancerous cells are being contributed by such tumour promotion than by the initial mutagenic event.

Clonal expansion makes multiple genetic hit cancer feasible. Geneticists do not usually worry about the mechanics of mutating multiple genes, but it is possible to calculate the likelihood of these events. Mutations after low UV doses occur in mammalian genes at a frequency of 10^{-5} per cell generation or less (McGregor *et al*, 1991). Spontaneous base substitutions are even rarer. Thus, the probability of mutating both alleles of two particular tumour suppressor genes is at best 10^{-20}. Because the number of proliferating keratinocytes in human skin is about $10^6/cm^2$, with about 0.1 m² of skin exposed, about 10^{-11} cells

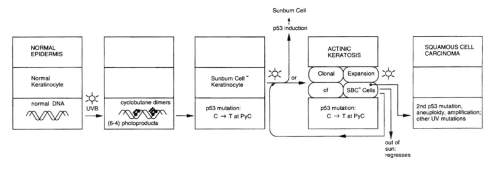

Fig. 5. A model for sunlight's role as a mutagen and as a selection pressure that drives clonal expansion of *TP53* mutated cells. Reproduced by permission of Macmillan Journals from Ziegler et al (1994), with permission from *Nature*

will be quadruply mutated. Even after 100 cell generations, only five people on the planet would have a skin tumour. For comparison, the lifetime expectancy of skin cancer in sunny climates is actually 20% or more. This discrepancy cannot easily be resolved by invoking mutator phenotypes and will grow worse if more than two genes are involved. Accounting for tumours in terms of multiple hits in one cell rapidly becomes impossible.

Clonal expansion, however, can easily increase by 1000-fold the number of targets for a subsequent mutation. The next mutation can then be quite rare, because only one cell in one of the clones must be hit. The number of clones can also be large, because apoptosis is a relatively high frequency physiological event that can facilitate the expansion of many *TP53* mutated keratinocytes simultaneously. Once both *TP53* alleles are mutated, the cell is prone to aneuploidy (Livingstone *et al*, 1992; Yin *et al*, 1992), increasing the likelihood of allelic loss.

CLONAL LINEAGES

The entire body is clonal. A clear statement of the cancer lineage problem is therefore the one given earlier: Is the same somatic mutation present in lesions of different morphology believed to belong to the same clone? Have the more advanced stages acquired additional mutations not present in the founder lesion? Of course, if one happens to be studying a gene that is mutated after the founder lesion, a lineage of lesions may seem unrelated. A single lesion may even appear polyclonal—and is, with respect to the late mutation.

The early appearance of *TP53* mutations in human skin cancer development has allowed lineage studies. Microdissecting skin specimens containing SCC, CIS and dysplasia reveals that each stage of the same lesion contains the same *TP53* mutation (Ren *et al*, 1996a). Thus invasive SCC and its precursors each derive from the same founder lesion. To show that these lesions fall on a lineage, as opposed to arising independently from the same founder, it will be necessary to find additional mutated genes that appear in succession. Within BCCs, such progression can be seen with respect to *TP53* mutations. Microdissection shows that one *TP53* mutation is present throughout the tumour, with the addition of a second mutation in parts of the tumour (Pontén *et al*, 1997). The second mutation can differ in different regions of the tumour.

In contrast, the tiny clones of morphologically normal *TP53* mutant keratinocytes never share a *TP53* mutation with adjacent SCCs, CISs, dysplasias or BCCs (Ren *et al*, 1996a, 1997a; Pontén *et al*, 1997). Any *TP53* mutant clone that gives rise to a more advanced lesion is evidently quickly overgrown by its offspring, or it regresses. Indeed, in the absence of a hybrid lesion it cannot be concluded that *TP53* mutant clones ever give rise to a more advanced lesion. Is it likely that hybrid lesions would have been missed? The frequency of *TP53* mutant clones in sun exposed skin is about 30/cm^2, so a lesion and its adjacent normal skin would contain 30 clones or more. Encountering a lesion's founder clone would require either luck or an exhaustive search, as well as the circumstance that the advanced lesion grew off to the side of the founder. Given the tendency of dysplasias to regress, it is perhaps more surprising that many epithelial tumours retain adjacent remnants of their CIS and dysplasia stages.

DRUGS

Dysplasias are often removed by treatment with 5-fluorouracil (5-FU). This drug inhibits thymidylate synthetase and thus DNA synthesis and DNA repair (Schwartz and Stoll, 1993). Treated actinic keratoses redden, encrust and then disappear over the course of several weeks. Arsenical keratoses are less responsive. Normal skin is unaffected, but is severely sensitive to sunlight or X-ray during treatment. As mentioned earlier, 2–10 mm diameter red spots also appear at sites not previously judged to be abnormal. These "latent actinic keratoses" undergo a similar course. Xeroderma pigmentosum patients treated for 4 weeks were free of dysplasias and cancers at the treated site for at least 11 months, suggesting that precancerous cells had been removed (Carter *et al*, 1968). Apoptosis inducing agents such as 5-FU may be effective on more minor sun damage as well. Many patients undergoing prolonged systemic chemotherapy seem to "show smoothening and general softening of the skin texture" (Falkson and Schulz, 1962); topical treatment of xeroderma pigmentosum patients relieved their xeroderma as well as their dysplasias (Carter *et al*, 1968).

The reddening and underlying immune response are not required for regression (Breza *et al*, 1976). 5-FU's specificity for dysplasias is instead thought to result from their cells' greater DNA replication (Eaglstein *et al*, 1970). In cell cultures 5-FU leads to *TP53* dependent apoptosis (Lowe *et al*, 1993). Approximately 1% of dysplasias are resistant to 5-FU (Klein, 1968), raising the possibility that these are a subset of lesions, perhaps $TP53^{-/-}$, that are most likely to progress to SCC.

Retinoic acid, which alters differentiation and immune function, causes complete regression of about 50% of dysplasias and partial regression of the remainder (Lippman *et al*, 1987). However, the lesions reappear once treatment ends. This response fits with the apparent role of retinoids in tumour promotion, that is clonal expansion of an already mutated cell (Lippman *et al*, 1987). A similar effect is seen with skin tumours in xeroderma pigmentosum patients (Kraemer *et al*, 1988), contrasting with the long term relief after 5-FU.

Sunscreens halve the frequency of precancers (Thompson *et al*, 1993; Naylor *et al*, 1995). This reduction is quite modest, however, compared to a sunscreen's 15 to 30-fold reduction in UV penetration. One reason may be that sun protection factor values are assigned on the basis of reducing skin reddening, rather than on their ability to reduce DNA damage or mutagenesis. "Mutation protection factor" has been proposed as an alternative measure (Ananthaswamy *et al*, 1997). A worrisome prospect is that reduced UV penetration is being offset by a sunscreen's carcinogenicity. For example both UVB and UVA excite *p*-aminobenzoic acid (PABA)—a UVB sunscreen—to a free radical that damages DNA and mutates cells (Knowland *et al*, 1993; McHugh and Knowland, 1997). Irradiating PABA with simulated sunlight generates singlet oxygen (Allen *et al*, 1996). Compounds related to Parsol 1789, which is used in UVA sunscreens, behave like PABA when irradiated and are known carcinogens (Knowland *et al*, 1993).

Immunosuppressive agents often lead to florid skin dysplasias (and multiple SCCs) in patients. As explained earlier, azathioprine and cyclophosphamide are DNA-damaging agents and potentially mutagenic (Penn, 1978). Cyclosporin inhibits keratinocyte proliferation (Urabe *et al*, 1989). By inducing apoptosis, these drugs may be introducing a selection pressure that favors the clonal outgrowth of apoptosis resistant cells. Thus the appearance of skin dysplasias may result from tumour promotion rather than from the drugs' immunosuppression.

Chemopreventive agents, usually antioxidants, can prevent the appearance of UV-induced tumours in mice. Some, such as geen tea polyphenols, can actually induce regression of papillomas already created (Wang *et al*, 1992). This regression may be related to the ability of green tea and chemopreventive antioxidants such as N-acetylcysteine to induce apoptosis of transformed cells without affecting normal cells (Ahmad *et al*, 1997; Liu *et al*, 1998).

ANIMAL MODELS FOR SKIN PRECANCER

In mice, SCCs can be generated on the skin of the back by irradiating with UVB daily for about 4 months (de Gruijl *et al*, 1983). Early in the process, reddish lesions appear that resemble dysplasias, both visibly and histologically (Winkelmann *et al*, 1963). The rate at which these lesions develop depends on UV dose (de Gruijl *et al*, 1983; de Gruijl and van der Leun, 1991), implying that initiation and clonal expansion of dysplasias are UV driven. In contrast, growth at the time dysplasias convert to SCC and thereafter is dependent on time but not UV dose. This result implies that conversion and subsequent tumour growth are due to spontaneous events. Subsequent UV only initiates new dysplasias. Many murine dysplasias regress, particularly once irradiation stops; SCCs do not (de Gruijl and van der Leun, 1991). These results suggest the sequence: initial mutation induced by UV; UV driven clonal expansion; and a spontaneous second mutation in one of the cells of the dysplasia. SCCs induced by UV often contain *TP53* mutations, although UV induced papillomas do not (Kress *et al*, 1992). The mutant cells begin to proliferate soon after irradiation begins (Berg *et al*, 1996).

In chronic exposure, UV acts as both initiator and promoting agent. A tumour promoter is defined as an agent that a) increases the frequency of cancer but does not itself cause cancer and b) is effective only when used after the initiator (Berenblum, 1975; Potter, 1984; Cerutti, 1985). UV is an initiator, because a single UV exposure generates tumours if it is followed by chronic treatment with a tumour promoting chemical (Epstein and Roth, 1968). Conversely, irradiating mice with UVB after treating with a chemical carcinogen increases the yield of tumours, apparently papillomas (Epstein and Epstein, 1962). UV's promoting effect leads to non-regressing lesions at high risk of progressing further.

It is widely believed that Blum's meticulous measurements of the kinetics with which ear sarcomas appeared under different irradiation conditions showed that UV solely stimulates the growth rate of already initiated tumours (Blum, 1959). This is a misconception based on two factors. First, Blum assumed a growth rate model and then adjusted the parameters to fit the data. The possibility that UV acted by generating mutations was excluded at the outset, on the grounds that tumours did not arise instantaneously. In the late 1950s, this was a plausible rationale. It was scarcely known that DNA was the hereditary material, and the experiments that showed that mutations do not arise instantaneously were still ongoing elsewhere. The concept of multiple genetic hits being required for a tumour was not even on the horizon. The second error was that the data never did fit the growth model. In refining the parameters, Blum found a particular equation that worked well. In a footnote he remarks that this equation arose as an algebraic error in evaluating the growth equation, but it worked so well that he retained it anyway. Reanalysing these data years later, Blum concluded that tumour growth was described by a mixture of irreversible genetic and reversible growth acceleration components (Blum, 1969).

Chemical carcinogens have been studied more intensely (DiGiovanni, 1992; Hennings *et al*, 1993; Yuspa, 1994; Greenhalgh *et al*, 1995). The classical Berenblum two stage procedure employs a single treatment with an initiator followed by multiple treatments with a promoter (Berenblum, 1975). The low toxicities involved were an advance in separating precancer and cancer from toxic or regenerative changes. This procedure generates papillomas, benign outgrowths whose cells proliferate rapidly and show delayed squamous differentiation. Dysplasia can then arise either in the papilloma or in flat epidermis. Papillomas usually regress when the tumour promoter is withdrawn, and fewer than 5% spontaneously convert to squamous cell carcinoma. Thus papillomas are precancers, or even preprecancers; murine precancer has been a major object of study for decades.

Several findings based on murine chemical carcinogenesis are particularly relevant to precancer. Initiation need not be accompanied by significant pathology, but individual cells are mutated during this stage. Initiation is essentially irreversible, since the first promoter exposure can be delayed for months with no reduction in eventual tumour yield. This dormancy suggests that the initiated cells are stem cells. Dormancy needs an explanation, since dysplasia clones and *TP53* mutant clones usually regress, and cells with aberrant cell cycles are often eliminated by apoptosis. It does seem that initiation proceeds as well in wild type mice as in *TP53* $^{-/-}$ mice (Kemp *et al*, 1993).

Papillomas can be divided into those at high or low risk for converting spontaneously to SCC (also referred to as "progression"). High risk papillomas arise shortly after promotion begins, are infrequent and have an unknown genetic basis, but they regress slowly and convert to SCC at a high rate. Continued pro-

moter treatment yields large numbers of low risk papillomas that carry mutations in *Hras1* and, on rare occasions, convert to SCC by losing the normal
Hras1 allele. Promotion beyond 5 weeks increases only the low risk papillomas
without increasing the number of SCCs (Hennings *et al*, 1993).

Papilloma regression shows rapid and slow components (half times of 24
and >140 days, respectively) (Burns *et al*, 1976). The rapid regression papillomas are the major component and the only ones affected by tumour promoters,
so they probably represent the low risk papillomas. Since the keratinocyte
turnover interval is about 21 days, one wonders whether the low risk papillomas
arise from the relatively harmless transit amplifying cells. In fact in transgenic
mice having suprabasal expression of a *RAS* oncogene, chemical carcinogenesis
generates only papillomas. Strikingly, papilloma regression tends to cluster at
multiples of 21 days after promoter treatment ends (Andrews, 1971). Lesions
that disappear on one of the higher multiples also underwent shrinkage on the
previous multiples. The 21 day figure again suggests that papilloma regression
relates to keratinocyte differentiation. Calculations indicate that a mere 5%
excess of cell production over cell loss would suffice to account for the observed
papilloma growth rates (Burns *et al*, 1976).

Conversion to SCC is associated with the appearance of *TP53* mutations.
The late role of *TP53* resembles its late appearance in human colon cancer and
differs from its early role in human skin cancer or UV induced murine SCC.
The difference thus appears to be related to the carcinogen rather than to tissue or species differences. In contrast, the role of *RAS* does differ between
species; activation is rare in humans or hamsters (Robles *et al*, 1993).
Papillomas can be made to progress more often to squamous cell carcinoma if
the mouse is treated again with a mutagenic carcinogen. Thus the mouse carcinogenesis model, extended to initiation–promotion–conversion, is beginning
to converge with the human multiple genetic hit model. In both species, mutagenic initiating events and non-mutagenic clonal expansion events probably
occur multiple times, often concurrently, and in different orders in different
tumours.

As with human tumours, important questions for the mouse model remain
unanswered. These include the number of genetic hits needed; possibilities of
hypermutability; mechanisms for clonal selection; and, in transgenic mice, the
interplay between oncogenes, tumour suppressor genes, growth or differentiation genes, and cellular phenomena such as wound repair.

SUMMARY

Squamous cell carcinoma of the skin and melanoma are the rare progeny of
precancerous lesions that usually remain stable or regress. For SCC the
sequence appears to include *TP53* mutant clones in normal skin; dysplasia; carcinoma in situ; and SCC. When such lesions are contiguous, their *TP53* mutations are consistent with a single clonal lineage. The set of *TP53* mutations in

tumours is more restricted than in precancers, suggesting additional selection. Melanoma lies at the end of a continuum including mole, dysplastic naevus, radial growth melanoma and vertical growth. The genetics of melanoma is less clear. Basal cell carcinomas seem to arise without a precancer and contain mutations in *TP53* and *PTCH*.

Childhood sunlight exposure directs the location and frequency of precancers. For melanoma, its effects on intermittently exposed body sites are superimposed on the effect at sites chronically exposed. SCC precancers and tumours, BCC tumours and melanoma cell lines contain UV induced mutations. Sun exposed skin of normal individuals contains thousands of small clones of *TP53* mutated cells. Predisposition to sunlight induced precancer is a multigenic trait involving factors such as hair and skin color, DNA repair proficiency and mole type and number. These each contribute a relative risk on the order of two to four. Familial predisposition to dysplastic naevi carries a larger risk.

The cell of origin for melanoma is uncontroversial, and the proposed hair follicle origin of BCC is consistent with the presence of stem cells in the bulge region. The origin of SCCs and the arrangement of interfollicular stem cell compartments are less clear. Clonal expansion of the initial mutated cell may also be driven by sunlight. When a mutation confers apoptosis resistance, as *TP53* mutations do, subsequent UV exposure will be more likely to kill normal cells than mutants. The latter can expand into a clone, only one cell of which need be mutated again. Immunosuppressant drugs may have the same effect as UV, facilitating the clonal expansion of precancers. In the absence of exogenous influences, mutant clones and precancers tend to regress. There is little evidence that regression of precancers is immunological, though regression of melanoma appears to be. The chemotherapeutic agent 5-FU causes regression of dysplasias by removing initiated cells, perhaps by enhancing apoptosis. In contrast, retinoic acid temporarily suppresses clonal expansion. Most sunscreens are mutagenic, with as yet unknown consequences.

Mice develop dysplasias and SCCs after UV irradiation. Initiation and clonal expansion of dysplasias is UV driven, but conversion to SCC and subsequent growth involve spontaneous events. With chemical carcinogens mice develop papillomas that usually regress and thus are precancers. Tumour promotion yields abundant low risk papillomas that contain *Hras1* mutations but rarely progress to SCC. High risk papillomas are infrequent but do convert to SCC, particularly if re-treated with mutagens. Conversion to SCC is associated with *TP53* mutations. The mechanisms of multiple mutation and clonal expansion observed in human and mouse systems, respectively, are beginning to converge into a coherent understanding of precancerous events in skin.

Acknowledgements

Research in our laboratory was supported by National Institutes of Health and American Cancer Society grants, Hull and Swebelius Cancer Research Awards, the Munson Foundation and fellowships from the Swiss National Foundation and Swiss Cancer League.

References

Abo-Darub JM, Mackie R and Pitts JD (1978) DNA repair deficiency in lymphocytes from patients with actinic keratosis. *Bulletin du Cancer* **65** 357–362

Agarwal ML, Taylor WR, Chernov MV, Chernova OB and Stark GR (1998) The p53 network. *Journal of Biological Chemistry* **273** 1–4

Ahmad N, Feyes DK, Nieminen AL, Agarwal R and Mukhtar H (1997) Green tea constituent epigallocatechin-3-gallate and induction of apoptosis and cell cycle arrest in human carcinoma cells. *Journal of the National Cancer Institute* **89** 1771–1886

Akiyama M, Dale BA, Sun TT and Holbrook KA (1995) Characterization of hair follicle bulge in human fetal skin: the human fetal bulge is a pool of undifferentiated keratinocytes. *Journal of Investigative Dermatology* **105** 844–850

Albino AP, Reed JA and McNutt NS (1997) Molecular biology of cutaneous malignant melanoma, In: DeVita VT, Hellman S and Rosenberg SA (eds). *Cancer: Principles and Practice of Oncology*, pp 1935–1946, Lippincott-Raven, Philadelphia, Pennsylvania

Alcedo J, Ayzenzon M, Von Ohlen T, Noll M and Hooper JE (1996) The *Drosophila* smoothened gene encodes a seven-pass membrane protein, a putative receptor for the hedgehog signal. *Cell* **86** 221–232

Allen JM, Gossett CJ and Allen SK (1996) Photochemical formation of singlet molecular oxygen ($^1O_2$) in illuminated aqueous solutions of *p*-aminobenzoic acid (PABA). *Journal of Photochemistry and Photobiology* **32** 33–37

Ananthaswamy HN, Loughlin SM, Cox P, Evans RL, Ullrich SE and Kripke ML (1997) Sunlight and skin cancer: inhibition of *p53* mutations in UV-irradiated mouse skin by sunscreens. *Nature Medicine* **3** 510–514

Andrews EJ (1971) Evidence of the nonimmune regression of chemically induced papillomas in mouse skin. *Journal of the National Cancer Institute* **47** 653–665

Barrandon Y and Green H (1987) Three clonal types of keratinocyte with different capacities for multiplication. *Proceedings of the National Academy of Sciences of the USA* **84** 2302–2306

Berenblum I (1975) Sequential aspects of chemical carcinogenesis: skin, In: Becker FF (ed). *Cancer. A Comprehensive Treatise*, pp 323–344, Plenum Press, New York

Berg RJW, van Kranen HJ, Rebel HG *et al* (1996) Early p53 alterations in mouse skin carcinogenesis by UVB radiation: immunohistochemical detection of mutant p53 protein in clusters of preneoplastic cells. *Proceedings of the National Academy of Sciences of the USA* **93** 274–278

Bergstresser PR, Pariser RJ and Taylor JR (1978) Counting and sizing of epidermal cells in normal human skin. *Journal of Investigative Dermatology* **70** 280–284

Blessing K and McLaren KM (1992) Histological regression in primary cutaneous melanoma: recognition, prevalence and significance. *Histopathology* **20** 315–322

Blum HF (1959) *Carcinogenesis by Ultraviolet Light*. Princeton University Press, Princeton, New Jersey

Blum HF (1969) Quantitative aspects of cancer induction by ultraviolet light: including a revised model, In: Urbach F (ed). *The Biologic Effects of Ultraviolet Radiation*, pp 543–549, Pergamon, Oxford, United Kingdom

Boyle J, Briggs JD, MacKie RM, Junor BJR and Aitchison TC (1984) Cancer, warts, and sunshine in renal transplant patients. *Lancet* **ii** 702–704

Brachman DG, Beckett M, Graves D, Haraf D, Vokes E and Weichselbaum RR (1993) *p53* mutation does not correlate with radiosensitivity in 24 head and neck cancer cell lines. *Cancer Research* **53** 3667–3669

Brash DE (1988) UV mutagenic photoproducts in *E. coli* and human cells: a molecular genetics perspective on human skin cancer. *Photochemistry and Photobiology* **48** 59–66

Brash DE (1996) Cellular proofreading. *Nature Medicine* **2** 525–526

Brash DE (1997) Sunlight and the onset of skin cancer. *Trends in Genetics* **13** 410–414

Brash DE, Rudolph JA, Simon JA *et al* (1991) A role for sunlight in skin cancer: UV-induced p53 mutations in squamous cell carcinoma. *Proceedings of the National Academy of Sciences of the USA* **88** 10124–10128

Brash DE, Ziegler A, Jonason A, Simon JA, Kunala S and Leffell DJ (1996) Sunlight and sunburn in human skin cancer: p53, apoptosis, and tumor promotion. *Journal of Investigative Dermatology Symposium Proceedings* **1** 136–142

Brauner GJ (1985) Cutaneous disease in the black races, In: Moschella SL and Hurley HJ (eds). *Dermatology*, pp 1904–1935, WB Saunders, Philadelphia, Pennsylvania

Braverman IM (1998) *Skin Signs of Systemic Disease*. WB Saunders, Philadelphia, Pennsylvania

Breza T, Taylor JR and Eaglstein WH (1976) Noninflammatory destruction of actinic keratoses by fluorouracil. *Archives of Dermatology* **112** 1256–1258

Brown K and Balmain A (1995) Transgenic mice and squamous multistage skin carcinogenesis. *Cancer and Metastasis Reviews* **14** 113–124

Brownstein MH and Rabinowitz AD (1979) The precursors of cutaneous squamous cell carcinoma. *International Journal of Dermatology* **18** 1–16

Burns FJ, Vanderlaan M, Sivak A and Albert RE (1976) Regression kinetics of mouse skin papillomas. *Cancer Research* **36** 1422–1427

Burton RC, Coates MS, Hersey P *et al* (1993) An analysis of a melanoma epidemic. *International Journal of Cancer* **55** 765–770

Cairns J (1975) Mutation selection and the natural history of cancer. *Nature* **255** 197–200

Campbell C, Quinn AG, Angus B, Farr PM and Rees JL (1993a) Wavelength specific patterns of *p53* induction in human skin following exposure to UV radiation. *Cancer Research* **53** 2697–2699

Campbell C, Quinn AG, Ro Y-S, Angus B and Rees JL (1993b) p53 mutations are common and early events that precede tumor invasion in squamous cell neoplasia of the skin. *Journal of Investigative Dermatology* **100** 746–748

Carter VH, Smith KW and Noojin RO (1968) *Xeroderma pigmentosum*: treatment with topically applied fluorouracil. *Archives of Dermatology* **98** 526–527

Cerutti PA (1985) Pro-oxidant states and tumor promotion. *Science* **227** 375–381

Chen Y and Struhl G (1996) Dual roles for patched in sequestering and transducing Hedgehog. *Cell* **87** 553–563

Chidambaram A, Goldstein AM, Gailani MR *et al* (1996) Mutations in the human homologue of the *Drosophila* patched gene in Caucasian and African-American nevoid basal cell carcinoma syndrome patients. *Cancer Research* **56** 4599–4601

Clark WH and Mihm MC (1969) Lentigo maligna and lentigo-maligna melanoma. *American Journal of Pathology* **55** 39–55

Clark WH, Elder DE, Guerry D, Epstein MN, Greene MH and van Horn M (1984) A study of tumor progression: the precursor lesions of superficial spreading and nodular melanoma. *Human Pathology* **15** 1147–1165

Clark WH, Elder DE and Guerry D (1990) Dysplastic nevi and malignant melanoma, In: Farmer ER and Hood AF (eds). *Pathology of the Skin*, pp 684–756, Appleton & Lange, Norwalk, Connecticut

Cooke KR and Fraser J (1985) Migration and death from malignant melanoma. *International Journal of Cancer* **36** 175–178

Dahmane N, Lee J, Robins P, Heller P and Ruiz i Altaba A (1997) Activation of the transcription factor Gli1 and the sonic hedgehog signalling pathway in skin tumors. *Nature* **389** 876–881

Danno K and Horio T (1987) Sunburn cell: factors involved in its formation. *Photochemistry and Photobiology* **45** 683–690

Dean M (1996) Polarity, proliferation and the *hedgehog* pathway. *Nature Genetics* **14** 245–247

de Gruijl FR and van der Leun JC (1991) Development of skin tumors in hairless mice after discontinuation of ultraviolet irradiation. *Cancer Research* **51** 979–984

de Gruijl FR, van der Meer JB and van der Leun JC (1983) Dose-time dependency of tumor formation by chronic UV exposure. *Photochemistry and Photobiology* **37** 53–62

DiGiovanni J (1992) Multistage carcinogenesis in mouse skin. *Pharmacology and Therapeutics*

54 63–128

Drobetsky EA, Grosovsky AJ and Glickman BW (1987) The specificity of UV-induced mutations at an endogenous locus in mammalian cells. *Proceedings of the National Academy of Sciences of the USA* **84** 9103–9107

Dumaz N, Drougard C, Sarasin A and Daya-Grosjean L (1993) Specific UV-induced mutation spectrum in the p53 gene of skin tumors from DNA repair deficient *Xeroderma pigmentosum* patients. *Proceedings of the National Academy of Sciences of the USA* **90** 10529–10533

Eaglstein WH, Weinstein GD and Frost P (1970) Fluorouracil: mechanism of action in human skin and actinic keratoses. *Archives of Dermatology* **101** 132–139

Elder DE and Clark WH (1986) Malignant melanoma, In: Thiers BH and Dobson RL (eds). *Pathogenesis of Skin Disease*, pp 445–457, Churchill Livingstone, New York

Elwood JM, Gallagher RP, Davison J and Hill GB (1985) Sunburn, suntan and the risk of cutaneous malignant melanoma—the Western Canada melanoma study. *British Journal of Cancer* **51** 543–549

Epstein JH and Epstein WL (1962) Cocarcinogenic effect of ultraviolet light on DMBA tumor initiation in albino mice. *Journal of Investigative Dermatology* **39** 455–460

Epstein JH and Roth HL (1968) Experimental ultraviolet light carcinogenesis. *Journal of Investigative Dermatology* **50** 387–389

Everson T and Cole W (1966) *Spontaneous Regression of Cancer*. WB Saunders, Philadelphia, Pennsylvania

Falkson G and Schulz EJ (1962) Skin changes in patients treated with 5-fluorouracil. *British Journal of Dermatology* **74** 229–236

Farber E and Rubin H (1991) Cellular adaption in the origin and development of cancer. *Cancer Research* **51** 2751–2761

Fisher DE (1994) Apoptosis in cancer therapy: crossing the threshold. *Cell* **78** 539–542

Florenes VA, Oyford T, Holm R *et al* (1994) TP53 allele loss, mutations and expression in malignant melanoma. *British Journal of Cancer* **69** 253–259

Gailani MR and Bale AE (1997) Developmental genes and cancer: role of patched in basal cell carcinoma of the skin. *Journal of the National Cancer Institute* **89** 1103–1109

Gailani MR, Leffell DJ, Ziegler A, Gross EG, Brash DE and Bale AE (1996a) Relationship between sunlight exposure and a key genetic alteration in basal cell carcinoma. *Journal of the National Cancer Institute* **88** 349–354

Gailani MR, Stahle-Backdahl M, Leffell DJ *et al* (1996b) The role of the human homologue of *Drosophila patched* in sporadic basal cell carcinomas. *Nature Genetics* **14** 78–81

Gatti RA and Good RA (1971) Occurrence of malignancy in immunodeficiency diseases. *Cancer* **28** 89–98

German J (1983) Patterns of neoplasia associated with the chromosome-breakage syndromes, In: German J (ed). *Chromosome Mutation and Neoplasia*, pp 97–134, AR Liss, New York

Glass AG and Hoover RN (1989) The emerging epidemic of melanoma and squamous cell skin cancer. *Journal of the American Medical Association* **262** 2097–2100

Gonzalez-Zulueta M, Bender CM, Yang AS *et al* (1995) Methylation of the 5′ CpG island of the *p16/CDKN2* tumor suppressor gene in normal and transformed human tissues correlates with gene silencing. *Cancer Research* **55** 4531–4535

Gorlin RJ (1995) Nevoid basal cell carcinoma syndrome. *Dermatologic Clinics* **13** 113–125

Graeber TG, Osmanian C, Jacks T *et al* (1996) Hypoxia-mediated selection of cells with diminished apoptotic potential in solid tumors. *Nature* **379** 88–91

Graham JH and Helwig EB (1964) Precancerous skin lesions and systemic cancer, In: *Tumors of the Skin*, pp 209–222, Year Book Medical Publishers, Chicago, Illinois

Green A (1992) A theory of site distribution of melanomas: Queensland, Australia. *Cancer Causes and Control* **3** 513–516

Green A, Beardmore G, Hart V, Leslie D, Marks R and Staines D (1988) Skin cancer in a Queensland population. *Journal of the American Academy of Dermatology* **19** 1045–1052

Green A, Siskind V, Bain C and Alexander J (1985) Sunburn and malignant melanoma. *British*

Journal of Cancer **51** 393–397

Green A, MacLennan R, Youl P and Martin N (1993) Site distribution of cutaneous melanoma in Queensland. *International Journal of Cancer* **53** 232–236

Green MH, Young TI and Clark WH (1981) Malignant melanoma in renal-transplant recipients. *Lancet* **i** 1196–1199

Greenblatt MS, Bennett WP, Hollstein M and Harris CC (1994) Mutations in the *p53* tumor suppressor gene: clues to cancer etiology and molecular pathogenesis. *Cancer Research* **54** 4855–4878

Greenhalgh DA, Wang XJ and Roop DR (1995) Multistage skin carcinogenesis in transgenic mice. *Proceedings of the Association of American Physicians* **107** 258–275

Gruis NA, Weaver-Feldhaus J, Liu Q *et al* (1995) Genetic evidence in melanoma and bladder cancers that p16 and p53 function in separate pathways of tumor suppression. *American Journal of Pathology* **146** 1199–1206

Gunz FW and Angus HA (1965) Leukemia and cancer in the same patient. *Cancer* **18** 145–152

Haake AR and Polakowska RR (1993) Cell death by apoptosis in epidermal biology. *Journal of Investigative Dermatology* **101** 107–112

Hahn H, Wicking C, Zaphiropoulos PG *et al* (1996a) Mutations in the human homologue of *Drosophila* patched in the nevoid basal cell carcinoma syndrome. *Cell* **85** 841–851

Hahn SA, Schutte M, Hoque AT *et al* (1996b) DPC4, a candidate tumor suppressor gene at human chromosome 18q21.1. *Science* **271** 350–353

Hall PA, McKee PH, Menage H, Dover R and Lane DP (1993) High levels of p53 protein in UV-irradiated normal human skin. *Oncogene* **8** 203–207

Harle-Bachor C and Boukamp P (1996) Telomerase activity in the regenerative basal layer of the epidermis in human skin and in immortal and carcinoma-derived skin keratinocytes. *Proceedings of the National Academy of Sciences of the USA* **93** 6476–6481

Healy E, Sikkink S and Rees JL (1996) Infrequent mutation of p16[INK4] in sporadic melanomas. *Journal of Investigative Dermatology* **107** 318–321

Hennings H, Glick AB, Greenhalgh DA *et al* (1993) Critical aspects of initiation, promotion, and progression in multistage epidermal carcinogenesis. *Proceedings of the Society for Experimental Biology and Medicine* **202** 1–8

Herbst RA, Gutzmer R, Matiaske F *et al* (1997) Further evidence for ultraviolet light induction of CDKN2 (p16[INK4]) mutation in sporadic melanoma *in vivo*. *Journal of Investigative Dermatology* **108** 950

Herman JG, Merlo A, Mao L *et al* (1995) Inactivation of the *CDKN2/p16/MTS1* gene is frequently associated with aberrant DNA methylation in all common human cancers. *Cancer Research* **55** 4525–4530

Hilgers JHC (1960) Pterygium: its incidence, heredity and etiology. *American Journal of Ophthalmology* **50** 635–644

Hogan B, Blessing M, Winnier G, Suzuki N and Jones C (1994) Growth factors in development: the role of TGF-beta related polypeptide signalling molecules in embryogenesis. *Development* **Supplement** 53–60

Holley EA, Kelly JW, Shpall SN and Chiu SH (1987) Number of melanocytic nevi as a major risk factor for malignant melanoma. *Journal of the American Academy of Dermatology* **17** 459–468

Holman CDJ and Armstrong BK (1984a) Cutaneous malignant melanoma and indicators of total accumulated exposure to the sun: an analysis separating histogenetic types. *Journal of the National Cancer Institute* **73** 75–82

Holman CDJ and Armstrong BK (1984b) Pigmentary traits, ethnic origin, benign nevi, and family history as risk factors for cutaneous malignant melanoma. *Journal of the National Cancer Institute* **72** 257–266

Holman CDJ, Mulroney CD and Armstrong BK (1980) Epidemiology of pre-invasive and invasive malignant melanoma in western Australia. *International Journal of Cancer* **25** 317–323

Hooper JE and Scott MP (1989) The *Drosophila* patched gene encodes a putative membrane protein required for segmental patterning. *Cell* **59** 751–765

Houghton AN and Viola MV (1981) Solar radiation and malignant melanoma of the skin. *Journal of the American Academy of Dermatology* **5** 477–483

Howell JB (1984) Nevoid basal cell carcinoma syndrome. *Journal of the American Academy of Dermatology* **11** 98–104

Howell JB and Mehregan AH (1970) Pursuit of the pits in the nevoid basal cell carcinoma syndrome. *Archives of Dermatology* **102** 586–597

Hussussian CJ, Struewing JP, Goldstein AM *et al* (1994) Germline p16 mutations in familial melanoma. *Nature Genetics* **8** 15–21

Hutchinson F (1994) Induction of tandem base change mutations. *Mutation Research* **309** 11–15

Hyde JN (1906) On the influence of light in the production of cancer of the skin. *American Journal of Medical Science* **131** 1–22

Johnson RL, Rothman AL, Xie J *et al* (1996) Human homolog of *patched*, a candiate gene for the basal cell nevus syndrome. *Science* **272** 1668–1671

Jonason AS, Kunala S, Price GJ *et al* (1996) Frequent clones of p53-mutated keratinocytes in normal human skin. *Proceedings of the National Academy of Sciences of the USA* **93** 14025–14029

Jones PH and Watt FM (1993) Separation of human epidermal stem cells from transit amplifying cells on the basis of differences in integrin function and expression. *Cell* **73** 713–724

Jones PH, Harper S and Watt FM (1995) Stem cell patterning and fate in human epidermis. *Cell* **80** 83–93

Kamb A, Gruis NA, Weaver-Feldhaus J *et al* (1994) A cell cycle regulator potentially involved in genesis of many tumor types. *Science* **264** 436–440

Kanjilal S, Pierceall WE, Cummings KK, Kripke ML and Ananthaswamy HN (1993) High frequency of p53 mutations in ultraviolet radiation-induced murine skin tumors: evidence for strand bias and tumor heterogeneity. *Cancer Research* **53** 2961–2964

Kao GF (1990) Precancerous lesions and carcinoma in situ, In: Farmer ER and Hood AF (eds). *Pathology of the Skin*, pp 550–567, Appleton & Lange, Norwalk, Connecticut

Kemp CJ, Donehower LA, Bradley A and Balmain A (1993) Reduction of p53 gene dosage does not increase initiation or promotion but enhances malignant progression of chemically induced skin tumors. *Cell* **74** 813–822

Kinzler K, Bigner S, Bigner D *et al* (1987) Identification of an amplified, highly expressed gene in a human glioma. *Science* **236** 70–73

Klein E (1968) Tumors of the skin. IX. Local cytostatic therapy of cutaneous and mucosal premalignant and malignant lesions. *New York State Journal of Medicine* **68** 886–899

Knowland J, McKenzie EA, McHugh PJ and Cridland NA (1993) Sunlight-induced mutagenicity of a common sunscreen ingredient. *FEBS Letters* **324** 309–313

Koh HK, Kligler BE and Lew RA (1990) Sunlight and cutaneous malignant melanoma: evidence for and against causation. *Photochemistry and Photobiology* **51** 765–779

Kopf AW, Rivers JK, Friedman RJ, Rigel DS and Heilman ER (1991) Dysplastic nevi, In: Friedman RJ, Rigel DS, Kopf AW, Harris MN and Baker D (eds). *Cancer of the Skin*, pp 125–141, WB Saunders, Philadelphia, Pennsylvania

Kraemer KH, Greene MH, Tarone R, Elder DE, Clark WH and Guerry D (1983) Dysplastic nevi and cutaneous melanoma risk. *Lancet* **ii** 1076–1077

Kraemer K, DiGiovanna JJ, Moshell AN, Tarone RE and Peck GL (1988) Prevention of skin cancer in *Xeroderma pigmentosum* with the use of oral isotretinoin. *New England Journal of Medicine* **318** 1633–1637

Kress S, Sutter C, Strickland PT, Mukhtar H, Schweizer J and Schwarz M (1992) Carcinogen-specific mutational pattern in the p53 gene in ultraviolet B radiation-induced squamous cell carcinomas of mouse skin. *Cancer Research* **52** 6400–6403

Kricker A, Armstrong BK, English DR and Heenan PJ (1991) Pigmentary and cutaneous risk factors for non-melanocytic skin cancer—a case-control study. *International Journal of Cancer* **48** 650–662

Kunala S and Brash DE (1992) Excision repair at individual bases of the *Escherichia coli lacI* gene: relation to mutation hotspots and transcription coupling activity. *Proceedings of the National Academy of Sciences of the USA* **89** 11031–11035

Lambert B, Ringborn U and Swanbeck G (1976) Ultraviolet-induced DNA repair synthesis in lymphocytes from patients with actinic keratosis. *Journal of Investigative Dermatology* **67** 594–598

Lear JT, Smith AG, Bowers B *et al* (1997) Truncal tumor site is associated with high risk of multiple basal cell carcinoma and is influenced by glutathione *S*-transferase, GSTT1, and cytochrome P450, CYP1A1 genotypes, and their interaction. *Journal of Investigative Dermatology* **108** 519–522

Lee JAH (1991) Epidemiology of cancers of the skin, In: Friedman RJ, Rigel DS, Kopf AW, Harris MN and Baker D (eds). *Cancer of the Skin*, pp 14–24, WB Saunders, Philadelphia, Pennsylvania

Levanat S, Gorlin RJ, Fallet S, Johnson DR, Fantasia JE and Bale AE (1996) A two-hit model for developmental defects in Gorlin syndrome. *Nature Genetics* 85–87

Lever WF and Schaumburg-Lever G (eds). (1990) *Histopathology of the Skin*. Lippincott, Philadelphia, Pennsylvania

Levine AJ (1997) p53, the cellular gatekeeper for growth and division. *Cell* **88** 323–331

Li G, Mitchell DL, Ho VC, Reed JC and Tron VA (1996) Decreased DNA repair but normal apoptosis in ultraviolet-irradiated skin of p53-transgenic mice. *American Journal of Pathology* **148** 1113–1123

Lippman SM, Kessler JF and Meyskens FL (1987) Retinoids as preventive and therapeutic anticancer agents. *Cancer Treatment Reports* **71** 493–515

Liu Q, Neuhausen N, McClure M *et al* (1995) CDKN2 (MTS1) tumor suppressor gene mutations in human tumor cell lines. *Oncogene* **10** 1061–1067

Liu M, Pelling JC, Ju J, Chu E and Brash DE (1998) Antioxidant action via p53-mediated apoptosis. *Cancer Research* **58** 1723–1729

Livingstone LR, White A, Sprouse J, Livanos E, Jacks T and Tlsty TD (1992) Altered cell cycle arrest and gene amplification potential accompany loss of wild-type p53. *Cell* **70** 923–935

Ljungman M and Zhang F (1996) Blockage of RNA polymerase as a possible trigger for UV light-induced apoptosis. *Oncogene* **13** 823–831

Lowe SW, Ruley HE, Jacks T and Houseman DE (1993) p53-dependent apoptosis modulates the cytotoxicity of anticancer agents. *Cell* **74** 957–967

Lund HZ (1965) How often does squamous cell carcinoma of the skin metastasize? *Archives of Dermatology* **92** 635–637

McGregor WG, Chen R-H, Lukash L, Maher VM and McCormick JJ (1991) Cell cycle-dependent strand bias for UV-induced mutations in the transcribed strand of excision repair-proficient human fibroblasts but not in repair-deficient cells. *Molecular and Cellular Biology* **11** 1927–1934

McHugh PJ and Knowland J (1997) Characterization of DNA damage inflicted by free radicals from a mutagenic sunscreen ingredient and its location using an *in vitro* genetic reversion assay. *Photochemistry and Photobiology* **66** 276–281

Mackenzie IC (1997) Retroviral transduction of murine epidermal stem cells demonstrates clonal units of epidermal structure. *Journal of Investigative Dermatology* **109** 377–383

MacKie RM (1992) Epidermal skin tumors, In: Champion RH, Burton JL and Ebling FJG (eds). *Textbook of Dermatology*, pp 1459–1504, Blackwell, Oxford, United Kingdom

McLelland J, Rees A, Williams G and Chu T (1988) The incidence of immunosuppression-related skin disease in long-term transplant patients. *Transplantation* **46** 871–874

Madsen A (1955) The histogenesis of superficial basal-cell epitheliomas. *Archives of Dermatology* **72** 29–30

Madsen A (1965) Studies on basal-cell epithelioma of the skin. *Acta Pathologica et Microbiologica Scandinavica* (**Supplement 177**) 9–63

Maestro R and Boiocchi M (1995) Sunlight and melanoma: an answer from MTS1 (p16). *Science* **267** 16–16

Maize JC (1977) Skin cancer in immunosuppressed patients. *Journal of the American Medical Association* **237** 1857–1858

Manusow D and Weinerman BH (1975) Subsequent neoplasia in chronic lymphocytic leukemia. *Journal of the American Medical Association* **232** 267–269

Marigo V, Davey RA, Zuo Y, Cunningham JM and Tabin CJ (1996) Biochemical evidence that patched is the Hedgehog receptor. *Nature* **384** 176–179

Marks R (1988) The relationship of basal cell carcinomas and squamous cell carcinomas to solar keratoses. *Archives of Dermatology* **124** 1039–1042

Marks R, Foley P, Goodman G, Hage BH and Selwood TS (1986) Spontaneous remission of solar keratoses: the case for conservative management. *British Journal of Dermatology* **115** 649–655

Marks R, Rennie G and Selwood TS (1988) Malignant transformation of solar keratoses to squamous cell carcinoma. *Lancet* **i** 795–797

Marks R, Jolley D, Dorevitch AP and Selwood TS (1989) The incidence of non-melanocytic skin cancers in an Australian population: results of a five-year prospective study. *Medical Journal of Australia* **150** 475–478

Marks R, Jolley D, Lectsas S and Foley P (1990) The role of childhood exposure to sunlight in the development of solar keratoses and non-melanocytic skin cancer. *Medical Journal of Australia* **152** 62–66

Marshall V (1974) Premalignant and malignant skin tumours in immunosuppressed patients. *Transplantation* **17** 272–275

Miller SJ (1991) Biology of basal cell carcinoma. *Journal of the American Academy of Dermatology* **24** 1–13, 161–175

Miller SJ, Lavker RM and Sun TT (1993a) Keratinocyte stem cells of cornea, skin and hair follicle: common and distinguishing features. *Seminars in Developmental Biology* **4** 217–240

Miller SJ, Sun TT and Lavker RM (1993b) Hair follicles, stem cells, and skin cancer. *Journal of Investigative Dermatology* **100** 288S–294S

Miller SJ, Wei ZG, Wilson C, Dzubow L, Sun TT and Lavker RM (1993c) Mouse skin is particularly susceptible to tumor initiation during early anagen of the hair cycle: possible involvement of hair follicle stem cells. *Journal of Investigative Dermatology* **101** 591–594

Mitchell DL and Nairn RS (1989) The biology of the (6-4) photoproduct. *Photochemistry and Photobiology* **49** 805–819

Moll I (1995) Proliferative potential of different keratinocytes of plucked human hair follicles. *Journal of Investigative Dermatology* **105** 14–21

Montgomery H (1939) Precancerous dermatosis and epithelioma in situ. *Archives of Dermatology and Syphilology* **39** 387–408

Moran DJ and Hollows FC (1984) Pterygium and ultraviolet radiation: a positive correlation. *British Journal of Ophthalmology* **68** 343–346

Morris RJ, Fischer SM and Slaga TJ (1985) Evidence that the centrally and peripherally located cells in the murine epidermal proliferative unit are two distinct cell populations. *Journal of Investigative Dermatology* **84** 277–281

Motzny CK and Holmgren R (1995) The *Drosophila* cubitus interruptus protein and its role in the wingless and hedgehog signal transduction pathways. *Mechanisms of Development* **52** 137–150

Nakano Y, Guerrero I, Hidalgo A, Taylor A, Whittle JR and Ingham PW (1989) A protein with several possible membrane-spanning domains encoded by the *Drosophila* segment polarity gene patched. *Nature* **341** 508–513

Nakazawa H, English D, Randell PL *et al* (1994) UV and skin cancer: specific p53 gene mutation in normal skin as a biologically relevant exposure measurement. *Proceedings of the National Academy of Sciences of the USA* **91** 360–364

Nathanson L (1976) Spontaneous regression of malignant melanoma: a review of the literature on incidence, clinical features, and possible mechanisms. *National Cancer Institute Monographs* **44** 67–76

Naylor MF, Boyd A, Smith DW, Cameron GS, Hubbard D and Neldner KH (1995) High sun protection factor sunscreen in the suppression of actinic neoplasia. *Archives of Dermatology* **131** 170–175

Nelson MA, Einspahr JG, Alberts DS *et al* (1994) Analysis of the *p53* gene in human precancerous actinic keratosis lesions and squamous cell cancers. *Cancer Letters* **85** 23–29

Nicholls EM (1968) Genetic susceptibility and somatic mutation in the production of freckles, birthmarks, and moles. *Lancet* **i** 71–73

Nicholls EM (1973) Development and elimination of pigmented moles, and the anatomical distribution of primary malignant melanoma. *Cancer* **32** 191–195

Nusse R (1994) The Wnt family in tumorigenesis and in normal development. *Journal of Steroid Biochemistry and Molecular Biology* **43** 9–12

Oro AE, Higgins KM, Hu Z, Bonifas JM, Epstein EH and Scott MP (1997) Basal cell carcinomas in mice overexpressing sonic hedgehog. *Science* **276** 817–821

Pearse AD and Marks R (1977) Actinic keratoses and the epidermis on which they arise. *British Journal of Dermatology* **96** 45–50

Penn I (1978) Tumors arising in organ transplant recipients. *Advances in Cancer Research* **28** 31–61

Perrimon N (1995) Hedgehog and beyond. *Cell* **80** 517–520

Pollock PM, Yu F, Parsons PG and Hayward NK (1995) Evidence for UV induction of *CDKN2* mutations in melanoma cell lines. *Oncogene* **11** 663–668

Pontén F, Berne B, Ren ZP, Nister M and Pontén J (1995) Ultraviolet light induces expression of p53 and p21 in human skin: effect of sunscreen and constitutive p21 expression in skin appendages. *Journal of Investigative Dermatology* **105** 402–406

Pontén F, Berg C, Ahmadian A *et al* (1997) Molecular pathology in basal cell cancer with p53 as a genetic marker. *Oncogene* **15** 1059–1067

Pott P (1771–75) *The Chirurgical Works of Percival Pott*, Volume 5, pp 60–68, Haes, Clarke and Collins, London, United Kingdom

Potten CS and Hendry JH (1973) Clonogenic cells and stem cells in epidermis. *International Journal of Radiation Biology* **24** 537–540

Potten CS and Morris RJ (1988) Epithelial stem cells *in vivo*, In: Lord BI and Dexter TM (eds). *Stem Cells*, pp 45–62, Company of Biologists Ltd, Cambridge, United Kingdom

Potter VR (1984) Use of two sequential applications of initiators in the production of hepatomas in the rat: an examination of the Solt-Farber protocol. *Cancer Research* **44** 2733–2736

Rehman I, Quinn AG, Healy E and Rees JL (1994) High frequency of loss of heterozygosity in actinic keratoses, a usually benign disease. *Lancet* **344** 788–789

Ren Z-P, Hedrum A, Pontén F *et al* (1996a) Human epidermal cancer and accompanying precursors have identical p53 mutations different from p53 mutations in adjacent areas of clonally expanded non-neoplastic keratinocytes. *Oncogene* **12** 765–773

Ren Z-P, Pontén F, Nister M and Pontén J (1996b) Two distinct p53 immunohistochemical patterns in human squamous cell skin cancer, precursors, and normal epidermis. *International Journal of Cancer* **69** 174–179

Ren Z-P, Ahmadian A, Pontén F *et al* (1997a) Benign clonal keratinocyte patches with p53 mutations show no genetic link to synchronous squamous cell precancer or cancer in human skin. *American Journal of Pathology* **150** 1791–1803

Ren Z-P, Pontén F, Nistér M and Pontén J (1997b) Reconstruction of the two dimensional distribution of p53 positive staining patches in sun exposed morphologically normal skin. *International Journal of Oncology* **11** 111–115

Riddle RD, Johnson RL, Laufer E and Tabin C (1993) Sonic hedgehog mediates the polarizing activity of the ZPA. *Cell* **75** 1401–1416

Robles AI, Gimenez Conti IB, Roop D, Slaga TJ and Conti CJ (1993) Low frequency of codon 61 Ha-ras mutations and lack of keratin 13 expression in 7,12-dimethylbenz[a]-anthracene-induced hamster skin tumors. *Molecular Carcinogenesis* **7** 94–8

Roelink H, Porter JA, Chiang C *et al* (1995) Floor plate and motor neuron induction by different concentrations of the amino-terminal cleavage product of sonic hedgehog autoproteolysis. *Cell* **81** 445–455

Rowan S, Ludwig RL, Haupt Y et al (1996) Specific loss of apoptotic but not cell-cycle arrest function in a human tumor derived p53 mutant. *EMBO Journal* 827–838

Rubinfeld B, Robbins P, El-Gamil M, Albert I, Porfiri E and Polakis P (1997) Stabilization of β-catenin by genetic defects in melanoma cell lines. *Science* **275** 1790–1792

Sato M, Nishigori C, Zghal M, Yagi T and Takebe H (1993) Ultraviolet-specific mutations in p53 gene in skin tumors in *Xeroderma pigmentosum* patients. *Cancer Research* **53** 2944–2946

Sbano E, Andreassi L, Fimiani M, Valentino A and Baiocchi R (1978) DNA-repair after UV-irradiation in skin fibroblasts from patients with actinic keratosis. *Archives of Dermatological Research* **262** 55–61

Schreiber MM, Moon TE and Bozzo PD (1984) Chronic solar ultraviolet damage associated with malignant melanoma of the skin. *Journal of the American Academy of Dermatology* **10** 755–759

Schwartz RA and Stoll HL (1993) Epithelial precancerous lesions, In: Fitzpatrick TB, Eisen AZ, Wolff K, Freedberg IM and Austen KF (eds). *Dermatology in General Medicine*, pp 804–807, McGraw-Hill, New York

Scotto J and Nam JM (1980) Skin melanoma and seasonal patterns. *American Journal of Epidemiology* **111** 309–314

Sekelsky J, Newfeld S, Raftery L, Chartoff E and Gelbart W (1995) Genetic characterization and cloning of mothers against dpp, a gene required for decapentaplegic function in *Drosophila melanogaster*. *Genetics* **139** 1347–1358

Shanley SM, Dawkins H, Wainwright BJ et al (1995) Fine deletion mapping on the long arm of chromosome 9 in sporadic and familial basal cell carcinomas. *Human Molecular Genetics* **4** 129–133

Sherley JL, Stadler PB and Johnson DR (1995) Expression of the wild-type p53 antioncogene induces guanine nucleotide-dependent stem cell division kinetics. *Proceedings of the National Academy of Sciences of the USA* **92** 136–140

Slichenmyer WJ, Nelson WG, Slebos RJ and Kastan MB (1993) Loss of a *p53*-associated G_1 checkpoint does not decrease cell survival following DNA damage. *Cancer Research* **53** 4164–4168

Sparrow LE, Soong R, Dawkins HJ, Iacopetta BJ and Heenan PJ (1995) p53 gene mutatiom and expression in naevi and melanomas. *Melanoma Research* **5** 93–100

Spencer WH (1996) Conjunctiva, In: Spencer WH (ed). *Ophthalmic Pathology*, pp 38–125, WB Saunders, Philadelphia, Pennsylvania

Springate JE (1986) The nevoid basal cell carcinoma syndrome. *Journal of Pediatric Surgery* **21** 908–910

Stone DM, Hynes M, Armanini M et al (1996) The tumour-suppressor gene patched encodes a candidate receptor for Sonic hedgehog. *Nature* **384** 129–134

Stretch JR, Gatter KC, Ralfkiaer E, Lane DP and Harris AL (1991) Expression of mutant p53 in melanoma. *Cancer Research* **51** 5976–5979

Strickland D and Lee JAH (1981) Melanomas of eye: stability of rates. *American Journal of Epidemiology* **113** 700–702

Taguchi M, Watanabe S, Yashima K, Murakami Y, Sekiya T and Ikeda S (1994) Aberrations of the tumor suppressor p53 gene and p53 protein in solar keratosis in human skin. *Journal of Investigative Dermatology* **103** 500–503

Tan CY and Marks R (1982) Lichenoid solar keratosis—prevalence and immunological findings. *Journal of Investigative Dermatology* **79** 365–367

Taylor HR, West SK, Rosenthal FS, Munoz B, Newland HS and Emmett EA (1989) Corneal changes associated with chronic UV irradiation. *Archives of Ophthalmology* **107** 1481–1484

Thiagalingam S, Lengauer C, Leach F et al (1996) Evaluation of candidate tumour suppressor genes on chromosome 18 in colorectal cancers. *Nature Genetics* **13** 343–346

Thomas SE, Pearse AD and Marks R (1985) Transplantation of human malignant and premalignant lesions of epidermis to nude mice. *European Journal of Cancer and Clinical Oncology* **21** 1093–1098

Thompson SC, Jolley D and Marks R (1993) Reduction of solar keratoses by regular sunscreen use. *New England Journal of Medicine* **329** 1147–1151

Tornaletti S and Pfeifer GP (1994) Slow repair of pyrimidine dimers at *p53* mutation hotspots in skin cancer. *Science* **263** 1436–1438

Ueda M, Ouhtit A, Bito T *et al* (1997) Evidence for UV-associated activation of telomerase in human skin. *Cancer Research* **57** 370–374

Unden AB, Holmberg E, Lundh-Rozell B *et al* (1996) Mutations in the human homologue of *Drosophila* patched (PTCH) in basal cell carcinomas and the Gorlin syndrome: different in vivo mechanisms of PTCH inactivation. *Cancer Research* **56** 4562–4565

Urabe A, Kanitakis J, Viac J and Thivolet J (1989) Cyclosporin A inhibits directly in vivo keratinocyte proliferation of living human skin. *Journal of Investigative Dermatology* **92** 755–757

Urbach F (1984) Ultraviolet radiation and skin cancer, In: Smith KC (ed). *Topics in Photomedicine*, pp 67–104, Plenum Press, New York

van den Heuvel M and Ingham PW (1996) smoothened encodes a receptor-like serpentine protein required for hedgehog signalling. *Nature* **382** 547–551

van Scott EJ and Reinertson RP (1961) The modulating influence of stromal environment on epithelial cells studied in human autotransplants. *Journal of Investigative Dermatology* **36** 109–117

Vitasa BC, Taylor HR, Strickland PT *et al* (1990) Association of nonmelanoma skin cancer and actinic keratosis with cumulative solar ultraviolet exposure in Maryland watermen. *Cancer* **65** 2811–2817

Walder BK, Robertson MR and Jeremy D (1971) Skin cancer and immunosuppression. *Lancet* **ii** 1282–1283

Waldmann TA, Strober W and Blaese RM (1972) Immunodeficiency disease and malignancy. *Annals of Internal Medicine* **77** 605–628

Wang ZY, Huang MT, Ho CT *et al* (1992) Inhibitory effect of green tea on the growth of established skin papillomas in mice. *Cancer Research* **52** 6657–6665

Weiss J, Heine M, Arden KC *et al* (1995) Mutation and expression of TP53 in malignant melanomas. *Recent Results in Cancer Research* **139** 137–154

White E (1994) p53, guardian of Rb. *Nature* **371** 21–22

Wicking C, Shanley S, Smyth I *et al* (1997) Most germ-line mutations in the nevoid basal cell carcinoma syndrome lead to a premature termination of the patched protein, and no genotype-phenotype correlations are evident. *American Journal of Human Genetics* **60** 21–26

Winkelmann RK, Zollman PE and Baldes EJ (1963) Squamous cell carcinoma produced by ultraviolet light in hairless mice. *Journal of Investigative Dermatology* **40** 217–224

Yamagiwa K and Ichikawa K (1914) Über die atypische epithelwucherung. *Verhandlungen Japonische Patholische Gesellschaft* **136**

Yamagiwa K and Ichikawa K (1918) Experimental study of the pathogenesis of carcinoma. *Journal of Cancer Research* **3** 1–21

Yin Y, Tainsky MA, Bischoff FZ, Strong LC and Wahl GM (1992) Wild-type p53 restores cell cycle control and inhibits gene amplification in cells with mutant p53 alleles. *Cell* **70** 937–948

Young AR (1987) The sunburn cell. *Photodermatology* **4** 127–134

Youngson RM (1972) Recurrence of pterygium after excision. *British Journal of Ophthalmology* **56** 120–125

Yuspa SH (1994) The pathogenesis of squamous cell cancer: lessons learned from studies of skin carcinogenesis. *Cancer Research* **54** 1178–1189

Ziegler A, Leffell DJ, Kunala S *et al* (1993) Mutation hotspots due to sunlight in the p53 gene of non-melanoma skin cancers. *Proceedings of the National Academy of Sciences of the USA* **90** 4216–4220

Ziegler A, Jonason AS, Leffell DJ *et al* (1994) Sunburn and p53 in the onset of skin cancer. *Nature* **372** 773–776

The authors are responsible for the accuracy of the references.

Molecular Alterations in Bladder Cancer

C CORDON-CARDO

Division of Molecular Pathology, Department of Pathology, Memorial Sloan-Kettering Cancer Center, 1275 York Avenue, New York, NY 10021

Introduction
Chromosomal alterations in bladder cancer
Alterations of oncogenes in bladder tumours
Alterations of tumour suppressor genes in bladder tumours
Bladder cancer as a model for the study of preneoplastic lesions and tumour
     progression
Summary

INTRODUCTION

Bladder cancer is one of the most common malignancies worldwide. The rates for these tumours are highest in developed countries, ranking as the sixth most frequent neoplasia. Bladder cancer develops more predominantly in males, with a sex ratio of more than 3:1, suggesting sex linked aetiological factors. In the USA, bladder cancer ranks as the fourth most common malignancy among men and sixth among women. Approximately 90% of malignant tumours arising in the urinary bladder are of epithelial origin, the vast majority being transitional cell carcinomas (Mostofi *et al*, 1973; Koss, 1975).

The association of specific risk factors and urothelial tumours has been revealed by a series of epidemiology studies (for a review see Zhang and Steineck, 1997). Cigarette smoking is considered the most important risk factor for bladder cancer (Prout, 1977). The two agents causally linked to human bladder cancer present in tobacco are 2-aminonaphthalene and 4-aminobiphenyl. Another proven bladder carcinogenic agent is the aromatic amine benzidine. Exposure to therapeutic agents such as potassium arsenite, high consumption of phenacetin, and *Schistosoma haematobium* infection are factors that should be accounted for in the context of the development of bladder cancer in certain circumstances. Other risk factors found to be inconsistent or non-causal include coffee, alcohol drinking, use of sweeteners and fat intake (Zhang and Steineck, 1997).

On the basis of morphological evaluation and natural history, urothelial neoplasms have been classified into two groups having distinct behaviour and prognosis: low grade tumours (always papillary and usually superficial) and high-grade tumours (papillary or non-papillary, and often invasive) (Koss, 1992). Clinically, superficial bladder tumours (stages T_a, T_{is}, and T_1) account for 75–85% of neoplasms, while the remaining 15–25% are invasive (T_2, T_3, T_4) or metastatic (N+,M+) lesions at the time of initial presentation (Prout, 1977). Over 70% of patients with superficial tumours will have one or more recurrences after initial treatment, and about one third of those patients will progress and eventually die from their disease (Reuter and Melamed, 1989). It is for these reasons that new methods are being developed to identify and monitor patients presenting with superficial tumours likely to develop recurrent and invasive carcinoma. In patients who present initially with invasive disease, we are faced with two major problems. First, despite aggressive surgical resection and adjuvant radiotherapy and/or chemotherapy, the overall cure remains in the range of 20–50%. In addition, distant micrometastatic disease, unrecognized at the time of initial diagnosis and treatment, occurs in an important percentage of patients and is the major cause of treatment failure and death. Since selection criteria to determine treatment for a particular tumour in a particular patient are incompletely defined, new biological determinants are needed for proper selection and monitoring of therapy.

As a corollary of the two pathways of urothelial neoplasms above mentioned, certain precursor lesions have been described. It must be emphasized that there are discrepancies among different clinical investigators regarding the significance of identifying such morphological changes. In addition, acceptance of nomenclature and reproducibility in interpretation have been difficult. It has been difficult to ascribe particular hyperplastic changes or everted papillomas as precursors to overt papillary transitional cell carcinomas of low stage and low grade. Even the term "papilloma", used to describe a benign uroepithelial neoplasm, has not achieved international acceptance (Reuter and Melamed, 1989; Johansson and Cohen, 1997). Other precursor lesions described relate more to the flat carcinoma in situ pathway of tumourigenesis, including the changes known as intraurothelial neoplasms (IUNs) (Koss, 1992). This latter group includes simple hyperplasia (IUN-I), atypical urothelial hyperplasia (IUN-II) and dysplasia or marked atypia (IUN-III). Multiple morphological criteria have been used in the diagnosis of dysplasia, which do not need to be present simultaneously. Some authors have used the terms "mild", "moderate" and "severe" dysplasia in analogy with the cervix (Johansson and Cohen, 1997). Others have suggested the term "carcinoma in situ" (CIS) grades 1 and 2 for mild and moderate dysplasia, respectively and grade 3 CIS for severe dysplasia and CIS (Mostofi and Sesterhenn, 1984). Several studies have revealed that identification of concomitant dysplasia increases the risk of tumour progression in patients with superficial bladder tumours (Kiemeney et al, 1994; Igawa et al, 1995). Regardless of terminology, it is becoming increasingly evident that morphological changes and their clinical manifestations are preceded by molecular and biochemical alterations.

Morphologically similar tumours may behave in radically different fashions, a fact that seriously hampers the ability to accurately predict clinical outcome and properly designed therapeutic intervention in a given case. The use of modern molecular and immunochemical techniques has led to remarkable progress in our understanding of cell growth and differentiation, these being key issues in tumour development and progression. Similarly, advances in analytical technology have substantially improved our knowledge of the clinically relevant question of how tumour progression relates to an accumulation of genetic disorders. Biological markers that correlate with tumour behaviour and response to therapy are constantly being identified. The addition of objective predictive assays to our armamentarium of diagnostic and prognostic tools will enhance our ability to assess tumour biological activities and to design effective treatment regimens. Regarding preneoplastic conditions, the need now is to conduct in depth molecular analyses utilizing well characterized lesions, including those described above. This, in turn, may provide the needed information to understand the clinical relevance of detecting genetic instability, as well as primary genetic or epigenetic alterations, in otherwise morphologically normal appearing urothelium and preneoplastic lesions.

CHROMOSOMAL ALTERATIONS IN BLADDER CANCER

Bladder tumours can be cultured successfully, thus allowing cytogenetic studies. However, preneoplastic lesions were not assessed as part of the early analyses. Nevertheless, these studies revealed non-random chromosomal aberrations, especially deletions. This is in contrast to the frequent translocations found in other malignant lesions, such as sarcomas, which appear to be specific for particular tumour types. Initial studies of bladder tumours identified monosomy of chromosome 9 (Gibas *et al*, 1984; Atkin and Baker, 1985) and interstitial deletions of chromosome 13 (Gibas *et al*, 1984) as frequent events. Other common abnormalities included trisomy of chromosome 7 and deletions affecting chromosomes 11p and 3p (Babu *et al*, 1987; Vanni *et al*, 1988).

More recent karyotype and interphase cytogenetic studies have confirmed previously reported data and provide evidence for novel alterations. For example, Tyrkus *et al* (1992) analysed 17 carcinomas in situ of the urinary bladder and found no chromosome 9 alterations but identified non-random chromosomal changes involving chromosomes 1, 5, 8 and 11. Hopman *et al* (1991) reported chromosomal alterations at 1q12, as well as numerical abnormalities of chromosomes 7, 9, 11 and 18. In an independent study, Waldman *et al* (1991) also reported numerical aberration of chromosomes 7, 9 and 11 in 27 bladder tumours. Fluorescence in situ hybridization (FISH) assays have been also utilized to assess gene amplification and copy number gains in bladder cancer. Moreover the use of gene specific probes has allowed interphase cytogenetics to evaluate particular molecular alterations in the context of tumourigenesis and progression. For example Sauter *et al* (1993) reported amplification of *ERBB2* (17q21) in 10 of 141 bladder tumours using a dual labelling hybridization assay. Gene amplification was associated with protein overexpression and was found only in tumours with aneusomy of chromosome 17, being more frequent in muscle invasive lesions. A similar approach was used for the analysis of *MYC* copy number on 87 bladder tumours (Sauter *et al*, 1995). Obvious amplification was found in three cases, while 32 of the remaining 84 tumours showed a low level *MYC* copy number increase. There was no association between low level copy number increase and protein overexpression. However, there was strong association between *MYC* gains and tumour grade, stage and Ki-67 labelling index, consistent with a role of chromosome 8 alterations in bladder cancer progression. FISH assays have been also used for analyses of specific gene losses. Physical *TP53* gene deletion (at 17p13) was examined in 151 bladder tumours (Sauter *et al*, 1994), and 17p deletion was found to be highly correlated with tumour stage and grade. Using centromeric probes, Y chromosome loss was reported as a frequent finding in bladder tumours (Sauter *et al*, 1995). Nullisomy and monosomy for chromosome Y was seen in 23 of 68 tumours (34%) and in 28 of 68 tumours, respectively. The use of gene specific probes for *CDKN2* and *IFNAα* genes, located at 9p21, revealed homozygous deletions for *CDKN2/INK4A* without homozygous *IFNA* deletion in 5 of 17 superficial (pT$_a$ or pT$_1$) tumours tested (29%) (Balazs *et al*, 1997). One additional case had both genes deleted and one tumour showed deletion of *IFNA* without deletion of *CDKN2*. These data confirmed the frequent and early nature of 9p21 alterations in bladder cancer (see below). FISH has been also used to assay bladder irrigation specimens (Wheeless *et al*, 1994). Labelled probes to centromeric sequences for chromosomes 1, 7, 9, 11, 15 and 17 were used on samples from 76 patients monitored for recurrent bladder tumours. Significantly, 24% of patients with a history of bladder cancer but no clinical evidence of disease exhibited monosomy of chromosome 9.

Comparative genomic hybridization has allowed the generation of a map of DNA sequence copy number to be assessed as a function of chromosomal location throughout the entire genome (Kallioniemi *et al*, 1992). With this technique, differentially labelled test DNA from tumour samples and normal reference DNA are hybridised simultaneously to normal chromosome spreads. Regions of gain or loss of DNA sequences are seen as changes in the ratio of the intensities of the fluorochromes along the target chromosomes. Using this innovative method, loci not previously recognized to be altered in bladder tumours have been identified. The analysis of genomic imbalances in 26 bladder cancers revealed losses on 11p, 11q, 8p, 9, 17p, 3p and 12q in more than 20% of the tumours (Kallioniemi *et al*, 1995). Bands involved in gains in over 10% of the cases were 8q21, 13q21-q34, 1q21, 3q24-q26 and 1p22 (Kallioniemi *et al*, 1995). Further molecular genetic studies may lead to the characterization of tumour suppressor genes and oncogenes residing in these regions that may have crucial roles in bladder tumourigenesis and tumour progression.

ALTERATIONS OF ONCOGENES IN BLADDER TUMOURS

The first mutation of the *RAS* family of oncogenes, a point mutation in codon 12 of the *HRAS* gene (11p15.1), was identified in the bladder cancer cell line T24 (Reddy *et al*, 1982). The mutation frequency of *RAS* genes in bladder cancer has been controversial. Before the advent of polymerase chain reaction (PCR) techniques, it was estimated that the rate of point mutations in *RAS* oncogenes ranged from 10 to 16% of samples analysed (Fujita *et al*, 1985; Nagatava *et al*, 1990). The predominant alteration identified was the codon 12 of *HRAS*, with few cases presenting *KRAS* mutations and no mutations detected affecting *NRAS*. However, more recent reports using a PCR based method revealed that approximately 40% of bladder tumours harbour *HRAS* codon 12 mutations (Czerniak *et al*, 1990, 1992). Other studies have confirmed this high frequency of *HRAS* point mutations. Ooi *et al* (1994) analysed a cohort of 124 patients with T_a or T_1 lesions and found that codon 12 G $\rightarrow$ T substitution was associated with non-recurring and recurring primary tumours, as well as with initial T_a/T_1 lesions from patients who suffered disease progression. Fitzgerald *et al* (1995) reported the detection of mutations in exon 1 of the *HRAS* gene in urine sediments from 44 of 100 prospectively evaluated patients presenting with bladder neoplasms.

Overexpression and/or amplification of epidermal growth factor receptor (EGFR) has been reported in bladder cancer. Neal *et al* (1985) observed increased expression of EGFR in invasive versus superficial bladder tumours, showing that overexpression was associated with high grade, high stage bladder cancer and was an independent prognostic factor (Neal *et al*, 1990). Messing *et al* (1990) noticed that EGFR was expressed at detectable levels in the basal layer of the normal urothelium, and increased expression in basal and suprabasal layers was identified in transitional cell carcinomas. Rao *et al* (1993) also found increased expression of EGFR in urothelial samples with dysplastic changes, postulating that overexpression of EGFR may be an early event in bladder carcinogenesis. In another study, Nguyen *et al* (1994) reported that overexpression of EGFR was not an independent prognostic marker in patients with advanced bladder cancer.

Amplification of the *ERBB2* gene was found in 1 of 14 bladder tumours in a study of Wood *et al* (1991). This case also displayed overexpression when analysed for mRNA and protein levels. In addition, 5 cases displayed high levels of mRNA with no signs of gene amplification and only 3 of these 5 cases had protein overexpression. Sato *et al* (1992) observed ERBB2 protein overexpression in 23 of 88 bladder tumours analysed and found a significant association with overexpression and poor clinical outcome, being an independent prognostic factor. Underwood *et al* (1995) studied *ERBB2* status in 236 bladder tumours. 16 of 89 patients with recurrent disease had evidence of *ERBB2* amplification; however, gene amplification was not observed in the non-recurrent tumours. There was a strong association with disease progression and *ERBB2* amplification. Nevertheless, protein overexpression could not be linked to disease progression. *ERBB2* gene amplification was of predictive value in multivariate analysis for overall bladder cancer death; however, stage and grade remained the most significant independent prognostic parameters. In a combined immunohistochemical and FISH study alterations in the genotype and phenotype of *EGFR* and *ERBB2* genes and encoded products were evaluated in premalignant lesions of the urinary bladder (Wagner *et al*, 1995). FISH analysis showed ERBB2 amplification in selected CIS. In addition, EGFR overexpression and diffuse ERBB2 positivity were associated with increased Ki67 proliferative index. However, only diffuse ERBB2 immunoreactivity was significantly associated with advanced dysplasia.

The analysis of the TP53 regulatory pathway has yielded a novel cellular proto-oncogene product, MDM2. This protein binds to TP53 and acts as a negative regulator, inhibiting its transcriptional activity (Oliner *et al*, 1992) and targeting its ubiquitin dependent degradation (Haupt *et al*, 1997). The *MDM2* gene is located on the long arm of chromosome 12 (12q13-14) and is transactivated by TP53 (Momand *et al*, 1992). Lianes *et al* (1994) characterized the frequency and clinical relevance of identifying *MDM2* and *TP53* alterations in patients with bladder neoplasms. This study revealed that 26 of 87 cases analysed had abnormally high levels of MDM2 proteins; however, only one case showed *MDM2* amplification. There was a striking association between MDM2 overexpression and low stage/low grade bladder tumours (p<0.01). Based on these results it was concluded that aberrant MDM2 phenotypes are common in bladder cancer and may be involved in tumourigenesis or early tumour progression in urothelial neoplasms. In an independent study that lacked clinicopathological correlations, Barbareschi *et al* (1995) reported MDM2 nuclear overexpression in 5 of 25 bladder tumours.

ALTERATIONS OF TUMOUR SUPPRESSOR GENES IN BLADDER TUMOURS

Although the aetiology of bladder cancer is largely unknown, the vast majority of patients do not have a family history of transitional cell carcinomas of the urinary tract. Nevertheless, a recent review of the literature has documented the clustering of transitional cell carcinoma in families, arguing in favour of a genetic component, albeit very unusual, to familial transitional cell carcinoma (Kiemeney and Schoenberg, 1996).

In the present review, however, we will centre in molecular genetic studies conducted in non-cultured, non-familial, bladder tumours. Through such analyses, abnormalities of certain known or candidate tumour suppressor genes involved in the development or progression of such neoplasms have been identified.

Confirming initial cytogenetic observations, loss of heterozygosity (LOH) of the short arm of chromosome 11 and 9q allelic losses were reported as frequent events in bladder tumours (Fearon *et al*, 1985; Tsai *et al*, 1990). 17p LOH was a common event (Olumi *et al*, 1990; Tsai *et al*, 1990) and was associated with high grade bladder cancer (Olumi *et al*, 1990).

A combined molecular genetics and immunopathology approach was used to survey five suspected or established tumour suppressor gene regions (3p21-25, 11p15, 13q14, 17p11-13 and 18q21) in 34 unselected patients by Presti *et al*, 1991. An immunohistochemical assay was also used for the analysis of the retinoblastoma gene product (RB). This study demonstrated that tumour grade correlated with deletions of 3p and 17p. Tumour stage was correlated with deletions of 3p and 17p and altered RB expression. This study also revealed that deletions of 17p (*TP53* locus) and 18q occur only in invasive tumours, whereas deletions of 3p and 11p occur in both superficial and invasive tumours. Dalbagni *et al* (1993) followed this study with the analysis of 60 paired bladder tumours and normal tissues using polymorphic DNA markers on 18 different chromosomal arms. Distinct genotypic patterns were associated with early and late stages of bladder cancer. Correlation of genetic alterations with clinico-pathological data suggested the existence of two different genetic pathways for the evolution of superficial bladder tumours. 9q deletions were found in 60% of the informative cases, confirming previous reports. Moreover 9q deletions were the sole abnormality found in some of the bladder lesions studied, suggesting the presence of a candidate tumour suppressor gene on chromosome 9, the alteration of which may lead to the genesis of a subset of superficial bladder tumours. None of the T_a lesions showed 5q alterations; however, 3 of 10 T_1 and 8 of 26 T_{2+} tumours presented with 5q LOH, indicating that 5q deletions may be involved in the transition from papillary superficial (T_a) to early invasive (T_1) tumours. Allelic loss of 17p was detected in 21 of 47 informative cases. Deletions were not identified among T_a lesions, whereas 21 of 38 invasive tumours exhibited 17p LOH. These findings support the involvement of 17p in the progression of bladder cancer. Allelic deletion of 3p was not present in any of the informative T_a neoplasms; however, 18 of 33 invasive tumours had such alterations. There was a statistically significant association with the various pathological parameters of poor outcome and 3p LOH. Other allelic losses (11p, 6q and 18q) were frequently detected, but no significant differences were observed when they were related to clinical and pathological parameters of poor outcome (Dalbagni *et al*, 1993).

Habuchi *et al* (1993) investigated the role of allelic losses of seven chromosomal arms (1p, 3p, 9q, 10q, 11p, 13q, 17p) in 49 urothelial cancers. They also found that 9q LOH was a common event in bladder tumours and that invasive tumours showed higher frequencies of 17p and 13q losses than non-invasive lesions. Deletions of the long arm of chromosome 13, including the *RB* locus (13q14), were independently reported by two groups (Cairns *et al* 1991; Ishikawa *et al*, 1991). In one of these studies, Cairns *et al* (1991) used intragenic *RB* probes and found 28 of 94 informative cases with LOH at the *RB* locus, with 26 of these 28 lesions being muscle invasive tumours.

Growth control in mammalian cells is accomplished largely by the action of RB protein, with regulates the exit from the G_1 phase of the cell cycle, and TP53 protein, which triggers growth arrest or apoptotic processes in response to cellular stress (for a review see Cordon-Cardo, 1995). In tumourigenesis RB and TP53 have collaborative roles, as evidenced by their frequent alterations in human tumours, the many tumour types that exhibit mutations in both *RB* and *TP53* and the need for both proteins to be inactivated by several oncoviruses for cell transformation to occur. The mechanistic basis for this dual requirement stems, in part, from the deactivation of a TP53 dependent cell suicide program that would normally be brought about as a response to unchecked cellular proliferation resulting from RB deficiency.

The potential relevance of RB alterations in bladder cancer was disclosed in two independent studies (Cordon-Cardo *et al*, 1992; Logothetis *et al*, 1992). Using a mouse monoclonal antibody and immunohistochemistry in frozen tissue sections of 48 primary bladder tumours, Cordon-Cardo *et al* (1992) found normal levels of RB expression in 34 cases. However, a spectrum of altered patterns of expression, from undetectable RB levels to heterogeneous expression of RB, was observed in 14 patients. 13 of 38 cases of muscle invasive tumours were categorised as RB altered, whereas only one of 10 superficial carcinomas had the altered RB phenotype. Survival was significantly decreased in patients with RB altered tumours compared with those with normal RB expression. Similarly, Logothetis *et al* (1992) found altered RB expression in locally advanced bladder cancer. 43 patients were evaluated using Rb-WL-1 polyclonal antiserum and immunohistochemistry. These investigators reported altered RB expression in 37% of the tumour specimens analysed. There was a significant decrease in disease free survival for patients with documented abnormal RB levels. Taken together, these data suggested that altered RB expression occurred in all grades and stages of bladder cancer, but was more commonly associated with muscle invasive tumours. Moreover altered patterns of RB may become an important prognostic variable in patients presenting with invasive bladder cancer.

The clinical implications of detecting *TP53* mutations and altered patterns of TP53 protein in bladder tumours was the focus of a series of early investigations (Sidransky *et al*, 1991; Fujimoto *et al*, 1992; Dalbagni *et al*, 1993). Such studies revealed that *TP53* mutations were common events in bladder cancer and were associated with tumour stage and grade. In a study designed to evaluate the sensitivity and specificity of different laboratory assays directed at the identification of *TP53* mutations (including immunohistochemistry with monoclonal antibody PAb1801, restriction fragment length polymorphism, PCR-SSCP [single-strand conformation polymorphism] and sequencing) a strong association was found between TP53 nuclear overexpression and 17p LOH, as well as TP53 nuclear overexpression and detection of *TP53* mutations by SSCP and sequencing (Cordon-Cardo *et al*, 1994a). Using receiver operating curve statistical analysis, the accuracy of detecting TP53 mutations by immunohistochemistry was estimated to be 90.3%. In addition, this study defined as an appropriate cut-off point for immunohistochemistry 20% tumour cells displaying nuclear immunoreactivities (TP53 positive phenotype) (Cordon-Cardo *et al*,

1994a). The aim of a group of analyses that followed was to investigate the hypothesis that altered patterns of TP53 expression correlated with tumour progression in patients with superficial bladder tumours (Sarkis *et al*, 1993, 1994; Esrig *et al*, 1994). These studies proved that detection of altered TP53 expression was associated with disease progression and death from bladder cancer. Moreover these aberrations were independent predictors of recurrence and survival. Alterations of *TP53* have been identified in dysplastic lesions of the urinary bladder, implying a potential prerequisite for a possible involvement of TP53 in bladder carcinogenesis (Soini *et al*, 1993; Schmitz-Drager *et al*, 1994).

The co-operative effects of TP53 and RB alterations in superficial bladder tumours was revealed in another study (Cordon-Cardo *et al*, 1997), in which nuclear overexpression of TP53 was identified in 37% of cases. A statistical significant association was observed between the TP53 positive phenotype and both disease progression and reduced survival. Undetectable levels of RB were observed in 19% of cases. An RB negative phenotype was associated with more frequent disease progression and decreased overall survival. A significant association was observed between altered TP53 and undetectable RB expression patterns. Nine tumours showed a TP53 positive, RB negative phenotype. There was an even more marked increase in progression and decreased overall survival in patients whose tumours had both alterations after controlling for tumour stage, tumour grade and suspicion of vascular invasion. These data suggest that alterations of TP53 and RB have a co-operative negative effect on both progression and survival in primary bladder cancer. As stated above, it may be postulated that aberrant TP53 and RB expression deregulate cell cycle control at the G_1 checkpoint and engender tumour cells with a reduced response to programmed cell death. The imbalance produced by enhanced proliferative activity and decreased apoptosis may underlie the aggressive clinical course of the bladder tumours harbouring both TP53 and RB alterations.

Loss of genetic material on chromosome 9 is an early abnormality detected in bladder tumours. The existence of two altered loci, one in each arm of chromosome 9, has been postulated (Cairns *et al*, 1993; Miyao *et al*, 1993). A detailed analysis by Orlow *et al* (1994) on 73 bladder tumours showed that two regions, one on 9p at the IFN cluster (9p21) and the other on 9q associated with the q34.1-2 bands, had the highest frequencies of allelic losses. The 9p21 region is mutated frequently in a wide variety of human tumour cell lines and the search for a putative tumour suppressor gene in this region led to the characterization of the so called multiple tumour suppressor 1 (*MTS1*) gene (Kamb *et al*, 1994). *MTS1* was confirmed to be the previously identified *CDKN2A* gene (Serrano *et al*, 1993). In addition, the *CDKN2B* (*INK4B*, *MTS2*) gene is found in tandem at 9p21 (Hannon and Beach, 1994). These genes encode members of a new family of negative cell cycle regulators, whose products function as cyclin dependent kinase inhibitory molecules (for a review see Cordon-Cardo, 1995). Additional complexity at this locus results from the discovery that exon 2 of *CDKN2A* is utilized, albeit in a different reading frame, by a second CDKN2A encoded gene product, termed p19[ARF] (ARF being the acronym of alternative reading frame) (Quelle *et al*, 1995). Thus, the *CDKN2A* gene contains two distinct exons 1 (1α and 1β), which assemble at the same acceptor site of exon 2 but produce two different proteins: p16 and p19[ARF], respectively. Overexpression of p19[ARF] has been shown to induce G_1 as well as G_2M arrest through mechanisms that do not involve inhibition of known cyclin dependent kinases. Several independent groups of investigators showed that genetic alterations, mainly of CDKN2A with concomitant effects on p19[ARF] and CDKN2B, are common events in bladder cancer. Orlow *et al* (1995) have reported an overall frequency of deletions and rearrangements for the *CDKN2A* and *CDKN2B* genes in bladder cancer of 19% and 18%, respectively. Moreover this study revealed that CDKN2A and CDKN2B alterations were associated with low stage, low grade bladder tumours. Only T_a and T_1, and not T_{is}, lesions showed deletions of either CDKN2A or CDKN2B. Since CDKN2A alterations occur independently of TP53 mutations (Gruis *et al*, 1995) and TP53 mutations are frequent events in T_{is} bladder tumours, data from that report further support the hypothesis that bladder carcinogenesis may develop through two distinct molecular pathways (Dalbagni *et al*, 1993; Spruck *et al*, 1994). Furthermore,

Fig. 1. (A) Proposed genetic model of bladder cancer progression as it relates to pathology staging. Two distinct presentations of early lesions can be described. T_a tumors are low grade, well differentiated, usually papillary neoplasms, which tend to recur but not to progress. T_{is} are high grade, poorly differentiated, flat lesions with a high progression rate. In T_a lesions, chromosome 9 alterations appear to be early events. Detailed analyses showed that two regions, one on 9p at the interferon cluster (9p21) and the other at 9q34.1-2, had the highest frequencies of mutations. It has been shown that two tumor suppressor genes (p16/INK4A and p15/INK4B), which reside on 9p21 and function as negative cell-cycle regulators, are altered in superficial bladder cancer. In T_{is} lesions, however, early genetic alterations have not been yet elucidated, even though deletions of 14q and 8p have been reported as harboring candidate suppressor genes. The transition from superficial non-invasive to early invasive T_1 lesions has been associated with several chromosomal abnormalities, including deletions of 5q, 3p and 17p. Late alterations, such as molecular abnormalities of TP53 (17p11.3) and RB (13q14), produce a selective advantage for tumor growth and an aggressive biological behavior. It is our premise that in tumor cells lacking both pRB and p53, activation of specific transcription factors (ie., E2F family members) may stimulate cell proliferation in the absence of apoptosis, leading to tumor progression. (B) Schematic representation of the proposed genetic model of bladder cancer (dotted lines represent alternative and infrequent pathways). In the earliest events in cellular transformation, normal appearing tissue may contain molecular abnormalities, such as altered patterns of DNA methylation and microsatellite abnormalities. Some of these alterations may account for the great degree of genetic instability found in neoplastic cells. "Primary" molecular aberrations can be defined as those directly related to the genesis of cancer. These are frequently found as the sole abnormality and are often associated with particular tumors. Primary abnormalities may have a dual nature: (1) events involved in the production of low-grade/well-differentiated neoplasms, destabilizing cellular proliferation but having minimal of no effects on cellular differentiation and apoptosis; and (b) events leading to high-grade/poorly differentiated tumors, severely disrupting growth control, apoptosis, and differentiation. "Secondary" abnormalities may be fortuitous or may determine the biological behavior of the tumor. Multiple molecular abnormalities are identified in most human cancers studied, including bladder neoplasms. It is the accumulation rather than the order of these genetic alterations which is most important, acting synergistically to produce an aggressive biological behavior.

evidence has accumulated revealing that the two products encoded by *CDKN2A* impact on the two prototype tumour suppressors, p16 through RB and p19[ARF] through p53, positioning the single gene *CDKN2A* at the nexus of the two most critical tumour suppressor pathways controlling neoplasia (Pomerantz *et al*, 1998). This in turn may explain the high frequency of mutations of the *CDKN2A* gene in human cancer.

BLADDER CANCER AS A MODEL FOR THE STUDY OF PRENEOPLASTIC LESIONS AND TUMOUR PROGRESSION

The molecular abnormalities reported to date, as well as the natural history of bladder cancer, have allowed the proposal of a working model for tumour development and progression of this group of neoplastic diseases (Dalbagni *et al*, 1993; Spruck *et al*, 1994; Cordon-Cardo *et al*, 1994b). It is the hypothesis of several groups of investigators that some specific chromosomal abnormalities and mutations of certain genes have a definite role in bladder tumour development and other alterations seem to correlate with tumour progression (Fig. 1). Other alterations affecting differentiation antigens have also been associated with tumourigenesis and tumour progression in bladder cancer (for a review see

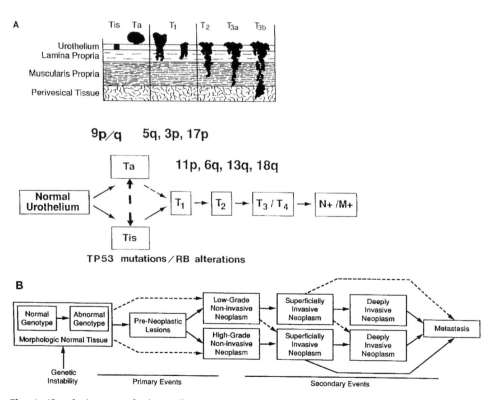

Fig. 1. (See facing page for legend)

Fradet and Cordon-Cardo, 1996). For example phenotypic biochemical markers, such as G-actin and M344 antigen, occur as early events in uroepithelial transformation (Bonner *et al*, 1993; Rao *et al*, 1993; Hemstreet *et al*, 1993). Blood group antigen alterations have been identified even in dysplasias of the urothelium (Yamada *et al*, 1991; Orlow *et al*, 1998). Similarly, unscheduled expression of cytokeratin 20 has been reported as a marker of urothelial dysplasia (Harnden *et al*, 1996). However, the analysis of changes occurring as part of potential field effects are not substantiated by in depth mapping studies of cystectomy specimens. Despite the significant progress made in the development and evaluation of various biological determinants, currently no solid recommendations can be made about most discovered markers in the management of bladder cancer. Most molecular and immunopathological analyses have been hampered by a series of obstacles and limitations. In molecular genetic analyses, normal tissue contaminating the tumour sample could be an important source of false negative results in, for example, assessments of tumour specific deletions. Another important concern is that different methodologies have been utilized on a variety of clinical samples, which may also account for discrepancies between reported studies. Specifically, varied results may be accounted for by the frequent grouping of superficial and muscle invasive lesions in a single analysis. Moreover many reports lack correlations between clinicopathological variables and laboratory data. Despite these limitations, the analysis of this group of neoplastic diseases, either as clinical entities or as molecular epidemiology systems, has served as a model for our understanding of tumourigenesis and cancer progression (Linehan *et al*, 1997).

SUMMARY

The molecular genetic changes reported in bladder tumours can be classified as primary and secondary aberrations. Primary molecular alterations may be defined as those directly related to the genesis of cancer. These are frequently found as the sole abnormality and often associated with particular tumours. We describe primary abnormalities as having a dual nature: those events involved in the production of low grade/well differentiated neoplasms, which would destabilise cellular proliferation but have minimal or no effects on cellular "social" interactions or differentiation or on rate of cell death or apoptosis; and others leading to high grade/poorly differentiated tumours, which would disrupt growth control, including cell cycle and apoptosis regulation and have a major impact on cellular differentiation. There is evidence that a target site(s) for a primary event(s) in low grade papillary superficial bladder tumours may reside on chromosome 9. However, a candidate for the initiation of high grade, flat carcinoma in situ lesions has not been yet elucidated. Novel approaches utilizing tissue microdissection techniques and molecular genetic assays are needed to shed light on this subject. Secondary genetic or epigenetic abnormalities may be fortuitous or may determine the biological behaviour of the tumour.

Multiple molecular abnormalities are identified in most human cancers studied, including bladder neoplasms. The accumulation, rather than the order, of these genetic alterations is the critical factor that grants synergetic activity. In this regard, it is noteworthy that most of the altered genes act upon the two recognized critical growth and senescence pathways, TP53 and RB. There is a major requirement for well designed, randomized, prospective trials evaluating the strongest candidate markers in order to validate many reported exploratory studies. Although great enthusiasm exists with the application of various tumour makers in the management of bladder cancer, concrete clinical recommendations must be tempered at this time. As with preoplastic conditions, the discrepancies that exist between clinical investigators regarding the significance of identifying such morphological changes have imposed crucial limitations. Another drawback has been the confusing nomenclature utilized and the lack of reproducibility in interpretation of morphological criteria. Molecular analyses utilizing well characterized preneoplastic lesions, including dysplasia samples, need to be pursued. This in turn may provide the needed information to realise the clinical relevance of detecting genetic instability, as well as molecular or epigenetic alterations, in otherwise morphologically normal appearing urothelium and preneoplastic lesions. The need now is to translate the newly developed scientific information into diagnostic and prognostic strategies, which in turn will prolong patient survival and quality of life.

References

Atkin NB and Baker MC (1985) Cytogenetic study of ten carcinomas of the bladder: involvement of chromosomes 1 and 11. *Cancer Genetics and Cytogenetics* **15** 253–268

Babu VR, Lutz MD, Miles BJ, Farah RN, Weiss L and Van DD (1987) Tumor behavior in transitional cell carcinoma of the bladder in relation to chromosomal markers and histopathology. *Cancer Research* **47** 6800–6805

Balazs M, Carroll P, Kerschmann R, Sauter G and Waldman FM (1997) Frequent homozygous deletion of cyclin-dependent kinase inhibitor 2 (MTS1, p16) in superficial bladder cancer detected by fluorescence in situ hybridization. *Genes, Chromosomes & Cancer* **19** 84–89

Barbareschi M, Girlando S, Fellin G, Graffer U, Luciani L and Palma PD (1995) Expression of mdm2 and p53 proteins in transitional cell carcinoma. *Urology Research* **22** 349–352

Bonner RB, Hemstreet GP III, Fradet Y, Rao JY, Min KW and Hurst RE (1993) Bladder cancer risk assessment with quantitative fluorescence image analysis of tumor markers in exfoliated bladder cells. *Cancer* **72** 2461–2469

Cairns P, Proctor AJ and Knowles MA (1991) Loss of heterozygosity at the RB locus is frequent and correlates with muscle invasion in bladder carcinoma. *Oncogene* **6** 2305–2309

Cairns P, Shaw ME and Knowles MA (1993) Preliminary mapping of the deleted region of chromosome 9 in bladder cancer. *Cancer Research* **53** 1230–1232

Cordon-Cardo C (1995) Mutation of cell cycle regulators: biological and clinical implications for human neoplasias. *American Journal of Pathology* **147** 545–560

Cordon-Cardo C, Wartinger D, Petrylak D *et al* (1992) Altered expression of the retinoblastoma gene product is a prognostic indicator in bladder cancer. *Journal of the National Cancer Institute* **84** 1251–1256

Cordon-Cardo C, Dalbagni D, Saez GT *et al* (1994a) TP53 mutations in human bladder cancer: genotypic versus phenotypic patterns. *International Journal of Cancer* **56** 347–353

Cordon-Cardo C, Dalbagni D, Sarkis A and Reuter VE (1994b) Genetic alterations associated with bladder cancer, In: DeVita VT, Hellman S and Rosenberg SA (eds). *Important Advances in Oncology*, pp 71–83, JB Lippincott Company, Philadelphia, Pennsylvania

Cordon-Cardo C, Zhang ZF, Dalbagni G *et al* (1997) Cooperative effects of p53 and pRB alterations in primary superficial bladder tumors. *Cancer Research* **57** 1217–1221

Czerniak B, Deitch D, Simmons H, Elkind P, Herz F and Koss LG (1990) Ha-*ras* gene codon 12 mutations and DNA ploidy in urinary bladder carcinomas. *British Journal of Cancer* **62** 762–763

Czerniak B, Cohen GL, Elkind P *et al* (1992) Concurrent mutations of coding and regulatory sequences of the Ha-*ras* gene in urinary bladder carcinomas. *Human Pathology* **23** 1199

Dalbagni G, Presti J, Reuter V, Fair WR and Cordon-Cardo C (1993) Genetic alterations in bladder cancer. *Lancet* **324** 469–471

Esrig D, Elmajian D, Groshen S *et al* (1994) Accumulation of nuclear p53 and tumor progression in bladder cancer. *New England Journal of Medicine* **331** 1259–1264

Fearon ER, Feinberg AP, Hamilton SH and Vogelstein B (1985) Loss of genes on the short arm of chromosome 11 in bladder cancer. *Nature* **318** 377–380

Fitzgerald JM, Ramchurren N, Rieger K *et al* (1995) Identification of H-*ras* mutations in urine sediments complements cytology in the detection of bladder tumors. *Journal of the National Cancer Institute* **87** 129–133

Fradet Y and Cordon-Cardo C (1996) Tumor markers in the management of bladder cancer, In: Raghavan D, Scher HI, Leibel SA and Lange P (eds). *Principles and Practice of Genitourinary Oncology*, pp 231–238, JB Lippincott Company, Philadelphia, Pennsylvania

Fujimoto K, Yamada Y, Okajima E *et al* (1992) Frequent association of p53 gene mutation in invasive bladder cancer. *Cancer Research* **52** 1393–1398

Fujita J, Srivastava SK and Kraus MH (1985) Frequency of molecular alterations affecting *ras* protooncogenes in human urinary tract tumors. *Proceedings of the National Academy of Sciences of the USA* **82** 3849–3853

Gibas Z, Prout GR, Connolly JG, Pontes JE and Sandberg AA (1984) Nonrandom chromosomal changes in transitional cell carcinoma of the bladder. *Cancer Research* **44** 1257–1264

Gruis NA, Weaver-Feldhaus J, Liu Q *et al* (1995) Genetic evidence in melanoma and bladder cancers that p16 and p53 function in separate pathways of tumor suppression. *American Journal of Pathology* **146** 1199–1206

Habuchi T, Ogawa O, Kakehi Y *et al* (1993) Accumulated allelic losses in the development of invasive urothelial cancer. *International Journal of Cancer* **53** 579–584

Hannon GJ and Beach D (1994) p15^{INK4B} is a potential effector of TGF-ß-induced cell cycle arrest. *Nature* **371** 257–261

Harnden P, Eardley I, Joyce AD and Southgate J (1996) Cytokeratin 20 as an objective marker of urothelial dysplasia. *British Journal of Urology* **78** 870–875

Haupt Y, Maya R, Kazaz A, and Oren M (1997) Mdm2 promotes the rapid degradation of p53. *Nature* **387** 296–299

Hemstreet GP III, Hurst RE, Bonner RB, Jones PL, Min KW and Fradet Y (1993) Alterations in phenotypic biochemical markers in bladder epithelium during tumorigenesis. *Proceedings of the National Academy of Sciences of the USA* **90** 8287–8291

Hopman AHN, Moesker O, Smeets W, Pauwels RPE, Vooijs GP and Ramaekers FCS (1991) Numerical chromosome 1, 7, 9, and 11 aberrations in bladder cancer detected by in situ hybridization. *Cancer Research* **51** 644–651

Igawa M, Urakami S and Shirakawa H (1995) A mapping of histology and cell proliferation in human bladder cancer: an immunohistochemical study. *Hiroshima Journal of Medical Science* **44** 93–97

Ishikawa J, Xu H-J, Hu S-X *et al* (1991) Inactivation of the retinoblastoma gene in human bladder and renal cell carcinomas. *Cancer Research* **51** 5736–5743

Johansson SL and Cohen SM (1996) Pathology of bladder cancer, In: Raghavan D, Scher HI, Leibel SA and Lange P (eds). *Principles and Practice of Genitourinary Oncology*, pp 207–213,

JB Lippincott Company, Philadelphia, Pennsylvania

Kallioniemi A, Kallioniemi OP, Sudar D *et al* (1992) Comparative genomic hybridization for molecular cytogenetic analysis of solid tumors. *Science* **258** 818–821

Kallioniemi A, Kallioniemi OP, Citro G *et al* (1995) Identification of gains and losses of DNA sequences in primary bladder cancer by comparative genomic hybridization. *Genes, Chromosomes & Cancer* **12** 213–219

Kamb A, Gruis NA, Weaver-Feldhaus J *et al* (1994) A cell cycle regulator potentially involved in genesis of many tumor types. *Science* **264** 436–440

Kiemeney LA and Schoenberg M (1996) Familial transitional cell carcinoma. *Journal of Urology* **156** 867–872

Kiemeney LA, Witjes JA, Heijbroek RP, Debruyne FM and Verbeek AL (1994) Dysplasia in normal-looking urothelium increases the risk of tumour progression in primary superficial bladder cancer. *European Journal of Cancer* **30** 1621–1625

Koss L (1975). *Atlas of Tumor Pathology: Tumors of the Urinary Bladder* (Fasicle 11), Armed Forces Institute of Pathology, Washington, DC

Koss L (1992) *Diagnostic Cytology and Its Histopathologic Bases*, JB Lippincott Company, Philadelphia, Pennsylvania

Lianes P, Orlow I, Zhang ZZ *et al* (1994) Altered patterns of MDM2 and TP53 expression in human bladder cancer. *Journal of the National Cancer Institute* **86** 1325–1330

Linehan WM, Cordon-Cardo C and Isaacs W (1997) Molecular biology of genitourinary cancers, In: DeVita VT, Hellman S and Rosenberg SA (eds). *Principles and Practice of Oncology,* pp 1253–1271, JB Lippincott Company, Philadelphia, Pennsylvania

Logothetis CJ, Xu H-J, Ro JY *et al* (1992) Altered retinoblastoma protein expression and known prognostic variables in locally advanced bladder cancer. *Journal of the National Cancer Institute* **84** 1257–1261

Messing EM (1990) Clinical implications of the expression of epidermal growth factor receptors in human transitional cell carcinomas. *Cancer Research* **50** 2530–2537

Miyao N, Tsai YC, Lerner SP *et al* (1993) Role of chromosome 9 in human bladder cancer. *Cancer Research* **53** 4066–4070

Momand J, Zambetti G, Olson D *et al* (1992) The mdm-2 oncogene product forms a complex with the p-53 protein and inhibits TP53-mediated transactivation. *Cell* **69** 1237–1245

Mostofi FK and Sesterhenn IA (1984) Pathology of epithelial tumors and carcinoma in situ of bladder. *Progress in Clinical Biological Research* **62** 55–74

Mostofi FK, Sobin LH and Torloni H (1973) Histologic typing of urinary bladder tumours, In: *International Histological Classification of Tumors*, Vol. 10, World Health Organization, Geneva

Nagatava Y, Abe M, Kobayashi K *et al* (1990) Point mutations of c-*ras* genes in human bladder cancer and kidney cancer. *Japanese Journal of Cancer Research* **81** 22–27

Neal DE, Marsh C, Bennet MK, Hall RR and Harris AL (1985) Epidermal growth-factor receptors in human bladder cancer: comparison of invasive and superficial tumors. *Lancet* **i** 366–368

Neal DE, Sharples L, Smith K, Fennelly J, Hall RR and Harris AL (1990) The epidermal growth factor receptor and the prognosis of bladder cancer. *Cancer* **65** 1619–1625

Nguyen PL, Swanson PE, Jaszcz W *et al* (1994) Expression of epidermal growth factor receptor in invasive transitional cell carcinoma of the urinary bladder: a multivariate survival analysis. *American Journal of Clinical Pathology* **101** 166–176

Oliner JD, Kinzler KW, Metlzer PS *et al* (1992) Amplification of a gene encoding a p53 associated protein in human sarcomas. *Nature* **358** 80–83

Olumi AF, Tsai YC, Nichols PW *et al* (1990) Allelic loss of chromosomes 17p distinguishes high grade from low grade transitional cell carcinoma of the bladder. *Cancer Research* **50** 7081–7083

Ooi A, Herz F, Setsuko I *et al* (1994) Ha-*ras* codon 12 mutation in papillary tumors of the urinary bladder: a retrospective study. *International Journal of Oncology* **4** 85–89

Orlow I, Lianes P, Lacombe L, Dalbagni G, Reuter VE and Cordon-Cardo C (1994) Chromosome 9 deletions and microsatellite alterations in human bladder tumors. *Cancer Research* **54** 2848–2851

Orlow I, Lacombe L, Hannon GJ *et al* (1995) Deletion of the p16 and p15 genes in human bladder tumors. *Journal of the National Cancer Institute* **87** 1524–1529

Orlow I, Lacombe L, Pellicer I, Delgado R, Szijan I and Cordon-Cardo C (1998) Genotype and phenotype characterization of the histoblood group ABO(H) in primary bladder tumors. *International Journal of Cancer* **75** 819–824

Pomerantz J, Schrieber-Agus N, Liegoeis N *et al* (1998) The INK4a tumor suppressor gene product, p19/Arf, interacts with MDM2 and neutralizes MDM2's inhibition of p53. *Cell* **92** 713–723

Presti JC, Reuter VE, Galan T, Fair WR and Cordon-Cardo C (1991) Molecular genetic alterations in superficial and locally advanced human bladder cancer. *Cancer Research* **51** 5405–5409

Prout GR (1977) Bladder carcinoma and a TNM system of classification. *Journal of Urology* **117** 583–588

Quell DE, Zindy F, Ashum RA, and Sherr CJ (1995) Alternative reading frames of the INK4A tumor suppressor gene encode two unrelated proteins capable of inducing cell cycle arrest. *Cell* **83** 993–1000

Rao JY, Hemstreet GP, Hurst RE *et al* (1993) Alterations in phenotypic biochemical markers in bladder epithelium during tumorigenesis. *Proceedings of the National Academy of Sciences of the USA* **90** 8287–8291

Reddy EP, Reynolds RK, Santos E and Barbacid M (1982) A point mutation is responsible for the acquisition of transforming properties by the T24 bladder carcinoma oncogene. *Nature* **300** 149–152

Reuter VE and Melamed MR (1989) The lower urinary tract, In: Sternberg SS (ed). *Diagnostic Surgical Pathology*, pp 1355, Raven Press, New York

Sarkis AS, Dalbagni G, Cordon-Cardo C *et al* (1993) Nuclear overexpression of p53 protein in transitional cell bladder carcinoma: a marker for disease progression. *Journal of the National Cancer Institute* **85** 53–59

Sarkis AS, Dalbagni G, Cordon-Cardo C *et al* (1994) Association of p53 nuclear overexpression and tumor progression in carcinoma in situ of the bladder. *Journal of Urology* **152** 388–392

Sato K, Moriyama M, Mori S *et al* (1992) An immunohistologic evaluation of c-erbB-2 gene product in patients with urinary bladder carcinoma. *Cancer* **70** 2493–2498

Sauter G, Moch H, Moore D *et al* (1993) Heterogeneity of erbB-2 gene amplification in bladder cancer. *Cancer Research* **53** 2199–2203

Sauter G, Deng G, Moch H *et al* (1994) Physical deletion of the p53 gene in bladder cancer. *American Journal of Pathology* **144** 756–766

Sauter G, Carroll P, Moch H *et al* (1995a) c-myc copy number gains in bladder cancer detected by fluorescence in situ hybridization. *American Journal of Pathology* **146** 1131–1139

Sauter G, Moch H, Wagner U *et al* (1995b) Y chromosome loss detected by FISH in bladder cancer. *Cancer Genetics and Cytogenetics* **82** 163–169

Schmitz-Drager BJ, van Roeyen CR, Grimm MO *et al* (1994) p53 accumulation in precursor lesions and early stages of bladder cancer. *World Journal of Urology* **12** 79–83

Serrano M, Hannon GJ and Beach D (1993) A new regulatory motif in cell-cycle control causing specific inhibition of cyclin D/CDK4. *Nature* **366** 704–707

Sidransky D, Von Eschenbach A, Tsai YC *et al* (1991) Identification of p53 gene mutations in bladder cancers and urine samples. *Science* **252** 706–709

Smeets W, Pauwels R, Laarakkers L, Debruyne F and Geraedts J (1987) Chromosomal analysis of bladder cancer, III, Nonrandom alterations. *Cancer Genetics and Cytogenetics* **29** 29–41

Soini Y, Turpeenniemi-Hujanan T, Kamel D *et al* (1993) p53 immunohistochemistry in transitional cell carcinoma and dysplasia of the urinary bladder correlates with disease. *British Journal of Cancer* **68** 1029–1035

Spruck CH, Ohneseit PE, Gonzalez-Zulueta M *et al* (1994) Two molecular pathways to transitional cell carcinoma of the bladder. *Cancer Research* **54** 784–788

Tsai YC, Nichols PW, Hiti AL, Williams Z, Skinner DG and Jones PA (1990) Allelic losses of chromosomes 9, 11, and 17 in human bladder cancer. *Cancer Research* **50** 44

Tyrkus M, Powell I and Fakr W (1992) Cytogenetic studies of carcinoma in situ of the bladder: prognostic implications. *Journal of Urology* **148** 44

Underwood M, Barlett J, Reeves J, Gardiner DS, Scott R and Cooke T (1995) C-erbB-2 gene amplification: a molecular marker in recurrent bladder tumors? *Cancer Research* **55** 2422

Vanni R, Scarpa RM, Nieddu M and Usai E (1988) Cytogenetic investigation on 30 bladder carcinomas. *Cancer Genetics and Cytogenetics* **30** 35

Wagner U, Sauter G, Moch H *et al* (1995) Patterns of p53, erB-2, and EGF-r expression in premalignant lesions of the urinary bladder. *Human Pathology* **26** 970–978

Waldman FM, Carroll PR, Kerschmann R, Cohen MB, Field FG and Mayall BH (1991) Centromeric copy number of chromosome 7 is strongly correlated with tumor grade and labeling index in human bladder cancer. *Cancer Research* **51** 3807

Wheeless LL, Reeder JE, Han R *et al* (1994) Bladder irrigation specimens assayed by fluorescence in situ hybridization to interphase nuclei. *Cytometry* **17** 319

Wood D, Wartinger DD, Reuter V, Cordon-Cardo C, Fair WR and Chaganti RS (1991) DNA, RNA and immunohistochemical characterization of the HER-2/neu oncogene in transitional cell carcinoma of the bladder. *Journal of Urology* **146** 1398–1401

Yamada T, Fukui I and Kobayashi T (1991) The relationship of ABH(O) blood group antigen expression in intraepithelial dysplastic lesions to clinicopathologic properties of associated transitional cell carcinoma of the bladder. *Cancer* **67** 1661–1666

Zhang Z-F and Steineck G (1996) Epidemiology and etiology of bladder cancer, In: Raghavan D, Scher HI, Leibel SA and Lange P (eds). *Principles and Practice of Genitourinary Oncology*, pp 215–222, JB Lippincott Company, Philadelphia, Pennsylvania

The author is responsible for the accuracy of the references.

Endpoint Markers for Clinical Trials of Chemopreventive Agents Derived from the Properties of Epithelial Precancer (Intraepithelial Neoplasia) Measured by Computer-assisted Image Analysis

C W BOONE • G J KELLOFF

Chemoprevention Branch, Division of Cancer Prevention, National Cancer Institute, Rockville, Maryland 20892-7322

INTRODUCTION

Cancer chemoprevention is generally defined as the prevention of cancer with diet supplements or drugs (Wattenberg, 1996). With regard to epithelia, chemoprevention seeks to prevent the onset of intraepithelial neoplasia (IEN) and the progression of established IEN to invasiveness across the epithelial basement membrane. The Chemoprevention Branch, NCI, is supporting over

80 clinical trials of chemopreventive agents and has dozens of drugs under development. It has not been possible to set up a rapid screen for these drugs using clinical trials with the endpoint of cancer incidence reduction because such trials are of such long duration (5–10 or more years), large scale of effort (tens of thousands of subjects) and great cost (many millions of dollars). To provide for rapid chemopreventive drug screening in humans, it has been necessary to develop endpoint markers that permit the trials to be shorter, smaller and less costly. Such markers must closely correlate with the risk of cancer incidence, so that reduction or elimination of the markers by a given test agent will reliably predict that the agent will also reduce cancer incidence. This article describes use of the morphological and functional properties of IEN to develop endpoint markers in short term clinical chemoprevention trials.

If cancer is defined as a continuously enlarging abnormal tissue mass which invades normal tissue, precancer may be simply defined as the same condition prior to the onset of invasiveness. Cancer is by convention divided into the carcinomas, involving epithelia derived from embryonal ectoderm and endoderm, and the sarcomas, derived from two types of embryonal mesodermal tissue, the mesenchyme (fat, muscle, fibrous tissue, cartilage and bone, which form soft tissue sarcomas, chondrosarcomas and osteosarcomas) and the haematolymphatic tissues (forming the leukaemias, lymphomas and lymphosarcomas). Since the great majority of adult cancers are of epithelial origin, the focus of this article will be restricted to precancer of epithelial tissues—IEN.

DIAGNOSTIC TERMINOLOGY OF EPITHELIAL PRECANCER (IEN) USED BY AMERICAN PATHOLOGISTS

In a landmark publication in 1969, "Neoplastic Development", Leslie Foulds presented evidence that the process of carcinogenesis is characterized by permanent, irreversible changes in one or more characters of the cellular phenotype that continue to appear within the growing neoplastic cell population. Foulds applied the term "neoplastic progression" to describe this evolving continuum (Foulds, 1969a,b). Soon after, using cytogenetic methods applied to haematologic malignancies, Nowell (1976, 1986, 1990) established that clonal evolution (continual formation of genetically variant clones within a neoplasm) is the basis for neoplastic progression. In accordance with the work of Foulds and Nowell, this article will apply the term "neoplasia" to the entire continuum of epithelial carcinogenesis, from the first clonal expansion of a mutated stem cell within the epithelium, through continuing clonal evolution with progressive increase in bulk of the neoplastic cell population, to invasion across the epithelial basement membrane and dissemination by local extension and distant metastases. Figures 1 and 2A,B illustrate the development of neoplasia in squamous epithelium such as the uterine cervix and in glandular epithelium such as colon; they also present the terminology used by American pathologists to describe various diagnostic features. The figures divide the continuum of neo-

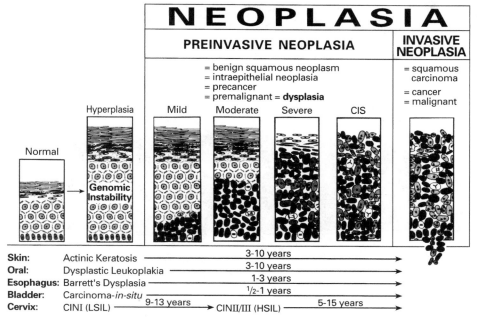

Fig. 1. Diagram of neoplasia of squamous epithelium, preceded by hyperplasia and genomic instability. Neoplastic progression is divided into two phases: preinvasive neoplasia, also called IEN, dysplasia and precancer and invasive neoplasia, which is by definition cancer. The name carcinoma in situ (CIS) is sometimes given to very severe preinvasive neoplasia. Individual neoplastic cell nuclei show abnormal variation in size, shape and staining intensity

plasia into two phases: preinvasive, or intraepithelial, neoplasia and invasive neoplasia, which is by general definition cancer. As shown in the figures, intraepithelial neoplastic disease frequently develops many years before the phase of invasiveness. The term "precancer" as applied to epithelia is equivalent to "intraepithelial neoplasia". The term IEN will therefore be used in the rest of this article.

CLARIFICATION OF PROBLEMATIC DIAGNOSTIC TERMS APPLIED TO IEN

There are four diagnostic terms frequently used to describe IEN that invite misunderstanding and defy replacement. They are "dysplasia", "atypia", "carcinoma in situ" and "preneoplasia". Figures 1 and 2A,B illustrate how the terms mild, moderate and severe dysplasia are used to grade IEN. The question frequently asked by non-specialists is, "Is dysplasia a neoplastic condition?" The most satisfactory answer is that moderate and severe grade dysplasia (defined as involvement by neoplastic cells of more than the lower third of the epithelium) are indeed neoplastic, but that mild dysplasia is frequently difficult to distinguish from an inflammatory reaction of the epithelium to infection, toxic agents or trauma (Wright *et al*, 1994).

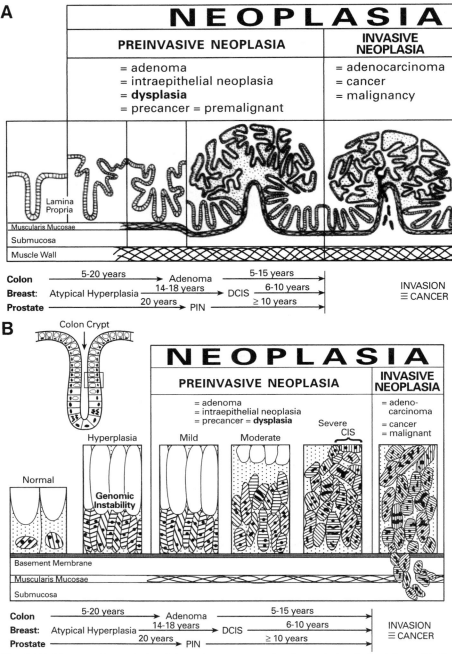

Fig. 2 (A) Diagram of neoplasia of the colon, an example of neoplasia of glandular epithelium. Proliferating stem cells develop outpockets from the upper crypt which form secondary and tertiary crypts that combine to produce an elevated adenomatous polyp. By convention, the diagnosis of cancer requires that invasion has occurred not only across the epithelial basement membrane but also across the muscularis mucosa, as shown in the figure. (B) Neoplasia of the colon at higher power. The crypt cell nuclei show crowding, stratification (multiple rows) and loss of vertical orientation (polarity). The individual nuclei show abnormal variation in size and shape in a manner similar to the nuclei of neoplastic squamous epithelium

The second problematic term, atypia, is used with the connotation of "neoplastic" by pathologists and particularly by cytopathologists, who must interpret cell smears without the benefit of tissue architecture as a guide. However, to non-pathologists the term is unclear and may have only the meaning, "not typical but within normal limits".

The third diagnostic term inviting misunderstanding is "carcinoma in situ". To attempt to make a diagnosis of carcinoma on the basis of abnormal cell and tissue morphology alone, without the irrefutable marker of invasiveness across the epithelial basement membrane, invites imprecision and disagreement. There is now well reviewed evidence that the diagnoses of severe dysplasia and carcinoma in situ of the cervix describe two generously overlapping ends of the same continuum of neoplastic change (Buckley *et al*, 1982). Ductal carcinoma in situ of the breast is a particularly imprecise diagnosis because this condition exhibits a variable mixture of five different architectural patterns that have differing invasive potential—for example, comedo versus micropapillary patterns (Boone and Kelloff, 1995).

Finally, use of the term "preneoplasia" to mean IEN, dysplasia or precancer is particularly confounding because to allude to intraepithelial *neoplasia* as *pre*neoplasia is clearly oxymoronic. In 1969, before the term intraepithelial neoplasia came into use, Foulds stated: "The most frustrating gap in the terminology of pathology of tumours in man is a lack of a satisfactory name for the so-called precancerous lesions. "Preneoplastic...can only mean that the lesions are not neoplastic whereas I maintain strongly that they are neoplastic and that this should be recognized in their designation" (Foulds, 1969b).

Following the lead of Richart (1973), who coined the name cervical intraepithelial neoplasia more than 20 years ago, there has been a gradual trend towards standardizing the terminology of precancer by using the words intraepithelial neoplasia preceded by the name of the organ involved. Examples are squamous intraepithelial neoplasia of head and neck (Crissman and Zarbo, 1989), intra-urothelial neoplasia (Koss, 1992), mammary intraepithelial neoplasia (Rosai, 1991) and prostatic intraepithelial neoplasia (Bostwick, 1992).

NON-NEOPLASTIC CONDITIONS DIFFUSELY AFFECTING THE EPITHELIUM THAT PRECEDE THE ONSET OF IEN AND HAVE A BEARING ON THE DEVELOPMENT OF ENDPOINT MARKERS FOR CHEMOPREVENTION CLINICAL TRIALS

Diffuse Epithelial Genomic Instability

Diffuse epithelial genomic instability (diffuse as compared to the focal genomic instability that develops within neoplastic populations) appears to be a very frequent if not obligatory precursor of the neoplastic process in epithelia. It may be defined as an abnormally increased rate of unrepaired DNA strand breakage with continual accumulation of genomic structural variations (ie somatic cell mutations) at all orders of magnitude. Somatic mutations may involve DNA segments that vary in size from point mutations, to oligonucleotide segments of 1–50 kilobases (eg microsatellites), to multiallelic segments (with loss of heterozygosity, amplification or recombination and formation of extranuclear acentric micronuclei), to karyotype chromosomal aberrations (eg double minutes, homogeneous staining regions, loss and gain of arm length, translocations and isochromosomes), to aneuploidy.

The special importance of diffuse epithelial genomic instability to the development of screening assays for chemopreventive agents is that the temporal accumulation of genetic lesions is directly reflected in the appearance of increasingly abnormal phenotypic heterogeneity (Fidler, 1987). Phenotypic heterogeneity is the basis for the large number of chemoprevention clinical trial endpoint markers at the cellular level listed as packages in Table 1, concerning nuclear morphology, proliferation, apoptosis, differentiation and inflammation.

Chronic Diffuse Epithelial Hyperplasia

Chronic diffuse epithelial hyperplasia, characterized by an increase in both cell density and mitotic rate and in the case of secretory glandular epithelia, some-

TABLE 1. Chemoprevention clinical trial endpoint marker packages

CAQIA nuclear morphology package: Cytonuclear size, shape, chromatin texture (many texture features, some specific for neoplastic change); variance of size, shape, texture; nucleolar size and frequency per 100 nuclei; DNA ploidy.

Genomic instability package: Identification by gel electrophoresis of: DNA breaks, adducts, hypomethylation, point mutations, microsatellite length polymorphisms, allelic loss (LOH) of tumour suppressor genes, allelic gain (amplification) of oncogenes. **Identification by cytogenetic analysis of:** aneusomy, aneuploidy, double minutes, homogenous staining regions, deletions, insertions, trans-locations, inversions, isochromosomes; cytologic identification of micronuclei and AgNORs.

Oncogene package: Cytoplasmic: RAS, RAF, MYC, SRC, MAD, MAX, BAX, BCL2, ERBB2. **Nuclear:** RB, TP53, APC, MCC, DCC, MSH2, MHL1

Proliferation package: Cell density (cells/mm^2), MF count (+/–stain for MF); Antibody probes for Ki-67, MIB-1, PCNA; uptake of ^{3}HT, BrdU.

Apoptosis package: Apoptotic figure count; TUNEL assay.

Differentiation package: Fibres: Actin microfilaments, keratins (molecular weight specified), microtubules, involucrin, filagrin, cornifin. **Adhesion molecules:** Cell-cell: gap junctions, cadherins, desmosomes; Cell-substrate: integrins, fibronectin, proteoglycans, laminins, collagen. **Glycoconjugates:** mucin core Ta, T, sialyl Tn, apomucins (*MUC 1,2,3* genes); brush border enzymes (sucrase, isomaltase), blood group substances (Le^y, extended Le^y), glycolipids. **Growth factors (receptors):** PDGF(R), EGF(R), TGF(R), FGF(R), IGF(R).

Inflammation package: Number and distribution of macrophages, lymphocytes, endothelial cells, and fibroblasts, using immunostaining or CAQIA.

CAQIA = computer-assisted quantitative image analysis; LOH = loss of heterozygosity; AgNORs = silver ion binding to fibrillar proteins of nucleolar organizing regions; MF = mitotic figures; TUNEL = Terminal deoxynucleotidyl transferase-mediated deoxyuridine triphosphate (UTP)-biotin nick end-labelling.

times associated with metaplasia to another type of epithelium, is commonly seen as a precursor to IEN. It may be caused by chronic infection, as in urinary bladder schistosomiasis (Ferguson, 1911), chronic mechanical irritation, as in urinary bladder stones (Kantor *et al*, 1988), indwelling catheters (Locke *et al*, 1985) and gall bladder stones (Yamagiwa, 1989) and toxic irritation, as with cigarette smoke effects on the respiratory epithelium (Boone *et al*, 1992) and with gastro-oesophageal acid reflux effects on the lower oesophagus (Barrett's Oesophagus) (Neshat *et al*, 1994).

Subepithelial Chronic Inflammation

Subepithelial chronic inflammation not infrequently accompanies the epithelial hyperplastic conditions referred to above, as described in the references given. Chronic inflammation subtending epithelial hyperproliferation is also seen in ulcerative colitis (Collins *et al*, 1987) and in actinic keratosis (Fielding and Allum, 1996).

PROPERTIES OF IEN RELATED TO DEVELOPMENT OF ENDPOINT MARKERS FOR CHEMOPREVENTION CLINICAL TRIALS

The detailed natural history of IEN has been described previously (Boone *et al*, 1992). Here the properties of IEN that apply to the development of endpoint markers for clinical trials of cancer chemopreventive agents will be summarized, with emphasis on properties that can be measured by computer-assisted quantitative image analysis (CAQIA).

A progressing IEN lesion develops accelerating genomic instability, abnormally high rates of proliferation and apoptosis and decreased differentiation. They are measured using the assays listed as packages in Table 1. Decreased differentiation is the least specific property, because many times it may simply represent the replacement of mature differentiated epithelial structures by ingrowing less differentiated neoplastic cells.

Multicentricity

Figure 3 illustrates an important characteristic of IEN, that against a background of diffuse genomic instability, neoplastic clonal expansions of IEN may begin at multiple sites, each site progressing at its own pace along an independent path of clonal evolution, every clone accumulating a unique set of somatic mutations. Slaughter, in a landmark paper in 1951 describing observations on 783 patients with oral cancer, was the first to focus attention on the multicentric origin of in situ (ie intraepithelial) neoplasms of the oral cavity, each neoplasm occurring as an independently progressing focus that ultimately developed invasive squamous cell carcinoma (Slaughter *et al*, 1951). Over 11% of

"Field Cancerization"

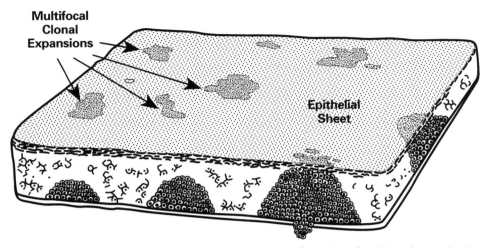

Fig. 3. Diagram showing an important property of IEN, the formation of multicentric neoplastic lesions which enlarge and progress independently of each other

Slaughter's patients simultaneously exhibited one or more independent squamous cell carcinomas involving the oesophagus or lung. He coined the term "field cancerization" to describe such an epithelium "preconditioned" by a carcinogenic agent. In modern terms, Slaughter's field cancerization represents diffuse epithelial genomic instability and associated development of multicentric IEN lesions.

Multiple actinic (solar) keratoses of the face is a common example of the multicentric development of IEN lesions. In one study (Nelson *et al*, 1994), 8 of 15 actinic keratoses exhibited *TP53* gene mutations and in another (Bito *et al*, 1995), 12 of 26 actinic keratoses showed overexpression of cyclin D and TP53 protein. As another example, in the same prostate with invasive adenocarcinoma, many separate multicentric lesions of prostatic IEN were found that exhibited individually unique patterns of aneuploidy (Qian *et al*, 1995). Adenomatous polyps of the colorectum are a final example of multicentric IEN lesions that progress independently (Mulder *et al*, 1992). In this case each lesion is supported by a fibrovascular stalk.

Multipath Genetic Progression

As is now well known, Vogelstein et al (1988) described four common genetic changes within the dysplastic (ie intraepithelial neoplastic) mucosa on the surface of colorectal polyps: a *Ras* gene mutation and allelic deletions on chromosomes 5q, 17p and 18q. The accumulation of all four lesions occurred in less than 10% of colorectal polyps, indicating that other gene changes exist that determine the development of colorectal neoplasia. In addition, his group found different numbers and combinations of genetic lesions, not only among different polyps, but also at different sites within the same polyp (Fearon and Vogelstein, 1990). The allelotyes of the different epithelial cancers show that they all exhibit a variable extent of allelic loss and gain both within and among the different chromosomes. At the level of whole chromosomes, it is well established that aneuploidy frequently develops during IEN in many organ epithelia, as shown for IEN of breast (Boone and Kelloff, 1995), cervix (Reid and Fu, 1986), prostate (Montironi *et al*, 1992), bladder (Koss, 1992), colon (Quirke, 1986), lung (Nasiell *et al*, 1978), oral leukoplakia (Grassel-Pietrusky, 1982), larynx (Crissman and Fu, 1986), oesophagus (Reid *et al*, 1987) and stomach (Macartney and Camplejohn, 1986). It appears that neoplasms in general may progress by means of multipath genetic progression—that is, by the accumulation of one or more abnormal gene changes in variable sequence and at variable times.

The approach of seeking to develop chemopreventive agents that block a given step in a proliferation related signal pathway may be frustrated by the occurrence of "clonal escape." Based on the redundancy of proliferation related signal pathways, clones mutated in pathways other than the one blocked by the chemopreventive agent could easily escape and give rise to further expansion of the neoplastic population by continuing clonal evolution. A preferable approach would be to seek agents that block non-redundant effector pathways related to synthesis of essential cell components—for instance, nucleic acids (methotrexate is an example). In this case the risk of toxicity to normal cells would be expected to increase as the number of possible alternative pathways became decreased or eliminated.

ENDPOINT MARKERS BASED ON THE MORPHOLOGICAL CRITERIA OF IEN MEASURED BY CAQIA

In present day histopathological diagnosis, the established pathologist's practice of subjectively estimating cancer risk by nuclear grading, using relatively imprecise descriptive terms such as "mild nuclear pleomorphism and hyperchromasia" or "moderately increased number of mitoses", will no doubt continue into the indefinite future. Nevertheless, CAQIA is being used increasingly to measure the morphometric and DNA densitometric parameters of IEN. Basically, two modalities are used in CAQIA. One, cyto*morph*ometry, measures geometric relationships, such as nuclear dimensions and nucleolar size, shape and position. The other, cyto*photo*metry, measures nuclear DNA optical density (DNA ploidy) and chromatin texture. The range of applications of image cytophotometry is wide because it can also be used to quantify the density and location in tissue sections of specific antibody or cDNA probes conjugated to a chromogen generating molecule (eg a fluorescent dye or horseradish peroxidase).

Selection of the Most Useful Clinical Trial Endpoint Markers

In searching for some property of early intraepithelial neoplastic progression that correlates with high cancer risk, the morphological changes of IEN, measured by CAQIA, immediately suggest themselves. Since the diagnostic properties of IEN are part of the early phase of the chronic disease of neoplasia, they are more correctly designated early disease markers rather than surrogate endpoint biomarkers (SEB), as they have been called in previous publications (Boone and Kelloff, 1994). Nuclear morphology based endpoint markers have been critically reviewed previously. Briefly, they are increased nuclear size, altered nuclear shape, increased variance of nuclear size and shape (pleomorphism), altered chromatin texture, increased mitotic index, abnormal mitoses and alteration or absence of differentiation and maturation. Measuring morphonuclear changes and proliferative behaviour of multicentric IEN lesions as predictors of later invasive neoplasia may be confounded by the fact that spontaneous regression of some of these lesions may occur, especially if the lesions are mild to moderate in extent. Therefore, in addition to evaluating IEN lesions quantitatively in biopsy samples from the same patient before and after intervention with a chemopreventive agent, comparison should also be made with lesions in control subjects given placebos. Although among a given set of multicentric IEN lesions some may remain stationary or regress, from established knowledge of the natural history of IEN it is assured that other lesions will of course progress. From the statistical point of view, the set of IEN lesions in an epithelium taken as a group have a negative predictive value approaching 100%. That is, the absence of any IEN lesions reliably predicts that cancer will not occur.

The core endpoints now being used in over 80 chemoprevention clinical trials monitored by the Chemoprevention Branch include morphonuclear markers (nuclear and nucleolar size, shape, variance of size and shape, frequency of number of nucleoli per 100 cells and, particularly, dozens of chromatin texture features) and DNA ploidy, all quantitated objectively with CAQIA. Also a core endpoint is the mean and variance of cellular proliferation rates, measured with antibody probes for proliferation (PCNA, Ki-67) or nucleic acid uptake (tritiated thymidine or bromodeoxyuridine uptake).

Design of Computer Software to Detect Nuclear Chromatin Texture Changes Relatively Specific for Neoplastic Epithelial Cells

Dozens of nuclear chromatin texture features have been measured in neoplastic cells, based on analysis of patterns of comparative change in optical density proceeding from one small pixel, 0.5 μm × 0.5 μm in size, to another in the digitized image of the nucleus. A new computer instrument with new software programs developed by Bacus Laboratories Imaging Systems, called the BLISS instrument, measures quantitatively and objectively many of the nuclear chromatin texture features used by pathologists to make a diagnosis of IEN. An example of the measurement of one chromatin texture feature will be presented here: the "Deep Valley Detector".

The Deep Valley Detector

The cell nuclei of IEN lesions are commonly described by the pathologist as showing "chromatin clumping". The edges of the chromatin clumps are said to be "sharply marginated". John Frost, the late chief of cytopathology at The Johns Hopkins Medical Center, coined the term "cookie cutter chromatin" to describe this characteristic sharp margination. He also emphasized that the space between chromatin clumps was lighter than normal and called this space, as others have, "parachromatin clearing". Figure 4 compares the nuclear chromatin pattern of a normal hyperplastic cell of the uterine cervix with a neoplastic cell from the same tissue. The sharply marginated chromatin clumps and lighter area between the clumps of the neoplastic cell can easily be seen. A software program was designed that directs the computer to identify the number and location within the nucleus of sets of three pixels in a row, the centre pixel of which has an optical density (OD) that is less than the optical density of either end pixel by at least 0.05 OD units. This program is called the Deep Valley Detector because it identifies the margins of chromatin clumps in neoplastic nuclei that have a steep and deep optical density "drop off". Figure 5B shows the computer image of a nucleus from a neoplastic cell of high grade cervical IEN, in which 111 deep valley sites were counted and their locations shown (by a red mark in the original image). By contrast, Fig. 5A is the nucleus of a non-neoplastic hyperplastic cell from adjacent cervical epithelium, which had only 16 sites. This large quantitative difference in number of deep

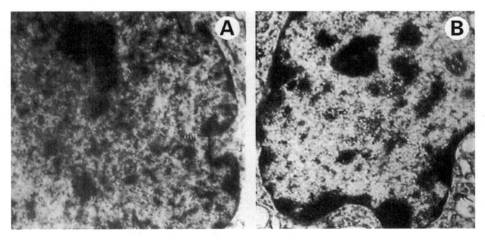

Fig. 4. High power images of nuclei from cells of the uterine cervix. (A) Hyperproliferating normal cell. (B) Neoplastic cell of cervical IEN (CIN) grade III. Note the formation of chromatin clumps with sharp margins bordering clear areas ("parachromatin") of lighter density

A

B

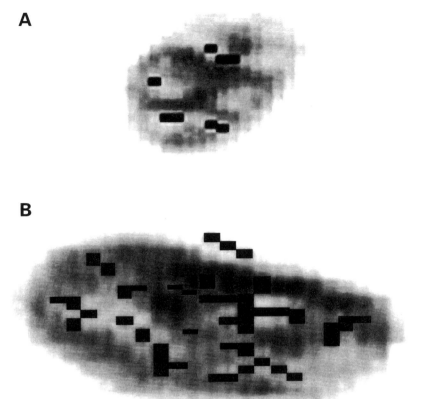

Fig. 5. Computer images of cell nuclei from the uterine cervix. A black rectangle marks the site of a "deep valley", i.e, a site with pixel optical density gradient of > .05 OD units. (A) Nucleus of a normal cell showing eight deep valley sites. (B) Nucleus of a neoplastic cell from cervical IEN (CIN) grade III showing over 115 deep valley sites

valley sites in normal hyperplastic as compared to neoplastic nuclei was generally found for all nuclei in the specimen.

The number of deep valley sites may be used to measure with precision the extent of neoplastic progression. In addition, the modulating effects of chemopreventive agents on IEN may be quantitated by the change they produce in the number of deep valley sites per nucleus.

SUMMARY

The Chemoprevention Branch, NCI, is supporting over 80 clinical trials of chemopreventive agents and has dozens of drugs under development. The structural and functional properties of epithelial precancer (also called preinvasive or IEN), such as increasingly aberrant nuclear size, shape and rates of cellular proliferation and apoptosis, measured by CAQIA, form the basis for specific and quantitative end markers in short term clinical trials of chemopreventive agents. IEN very frequently, if not invariably, is preceded by two conditions diffusely affecting the epithelium: genomic instability and chronic hyperplasia. Chronic subepithelial inflammation is also commonly present. Multicentricity and multipath genetic progression of individual lesions are important characteristics that must be considered when designing endpoint markers and planning for adequate biopsy sampling in clinical trials of chemopreventive agents. Use of CAQIA provides increased sensitivity and specificity when measuring the cellular changes of IEN, such as increasingly aberrant nuclear size, nuclear shape, integrated optical density of nuclear DNA and nuclear chromatin texture features. A software program called the Deep Valley Detector, which measures the optical density gradient at the margins of chromatin clumps in cell nuclei of histological sections stained for DNA, is one example of many nuclear chromatin texture features measured. In the image of the nucleus of a neoplastic cell from high grade IEN of the cervix, 111 deep valley sites were counted, whereas the nucleus of a non-neoplastic hyperplastic cell showed only 16 sites. The modulating effects of chemopreventive agents on IEN may be quantitated by the change they produce in the average number of deep valley sites per nucleus.

References

Bito T, Ueda M, Ahmed NU *et al* (1995) Retinoblastoma gene product expression in actinic keratosis and cutaneous squamous cell carcinoma in relation to p53 expression. *Journal of Cutaneous Pathology* **22** 427–434

Boone CW and Kelloff GJ (1993) Intraepithelial neoplasia, surrogate endpoint biomarkers and cancer chemoprevention. *Journal of Cellular Biochemistry* **Supplement 17F** 37–48

Boone CW and Kelloff GJ (1994) Development of surrogate endpoint biomarkers for clinical trials of cancer chemopreventive agents: relationships to fundamental properties of preinvasive (intraepithelial) neoplasia. *Journal of Cellular Biochemistry* **Supplement 19** 10–22

Boone CW and Kelloff GJ (1995) Biomarkers of premalignant breast disease and their use as surrogate endpoints in clinical trials of chemopreventive agents. *The Breast Journal* **1** 228–235

Boone CW, Kelloff GJ and Steele VE (1992) Natural history of intraepithelial neoplasia in humans with implications for cancer chemoprevention strategy. *Cancer Research* **52** 1651–1659

Bostwick DG (1992) Prostatic intraepithelial neoplasia (PIN): current concepts. *Journal of Cellular Biochemistry* **Supplement 16H** 10–19

Buckley CH, Butler EB and Fox H (1982) Cervical intraepithelial neoplasia. *Journal of Clinical Pathology* **35** 1–13

Collins RH, Feldman M, Fordtran JS (1987) Colon cancer, dysplasia and surveillance in patients with ulcerative colitis: A critical review. *New England Journal of Medicine* **316** 1654–1658

Crissman JD and Fu YS (1986) Intraepithelial neoplasia of the larynx. A clinicopathological study of six cases with DNA analysis. *Archives of Otolaryngological—Head and Neck Surgery* **112** 522–528

Crissman JD and Zarbo RJ (1989) Dysplasia, in situ carcinoma and progression to invasive squamous cell carcinoma of the upper aerodigestive tract. *American Journal of Surgical Pathology* **13(Supplement 1)** 5–16

Fearon ER and Vogelstein B (1990) A genetic model for colorectal tumorigenesis. *Cell* **62** 759–767

Ferguson AR (1911) Associated bilharziosis and primary malignant disease of the urinary bladder, with observations on a series of forty cases. *Journal of Pathology and Bacteriology* **16** 76–94

Fidler IJ (1987) Biological heterogeneity of cancer metastases. *Breast Cancer Research and Treatment* **9** 17–26

Fielding JWL and Allum WH (1996) *Premalignancy and Early Cancer in General Surgery*, p 167, Oxford University Press, New York

Foulds L (1969a) *Neoplastic Development*, **vol 1,** p 45, Plenum Press, New York

Foulds L (1969b) *Neoplastic Development*, **vol 1,** p 19, Plenum Press, New York

Grassel-Pietrusky R, Deinlein E and Hornstein OP (1982) DNA-aneuploidy rates in oral leukoplakias determined by flow cytometry. *Journal of Oral Pathology* **11** 434–438

Kantor AF, Hartge P, Hoover RN and Fraumeni JF (1988) Epidemiological characteristics of squamous cell carcinoma and adenocarcinoma of the bladder. *Cancer Research* **48** 3853–3855

Koss LG (1992) Bladder cancer from a perspective of 40 years. *Journal of Cellular Biochemistry*, **Supplement 16I** 23–29

Locke JR, Hill DE and Walzer Y (1985) Incidence of squamous cell carcinoma in patients with long-term catheter drainage. *Journal of Urology* **133** 1034–1035

Montironi R, Scarpelli M, Galluzzi CM and Diamanti L (1992) Aneuploidy and nuclear features of prostatic intraepithelial neoplasia (PIN). *Journal of Cellular Biochemistry*, **Supplement 16H** 47–53

Macartney JC and Camplejohn RS (1986) DNA flow cytometry of histological materials from dysplastic lesions of human gastric mucosa. *Journal of Pathology* **150** 113–118

Mulder JW, Offerhaus GJ, de Feyter EP, *et al* (1992) The relationship of nuclear morphology to molecular genetic alterations in the adenoma-carcinoma sequence of the large bowel. *American Jounal of Pathology* **141** 797–804

Nasiell M, Kato H, Auer G *et al* (1978) Cytomorphological grading and Feulgen DNA analysis of metaplastic and neoplastic bronchial cells. *Cancer* **41** 1511–1521

Nelson MA, Einspahr JG, Alberts DS *et al* (1994) Analysis of p53 gene in human precancerous actinic keratosis lesions and squamous cell cancers. *Cancer Letters* **85** 23–29

Neshat K, Sanchez CA, Galipeau PC *et al* (1994) Barrett's esophagus: a model of human neoplastic progression. *Cold Spring Harbor Symposia on Quantitative Biology* **59** 577–583

Nowell PC (1976) The clonal evolution of tumor cell populations. *Science* **194** 23–28

Nowell PC (1986) Mechanisms of tumor progression. *Cancer Research* **46** 2203–2207

Nowell PC (1989) Chromosome and molecular clues to tumor progression. *Seminars in Oncology* **16** 116–127

Qian J, Bostwick DG, Takahashi S *et al* (1995) Chromosomal anomalies in prostatic intraepithelial neoplasia and carcinoma detected by fluorescence hybridization. *Cancer Research* **55** 5408–5414

Quirke P, Fozard JB, Dixon MF *et al* (1986) DNA ploidy in colorectal adenomas. *British Journal of Cancer* **53** 477–481

Reid BJ, Habbitt RC, Rubin CE and Rabinovich A (1987) Barrett's esophagus. Correlation between flow cytometry and histology in detection of patients at risk for adenocarcinoma. *Gastroenterology* **93** 1–11

Reid R and Fu YS (1986) Is there a morphologic spectrum linking condyloma to cervical cancer? In: Peto R and Zur Hausen H (eds) *Viral Etiology of Cervical Cancer*, pp 91–113, Cold Spring Harbor Laboratory, New York

Richart RM (1963) A radioautographic analysis of cellular proliferation in dysplasia and carcinoma in situ of the uterine cervix. *American Journal of Obstetrics and Gynecology* **86** 925–930

Rosai J (1991) Borderline epithelial lesions of the breast. *American Journal of Surgical Pathology* **15** 209–221

Slaughter DP, Southwick HW and Smejkal W (1951) Field cancerization in oral stratified squamous epithelium: clinical implications of multicentric origin. *Cancer* **6** 963–968

Vogelstein B, Fearon ER, Hamilton SR *et al* (1988) Genetic alterations during colorectal tumor development. *New England Journal of Medicine* **319** 525–532

Wattenberg LW (1996) Chemoprevention of cancer. *Preventive Medicine* **25** 44–45

Wright TC, Kurman RJ and Ferenczy A (1994) 7 Precancerous lesions of the cervix, In: Kurman RJ (ed). *Blaustein's Pathology of the Female Genital Tract*, pp 229–256, Springer-Verlag, New York

Yamagiwa H (1989) Mucosal dysplasia of gallbladder: isolated and adjacent lesions to carcinoma. *Japanese Journal of Cancer Research* **80** 238–243

The authors are responsible for the accuracy of the references.

Precancer of the Prostate

P C BUSCH[1] • L EGEVAD[2] • M HAGGMAN[3]

[1]Department of Pathology, University Hospital, N-9037 Tromsø, Norway; [2]Department of Pathology, Karolinska Hospital, S-171 76 Stockholm; [3]Department of Urology, University Hospital, S-751 85 Uppsala, Sweden

INTRODUCTION

The ductoacinar epithelium of the prostate is no exception from the rule that cells of epithelial compartments can announce their potential to develop invasive neoplasia by expressing morphological, cytogenetic and molecular genetic abnormalities. Originally, and still mainly, recognition of precancer is based on visual interpretation of structural deviations, ranging from very subtle to marked. Various labels have been attached to these images, long familiar to pathologists (see below). The presently most widely used is prostatic intraepithelial neoplasia (PIN) (Bostwick and Brawer, 1987). Before discussing the specific pathobiology and clinical implications of PIN we will highlight and try to define the basic concepts "malignancy" and "malignancy grade".

MALIGNANCY

Malignancy is a biological phenomenon, which could be characterized as behavioural. It is generally believed to be the consequence of accumulated mutations. Tumour behaviour is the net result of hits in three hypothetical sets of genes:

- genes involved in the regulation of proliferation and programmed cell death(cell cycle and apoptosis regulating genes)
- genes that regulate cellular "social behaviour", ie genes involved in intercellular signalling and/or contacts, cell matrix interrelations and cell motility
- genes involved in the specialized functions of the tissue, ie differentiation genes. These include genes organizing the nuclear matrix and chromatin structure, which are also believed to be important for the regulation of normal differentiation. Structural changes of the nuclear matrix and chromatin are early indicators of precancer, and the degree of deviation also reflects grade of malignant potential as discussed below.

Definitions

Malignancy in epithelium may be defined as the consequence of the sum of many functional disturbances of the cell, together constituting the requirements for invasion and metastasis. This behavioural disturbance is very complex. Some changes represent enhanced or added functions, others reduced or lost functions.

Requirements for Invasive and Metastatic Cancer

The net of the changes gives the cell a whole range of capacities, all necessary for invasion and metastasis (see Fig. 1):

- to proliferate, ie to form a clone
- to survive, ie to escape immunological and other host defence mechanisms
- to change its immediate environment (break down basement barriers, change the composition of the matrix)
- to downregulate its own sensors for neighbouring cells and matrix

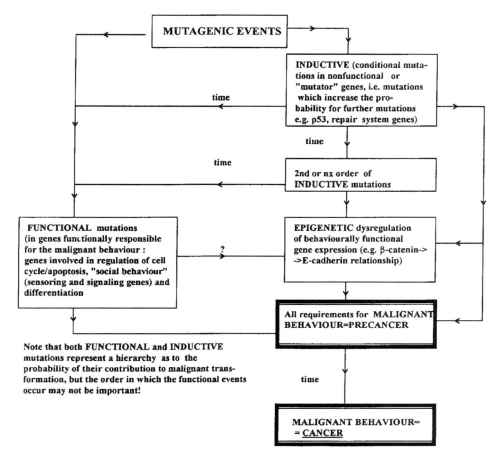

Fig. 1. A model for the evolution of precancer and cancer

- to form a new environment, ie matrix, blood vessels and new cell contacts
- to change its motility (probably most often to become dysregulated and disharmonic)
- to migrate, implying combined motility and adhesiveness
- to allow itself to travel to distant organs by various routes
- to express homing receptors
- to settle in the new places and sometimes to start the metastasising sequence again.

In other words, malignant behaviour requires a whole range of conditions if it is to emerge in its full capacity, and invasiveness is only one of the initial steps.

The hits accumulate, not necessarily in a certain order but with varying degrees of probability. The composition of the hit pattern, rather than the sequence, determines the behaviour.

We also postulate that structural disorganization and functionally disharmonic regulation of cell life are more important for the malignant behaviour than suppression or enhancement of single, discrete functions. This does not mean that there may not exist a hierarchy of candidate genes, mutations of which contribute different degrees of probability to the eventual asocial behaviour. The mutations may contribute by being either functional or inductive. If this concept holds true, correction of the last mutational event before the malignancy threshold is passed may be either unnecessary or the only possible correction that could lead to normalization of the behaviour of the cell. Many hits may be equally important for maintenance of the malignant phenotype regardless of the order in which they occur.

MALIGNANCY GRADE

Definitions

The concept of malignancy grade emanates from the recognition that certain microscopical structural patterns are associated with particularly fast progression to higher tumour stage. Morphological features indicative of high malignancy grade are associated with high proliferation rates and dysplasia. The latter term includes architectural derangement, ie impaired formation of normal tissue structures and cellular atypia (abnormalities in size, shape, texture and isometry of individual cells).

Traditionally, the grading of dysplasia and proliferation relies on morphological variables and DNA ploidy aberrations. Theoretically, however, many other, more dynamic expressions of cell life, such as pattern of motility, signal transduction disturbances, energy consumption and heat production, may relate to malignancy grade. In prostate pathology subgrading of PIN is a matter of controversy.

The complexity of the malignancy and malignancy grade implies several things. First, malignant transformation requires many events to occur. These events accumulate over time. Some events are functional, ie they contribute to an actual functional disturbance which is a component of the malignant behaviour. Others are inductive or conditional, ie they predispose to the development of truly functional mutations. *TP53* mutations could be regarded as inductive in the sense that they may contribute to enhanced risk for mutations in cell cycle regulatory or other "functional" genes. Mutations in genes involved in DNA repair (mutator genes) could serve as another example. Thus, there may be first, second or any order of inductive changes in the sense that they pave the way for new inductive changes, which in turn increase the probability of new functional events.

Second, changes could also occur in an already malignant cell population, enhancing their probability of developing functional changes that increase the malignancy grade (escape from repair and other defence mechanisms). This has frequently been described as tumour progression, but actually means progression of malignancy grade (Table 1).

TABLE 1. Different uses of the term "progression"

Term	Key feature	Signs	Remarks
Morphological progression	Microscopic assessment	Increased cellular atypia and decreased differentiation	Genetic or epigenetic mechanisms
Genetic progression	Addition of new mutations	Not obligate. Can be "clandestine"	All genes in principle susceptible. Most mutations probably lethal
Tumour progression; progression of malignancy grade	Selection of increasingly malignant phenotypes. Mutations in oncogenes or suppressor genes	Increased clinical malignancy with metastasis, rapid growth, resistance to treatment	Selected genotypes may pre-exist or be acquired through genetic instability
Clinical progression	Continued tumour growth	Increased tumour volume, metastases, local recurrence	Not shown to depend on mutations

Finally, it should also be kept in mind that genetic changes might lead to epigenetic downstream functional imbalances, which are in fact also operational in the malignant behaviour. Mutations in the catenin genes (Morton *et al*, 1993), leading to downregulation of E-cadherin, could serve as an example of this category (Giroldi *et al*, 1995). Of course it may be difficult to categorize disturbances as genetic or epigenetic and as inductive or functional, since they are links in chains and networks of cellular events, which are interdependent.

Thus markers used to characterize precancer may be qualitatively very different with respect to the precise nature of their contribution to malignancy and its grade. Recognition of this fact could possibly help an understanding of the precancer→ cancer transition and clarify some aspects of the "tumour marker" concept.

Implications for Precancer of the Prostate

It would be useful to define the description of any feature found to be associated with simultaneous or later invasive and metastatic cancer as inductive (or conditional) of first or any order, or as functional. Functional markers should be further defined as genetic or epigenetic.

In the end, the task is to identify sufficient numbers of predictive features and to organize and combine them into practically useful information. In this process it is wise to be open minded about the aspects of cell life that should be studied and critical about the technique used.

MORPHOLOGICAL SUBTYPES

The first study to define precancer in the prostate was that of Miller and Seljelid in 1971.

They named the changes "slight" or "marked" atypia. A large amount of material from transvesical prostatectomies after a clinical diagnosis of hyperplasia was examined. Carcinomas and cases with marked atypia were unexpected findings at microscopy. At seven years of follow-up no difference in crude survival between cases with marked atypia (and carcinoma) and the normal population was found (Miller and Seljelid, 1971).

Later descriptions of preinvasive epithelial changes in the prostate have used many labels, such as atypical primary hyperplasia (Kastendieck, 1980), hyperplasia with malignant change (Mostofi 1984; Mostofi et al, 1989), intraductal dysplasia (McNeal and Bostwick, 1986), large acinar atypical hyperplasia (Kovi et al, 1988), atypia in hyperplasia (Srigley et al. 1989), duct-acinar dysplasia (McNeal et al, 1988a,b, 1991), and prostatic dysplasia/atypical hyperplasia (Kastendieck and Helpap, 1989).

In analogy to precancerous lesions of the uterine cervix, the term "prostatic intraepithelial neoplasia" was introduced (Bostwick and Brawer, 1987) and has since been generally accepted (Anonymous, 1989; Troncoso et al 1989; Amin et al, 1993a; Bostwick 1995; Bostwick et al, 1995). PIN was originally graded 1–3, based on graded architectural deviations in both tissue and cellular compartments.

It was soon realized that inter and intraobserver reproducibility for the diagnosis of PIN grade 1 was low (Epstein et al, 1995), and the present consensus divides PIN into "low grade" (PIN 1=LGPIN) and "high grade" (PIN2+PIN3=HGPIN) (Drago et al, 1989). In a recent study of the interobserver variability in the diagnosis of HGPIN it was considered "moderate" with a κ value of 0.41–0.60, whereas that for the diagnosis of invasive cancer was "almost perfect" (κ=0.81–1.0) (Allam et al, 1996).

Tissue Architecture

Bostwick et al have described four common patterns of HGPIN: tufting (87%), micropapillary (85%), cribriform (32%) and flat (28%) (Fig. 2) (Bostwick et al, 1993). Several of these patterns may exist simultaneously even in the same duct-acinus (Fig. 2). They probably represent morphological variants of the same process rather than independent lesions.

The case illustrated in Fig. 2 is from a patient operated on for bladder carcinoma. In the cysto-prostatectomy specimen a small low grade invasive carcinoma was found. One such focus emanated from a large acinus in which flat, tufting and micropapillary patterns could be seen. The micropapillary pattern was in this case associated with similar protrusions into the surrounding stroma, with adjacent separate one cell layered microglandular elements. The detachment from the acinus was proven by serial sectioning and supported by the lack

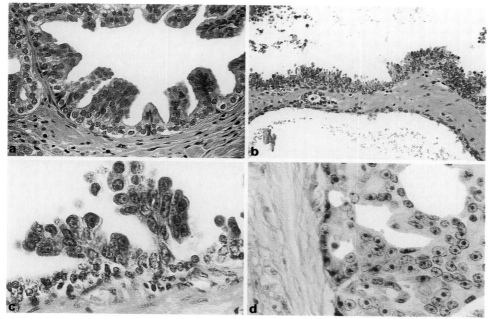

Fig. 2. Morphological subtypes of PIN: (a) tufting, (b) flat, (c) micropapillary, (d) cribriform

of basal cells on immunohistochemical staining of high molecular weight cytokeratins (Hedrick and Epstein, 1989; Shah *et al*, 1991).

Parallel to the increasing complexity of the pattern of PIN, the basal cells became discontinuous and eventually disappeared (Fig. 3). This single acinus can be used to illustrate not only HGPIN but also LGPIN along with normal cells in the same acinus. This shows the complexity and probably also reflects the dynamics of progression from normal to invasive cancer.

Microdissection and detailed analysis of phenotypical features as well as of molecular genetic characteristics of lesions like those in Fig. 3 will enhance our understanding of similar lesions.

Cytological Architecture

The original recognition of three grades of PIN was based mainly on nuclear atypia and nuclear interrelationships (McNeal and Bostwick, 1986). Thus grade 1 requires anisokaryosis along with nuclear enlargement and irregularity of cell spacing. Its recognition is difficult. Grade 2 includes the criteria for grade 1 plus moderate nuclear hyperchromasia and an increasing number of moderately enlarged nucleoli. It is commonly accompanied by dark staining of the cytoplasm. Grade 3 is distinguished by further enlargement of nuclei and nucleoli. Quantitative assessment of cytological features supports the grading concept (Oayasu *et al*, 1986; Helpap, 1988; Petein *et al*, 1991; Montironi *et al*, 1992).

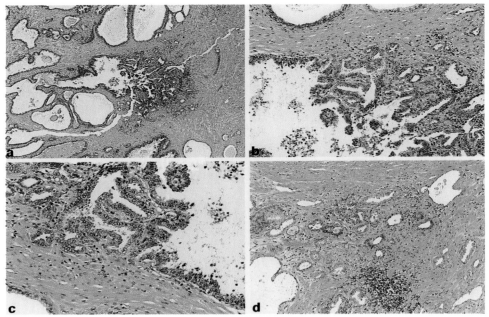

Fig. 3. A glandular acinus showing various forms of PIN and transition to invasive carcinoma: (a) Overview of the acinus with associated microglandular invasive carcinoma in its right end; (b) higher magnification of the transition from PIN to invasive cancer; (c) still higher magnification of the transition; (d) section serially cut 30 sections deeper in the block than the previous ones

MORPHOMETRY

Two Dimensional

Montironi and Bartels have developed quantitative methods for assessing PIN using image analysis (Montironi *et al*, 1990, 1994a, 1995; Bartels *et al*, 1995a,b).

One approach was to quantify the epithelial components of PIN using a fully automated procedure. First the system located and identified the duct and segmented the scene, followed by a process in which the lumen and darkly and lightly stained epithelial components were assembled.

Following this, histometric measurements were made of the reconstructed scene. The percentage of the duct contour with basal cells and the number and length of gaps between the basal cells were computed.

Second, the group has described a diagnostic decision support system for prostate lesions. A morphological diagnosis is based on the combination of morphological features registered by the eye. The diagnostic decision depends on our knowledge and experience from previous cases. In a given diagnostic category there is a certain probability for the occurrence of each feature individually and in combination. In the diagnostic decision we therefore take into account the general probability for a certain diagnosis based on previous experience.

When an unknown slide is read the probability of a certain diagnosis thus has to be calculated, given the observation of a combination of features and given our knowledge of the relative distribution of these features in the diseases.

This process can be automated in a decision flow chart based on probability matrices. The operation is an example of a Bayesian belief network (BBN). BBN has been used to identify prostate cancer and PIN. When BBN was used to classify a test set of slides including PIN lesions, the system gave high probabilities for the subjectively assumed correct categories (Montironi *et al*, 1995a).

An inference network in which a number of diagnostic outcomes were specified (eg grades or benign-malignant) was created.

The diagnostic decision is developed at a decision node and expressed as a belief vector. The diagnostic evidence is entered via evidence nodes. One such node is developed for each feature (eg nuclear chromatin appearance). To assist in making a consistent assessment, the system displays images showing ranked examples (eg chromatin textures from finely granular to clumped). Furthermore the system utilizes the concept of membership functions measuring the degree of membership to a category such as small, medium or large. The authors expand the technique using a BBN as the diagnostic decision network for PIN testing five diagnostic outcome alternatives: benign prostatic hyperplasia, low grade PIN, high grade PIN, cribriform prostatic adenocarcinoma and large acinar prostatic adenocarcinoma. Seven diagnostic features were used: the first three diagnostic categories were identified by four or more of the seven features.

The authors conclude that diagnostic reasoning as generally practised can now be supported by quantitation and analysis, and that we are only at the beginning of an era using expert systems, inference networks, neuronal networks and other artificial intelligence. One is tempted to suggest that a technique of this kind may help to explore the interdependence structure of various tumour markers comprising very rich data sets with both functional and inductive markers for precancer and its grade.

Three Dimensional

In extensive studies of the distribution of PIN and accompanying invasive cancer we have arrived at the following perception of their evolution (de la Torre *et al*, 1993):

Regional Distribution, Multicentricity

PIN lesions show the same distribution pattern as invasive cancer, ie they occur preferentially in the peripheral and central zones and they are multifocal. PIN is rarely found in the transitional zone.

Volume Distribution of PIN and Relation to Volumes of Invasive Cancer

There is an inverse relationship between the total volume of PIN and the total volume of invasive cancer (de la Torre *et al*, 1993). This means that at very small total volumes of invasive cancer (~<3 ml) the total volume of PIN will exceed that of the invasive cancer. At invasive cancer volumes above 10 ml PIN tends to vanish. Qian *et al* found the relative amount of flat PIN to be too small to be accounted for (Qian *et al*, 1995, 1997). This is interesting and might reflect a quick transformation of the flat PIN to the other patterns, as illustrated in the single acinus of the case shown in Fig. 3.

It was found that the number of invasive cancer foci decreased with larger total invasive cancer volume (de la Torre *et al*, 1993). This, taken together with the commonly described heterogeneity regarding grade, ploidy pattern, immunohistochemical and molecular genetic features, may imply that the large tumours represent a fusion product of many invasive cancers originally emanating from one PIN focus each.

This is supported by the finding of a marked genetic heterogeneity in PIN favouring a non-monoclonal origin of the different foci (Cheng *et al*, 1998).

Relation to Invasive Cancer

As stated above, there is a close spatial relationship between PIN and invasive cancer. Previous studies indicate that the higher the grade of PIN, the closer or more adjacent will an invasive cancer be expected (Bostwick and Brawer, 1987; Epstein *et al*, 1990; Quinn *et al*, 1990; Qian *et al*, 1995, 1997).

EPIDEMIOLOGY

Reliable epidemiological studies of the prevalence of PIN have so far been carried out only in the West. Geographical and racial differences elsewhere remain to be examined.

Prevalence of PIN parallels that of latent invasive cancer but precedes it by 5–10 years (Sakr *et al*, 1993a, 1994, 1996). In the last study of autopsy cases, HGPIN was first encountered in the third decade and increased with age, as did latent cancer. A comparison between Afro-American and Caucasian males showed no significant difference in the prevalence of latent cancer, whereas HGPIN was more prevalent in Afro-American men in each age group, starting in the fourth decade. The same study examined the occurrence of HGPIN in a series of radical prostatectomies in both Afro-American and Caucasian men. Again, the Afro-Americans aged 60 years or younger showed a higher prevalence of HGPIN than the Caucasians. In both races the mean percentage of the gland involved by HGPIN decreased with advancing age and with increasing volume of the concomitant invasive cancer. These results tend to support the volume distribution data quoted above (de la Torre *et al*, 1993).

HEREDITY

Family studies of malignancy of the prostate have so far been almost entirely restricted to clinically diagnosed invasive cancer, and hence specific information on hereditary features of PIN is sparse (Woolf 1960). It might be useful, however, to review recent observations regarding some genes associated with familial predisposition to prostate cancer. This is so, because study of cases with a family history and eventually displaying candidate genes will be ideal to throw further light on the relationship between PIN and invasive cancer.

Three types of studies have been conducted: family aggregation of prostate cancer, segregation analysis of family aggregation and twin studies.

Family Aggregation

Studies of the records of first and second degree relatives of Mormons with cancer collected by the Genealogical Society of Utah resulted in a ranking of all cancers. Prostate cancers were among the most familial, more so than breast cancer or bowel cancer (Cannon *et al*, 1982; Bishop and Skolnick, 1984). First degree relatives (brother, father or son) of a patient with prostatic cancer have double the risk of contracting the disease (Goldgar *et al*, 1994). Men with such an increased susceptibility are more likely to be diagnosed at an early age (Carter *et al*, 1990a, 1993a,b,c). The studies imply that any inherited susceptibility is relatively rare.

On the basis of the results of segregation analysis the following criteria have been defined for diagnosing hereditary prostate cancer: a cluster of three or more first degree relatives with prostate cancer; or prostate cancer in each of three generations in the paternal or maternal lineage; or two or more first or second degree relatives with prostate cancer under age 55.

Twin Studies

In a study from Sweden the national twin registry was linked with the national cancer registry. The concordance rate for prostate cancer was five times higher for monozygotic twins than for dizygotic twins (Gronberg *et al*, 1994, 1997). In another twin study, from the US, a similar difference between dizygotic and monozygotic twins was found (9% vs 26%)(Braun *et al*, 1995).

In a study of patients with a family history but not fulfilling the above criteria and also sporadic cases, no significant differences were found with respect to clinical stage, pathological stage, multifocality of invasive cancer, multifocality of HGPIN, Gleason score, tumour volume, preoperative prostate specific antigen (PSA) value and association with unusual non-neoplastic and neoplastic features (Bastacky *et al*, 1995).

Men carrying a *BRCA1* mutation run a 3.3 (95% confidence interval:1.8–6.2) times higher risk of prostate cancer than the general population.

Similarly, a germline *BRCA1* mutation has been identified in a male with hereditary prostate cancer (Langston *et al*, 1996). In other patients with a first degree relative with prostate cancer no *BRCA1* mutations were detected, and therefore the role of germline *BRCA1* mutations in prostate cancer susceptibility is probably minor.

A report of mapping of a prostate cancer susceptibility gene to chromosome 1 is interesting but requires further confirmation (Smith *et al*, 1996) The location of a putative prostatic cancer suppressor gene (*PRCA1*) is controversial (Gronberg *et al*, 1997; McIndoe *et al*, 1997).

Other genes suggested as candidates for susceptibility, if germline mutated, are the androgen receptor gene and the vitamin D receptor gene. Furthermore a non-significant association between polymorphisms in the 5á-reductase gene and prostate cancer has been claimed (Kanthoff *et al*, 1997).

As indicated above, any genetic changes suggested to be associated with hereditary susceptibility for prostate cancer should be examined regarding their presence in both LGPIN and HGPIN lesions, again using microdissection techniques. This could cast further light on the relationship between PIN and invasive cancer.

DNA PLOIDY AND CYTOGENETICS

Studies of the chromosomal aberrations of cancer were long restricted to DNA ploidy analysis and karyotyping of metaphase figures from explanted or cultured tumour cells. Considerable information has accumulated from such studies in spite of the technical limitations (for example selection problems, difficulties in cell culture). The development of fluorescent in situ hybridization (FISH) and comparative genomic hybridization techniques promises to speed up the collection of data.

DNA Ploidy Analysis

Numerous studies of DNA ploidy of PIN and concomitant cancer have been carried out using both static image analysis of tissue sections and analysis of isolated cell nuclei after microdissection (O'Malley *et al*, 1991; Montironi *et al*, 1992; Sakr *et al*, 1992; Amin *et al*, 1993b; Berner *et al*, 1993; Crissman *et al*, 1993; Weinberg *et al*, 1993; Baretton *et al*, 1994).

LGPIN lesions are near diploid, whereas HGPIN is characterized by an increasing occurrence of tetraploid and aneuploid cell lineages. Comparisons of PIN lesions with concomitant cancer tend to show similar ploidy patterns, mostly more aneuploid in invasive cancer than in adjacent PIN (Baretton *et al*, 1994). The incidence of aneuploidy in HGPIN ranges from 32% to 68%, hence slightly lower compared to invasive cancer (55% to 62%) (Amin *et al*, 1993b; Baretton *et al*, 1994; Crissman *et al*, 1993).

Chromosomal Changes

The studies of DNA ploidy are probably all hampered by sampling and selection difficulties and it is reasonable to pay more attention to studies using in situ techniques such as FISH, for example with multiple centromeric probes. Gross deviations of chromosomal numbers are not necessary requirements for invasive cancer to develop, and there are therefore bound to exist near diploid, low grade precancer lesions in spite of our limited accuracy regarding their visual recognition. Several studies indicate a relationship between PIN and invasive cancer, however (Brothman *et al*, 1990; Carter *et al*, 1990b,c; Bova *et al*, 1993; Brown *et al*, 1994; Macoska *et al*, 1994; Zenkiusen *et al*, 1994; Zitzesberger *et al*, 1994; Emmert-Buck *et al*, 1995; Qian *et al*, 1995; Walker Daniels *et al*, 1996). With the use of centromeric probes and an interphase FISH technique a 52% frequency of numerical aberrations of at least one investigated chromosome in prostate cancer was established. Adjacent PIN had largely normal karyotypes. Only 2 of 17 cases displayed loss of the Y chromosome (Alers *et al*, 1995). FISH studies of chromosomes 7, 8, 10, 12 and Y revealed similar chromosomal numerical anomalies in PIN and cancer, again supporting the precancer status of PIN. The most common alteration was a gain on chromosome 8 (Qian *et al*, 1995).

Chromosomal mapping studies by FISH and polymerase chain reaction (PCR) techniques have revealed allelic losses involving chromosomes 8, 10 and 16 in prostatic cancer (Carter *et al*, 1990b,c). Chromosomes 8p,16p and 10q appear to be particularly affected. Sequences that map within or near 8p22 appear to be affected in PIN and prostate cancer of localized and locally metastatic primary tumours, as well as in the lymph node metastases—8p losses have therefore been suggested to be early events in prostate tumourigenesis. Allelic losses involving 8p sequences occur in various degrees in different PIN foci, suggesting an identity between PIN and invasive cancer at the genetic level and that a subset of PIN lesions develop into invasive cancer.

The significant genetic changes for prostate cancer include losses for chromosomes 8p, 5q and 13q; gains for chromosomes 8q, 11p and 3q; aneusomies of chromosomes 7 and 8; and allelic losses at chromosome regions 8p 12-21, 10q23-24, 16q22.1-24 and 7q31.1-31.2 (Dong *et al*, 1997).

HGPIN gains, most frequently of chromosome 8, occur in both PIN and invasive cancer. The role of trisomy 7 is a matter of controversy. Its occurrence both in PIN and invasive cancer is usually multifocal, and several studies have described heterogeneity between individual foci of both categories (Alers *et al*, 1995; Emmert-Buck *et al*, 1995; Qian *et al*, 1995).

The role of trisomy 7 is a matter of controversy (Alcaraz *et al*, 1994; Bandyk *et al*, 1994; Brown *et al*, 1994; Takahashi *et al*, 1994; Alers *et al*, 1995). The frequency of trisomy 7 was higher in invasive cancer than in PIN, suggesting that gain on chromosome 7 may be operational in the progression of PIN to invasive cancer.

MOLECULAR GENETICS

Oncogenes

Enhanced expression of the epidermal growth factor receptor gene family *ERBB2* and *ERBB3* and its associated oncoproteins (ERBB2, ERBB3) reflect increased proliferative activity. Immunohistochemical studies tend to demonstrate positive staining of basal cells of benign prostate epithelium, in basal and secretory luminal cells of PIN and in the cells of carcinoma (Meilon *et al*, 1992; Zhau *et al*, 1992; Giri *et al*, 1993; Kuhn *et al*, 1993; Ware, 1993). Transfection experiments introducing the rat *Neu* activated gene into the rat ventral prostatic epithelial cell line NbE-1.4 resulted in the acquisition of a tumorigenic phenotype (Sikes and Chung, 1992).

The expression of *ERBB2* is androgen dependent, as is the presence of luminal secretory layer of epithelium in normal glands and in PIN (Bostwick, 1994). These cell types are also known to be sensitive to androgen deprivation, and more so than the accompanying basal cells. Both the absolute and relative volumes of PIN decrease after androgen deprivation (Hellstrom *et al*, 1993; Ferguson *et al*, 1994; Montironi *et al*, 1994b), which also has been suggested as an ablative or chemopreventive agent for PIN and perhaps early prostate cancer (Bostwick 1994). A word of caution may be justified, however: What about the androgen insensitive basal cells? Maybe some of them are already transformed stem cells now left without a need to compete with their aborted neighbours.

Another oncoprotein, BCL2, influences the other quality of the first of the three sets of genes indicated as targets for changes in the introduction of this chapter, namely apoptosis. BCL2 overexpression suppresses apoptosis and is observed in PIN and invasive cancer, whereas it is expressed only in the basal cells of normal and hyperplastic epithelium (Stattin *et al*, 1996).

Tumour Suppressor Genes

The concept of tumour suppressor genes originally referred to genes involved in the regulation of proliferation. The concept has been extended to refer to genes that suppress metastasis. This is in line with hits in the "signalling or social behaviour" set of genes, which if dysregulated lead to the evolution of malignancy.

TP53

The two most commonly studied tumour suppressor genes, *TP53* and *RB*, appear to be less commonly affected in the early development of prostate cancer than at late stages (Bookstein *et al*, 1990; Kubota *et al*, 1995).

Mutations in the *TP53* gene, serving as a "guardian of the cell cycle" (and apoptosis), could be labelled "inductive" rather than "functional". Consequently, overexpression of its mutated protein product as judged by immunohistochemistry seems to be restricted to high grade and high stage invasive cancer (Bookstein *et al*, 1993; Effert *et al*, 1993). Thus Myers *et al* (1994a) reported *TP53* mutations in only 6% in PIN, 11% in primary cancer and 56% in metastases.

Humphrey and Swanson (1995) found *TP53* immunopositivity in nuclei of PIN in 22.5% and a concordance between HGPIN and carcinoma for cases with an intense signal for *TP53*. In 70% of carcinomas with an intense *TP53* signal a similar strong signal was found in adjacent HGPIN. This may illustrate that inductive mutations may follow previous both functional and inductive genetic and epigenetic alterations as stage and grade progression proceed. This is probably illustrated by the findings of Mirchandani *et al* (1995), who demonstrated a pronounced intratumoural heterogeneity in primary cancers and metastases as to the pattern of *TP53* mutation.

Salem *et al* (1997) demonstrated *TP53* nuclear immunopositivity in ten tumours (10.4%), including six with high and four with low level reactivity. Of the tumours, 86 (89.6%) had no evidence of *TP53* immunoreactivity. Each of the six tumours with high level *TP53* reactivity had associated areas of prostatic intraepithelial neoplasia that also showed *TP53* nuclear reactivity (Salem *et al*, 1997). Similarly, Humphrey and Swanson (1995) found *TP53* immunoreactivity in high grade PIN lesions accompanying all cases of *TP53* immunopositive localized invasive carcinomas.

A word of caution regarding the potential role of *TP53* mutations as well as other initially rare events is justified. They may represent early inductive events and may be selected in the process of progression. Therefore even sparse occurrence of nuclei with proven *TP53* mutations in PIN could turn out to be prognostically unfavourable, because they may contribute to functional mutations, gradually increasing the probability for survival also of the original *TP53* mutation. The relative number of *TP53* mutated cells could then increase with increasing grade and stage.

RB

There seems to be consensus as to the lack of relationship between *RB* inactivation in the evolution of early prostate cancer (Bookstein *et al*, 1990; Sarkar *et al*, 1992; Sakr *et al*, 1992; Brooks *et al*, 1995). Loss of heterozygosity (LOH) has been demonstrated in 27% of invasive prostate cancers with no relationship with grade or stage, and the authors concluded that LOH of *RB* was not involved in multistep prostate carcinogenesis (Brooks *et al*, 1995).

Metastasis Suppressor Genes

Cell Adhesion Molecules

E-cadherin is a member of a family of Ca^{2+} dependent homophilic cell adhesion molecules (CAMs). CAMs are involved in the morphogenesis and maintenance of the epithelial phenotype (fitting both the social behaviour and the differentiation sets of genes discussed above). Loss of expression of E-cadherin is associated with increasing grade and invasiveness in prostate carcinoma (Giroldi and Schalken 1993, Giroldi *et al*, 1994–1995; Murant *et al*, 1997). It is not entirely clear how much of E-cadherin downregulation depends on downregulation of β-catenin, a cytoplasmatic molecule to which E-cadherin is linked. The relative frequency of disturbances in the processing of these two important players remains to be clarified.

C-CAM1 is a member of the immunoglobulin superfamily. Transfection and selection of PC-3 prostate adenocarcinoma cells with C-CAM1 produced clones showing slower growth rates, increased anchorage dependent growth and reduced tumorigenicity in vivo compared with control cells (Hsieh *et al*, 1995).

A discontinuous staining pattern of C-CAM1 was observed in the basal layer of benign prostatic tissue. Complete absence of staining was observed in Gleason score 5–10 prostate carcinomas (Kleinermann *et al*, 1995). It was concluded that downregulation of C-CAM1 occurs early and is associated with morphological transition from PIN to carcinoma.

Non-CAM Genes

CD44 is the cell surface receptor for hyaluronan. It exists in at least 12 different splice forms. In tumours, CD44 is upregulated, which in turn is claimed to be associated with propensity to metastasize (Gunthert *et al*, 1995).

Murant *et al* (1997) found a reciprocal expression pattern for E-cadherin and CD44 between moderately and poorly differentiated tumours. The precise relationship between CD44 expression in PIN and invasive prostate cancer, including the presence of hyaluronan, remains to be studied.

KAI1 (CD82) is a type III integral membrane protein of approximately 30kDa, which is expressed in normal prostate epithelium (Dong *et al*, 1997). Immunohistochemical analysis showed reduced KAI1 specific staining in 70% of the cases and in all metastases. Absence of KAI1 immunoreactivity was not associated with point mutations in the gene or allelic loss at chromosome 11p11, where the gene is located. Its expression in PIN has not yet been investigated.

Another metastasis suppressing gene, *maspin*, was identified by subtractive hybridization and differential display methods. With regard to prostate cancer maspin protein is present in PC-3 prostate carcinoma cells but absent from LNCAP and DU145 cells (Sheng *et al*, 1996). Maspin shares significant sequence similarity to the serine protease inhibitor superfamily, including plasminogen activator inhibitors (PAI) 1 and 2, which have been proposed to inhibit tumour invasion and metastasis (Zou *et al*, 1994). The relationship between PIN and invasive and metastasizing prostate carcinoma regarding maspin expression remains to be established.

IMMUNOHISTOCHEMISTRY AND HISTOCHEMISTRY

Numerous studies have established progressive differences between normal prostate gland and hyperplasia on the one hand and PIN and invasive cancer on the other. The markers range from those involved in growth regulation to those indicating social behaviour status and/or differentiation. Some of the markers are claimed to be associated with metastatic phenotypes (Nagle *et al*, 1991; Maygarden *et al*, 1994; Macoska *et al*, 1995).

Table 2 compares the differential expressions of some markers in basal cells and luminal cells in PIN with those in invasive cancer.

It can be concluded that proliferation and regulators of apoptosis are normally expressed in basal cells. Thus Ki67 (Berges *et al*, 1995; Leav *et al*, 1996), proliferating cell nuclear antigen (Montironi *et al*, 1993c; Helpap, 1995a,b), epidermal growth factor receptor (Bonkhoff, 1996), AgNORs (Deschenes *et al*, 1990; Min *et al*, 1990; Helpap and Riede, 1995; Sesterhenn *et al*, 1991), BCL2 appears and is increased in non-basal cells of PIN, to become further enhanced in carcinoma (Myers and Grizzle, 1996; Stattin *et al*, 1996). These categories could mostly be classified as functional or they represent epigenetic changes as a consequence of mutations of genes, "upstream" in the regulatory chain of events.

Other factors which are strongly expressed by the dysplastic luminal cells include neuroendocrine cells (di Sant Agnese, 1992; Algaba *et al*, 1995; Bonkhoff *et al*, 1995; Bostwick *et al*, 1994a; Iwamura *et al*, 1995) the nm23-H1 gene product (Myers and Grizzle, 1996), tumour associated glycoprotein-72 (TAG-72) (fatty acid synthetase) and proteolytic enzymes (Myers and Grizzle, 1996). These findings suggest that PIN lesions are derived from an impairment of the differentiation of basal cells (Bonkhoff, 1996). Studies of the microvascular architecture in PIN lesions promise to represent a new and important angle in future research (Bigler *et al*, 1993; Montironi *et al*, 1993a). The majority of biomarkers, which are strongly expressed in PIN lesions are also expressed in prostatic adenocarcinoma, supporting the concept that PIN is a preinvasive lesion (Myers and Grizzle, 1997).

Nagle and colleagues have demonstrated the implication of changes in the composition of the basement membrane as well as of extracellular matrix proteins (Knox *et al*, 1994; Nagle *et al*, 1995; Hao *et al*, 1996), and several studies of the expression of metalloproteinases such as cathepsin D and type IV collagenase indicate the role of a breakdown of normal boundaries in the progression of PIN (Boag and Young, 1993, 1994; Stearns *et al*, 1993; Hamdy *et al*, 1994; Kuczyk *et al*, 1994; Makar *et al*, 1994; Sinha *et al*, 1995).

DEVELOPMENT OF PRECANCER AND TRANSITION TO INVASIVE CANCER

Overwhelming amounts of data indicate that PIN is a precursor to invasive cancer. PIN is originally multifocal, probably mainly multiclonal, located mostly in

TABLE 2. Immunohistochemical and histochemical markers in PIN[a]

Marker	Normal			Hyperplasia			PIN		Cancer	Reference
	BC	NS	LC	BC	NS	LC	BC	LC		
Ki-67	+		−	+		−	+	+	+	Leav et al, 1996
PCNA	+		−	+		−	+	+	+	Myers and Grizzle, 1997; Helpap, 1995
EGFR	+		−	+		−	+	+	+	Turkeri et al, 1994; Bonkhoff, 1996; Ibrahim et al, 1993; Maygarden et al, 1992; Myers et al, 1993; Montone and Tomaszewski, 1993
ERBB2	+		−	+		−	+	+	+	Myers and Grizzle, 1994; Bostwick, 1994
ERBB3	+		−	+		−	+	+	+	Meilon et al, 1992
BCL2	+		−	+		−	←	←	←	Stattin et al, 1996; Myers and Grizzle, 1997
AB		+			+		+	+		Montironi et al, 1993
IGFBP2	+		+	+		+	←	←	←	Tennant et al, 1996
IGFBP3	+		+	+		+	←	←	→	Tennant et al, 1996
AgNOR	(+)		(+)	(+)		(+)	←	←	←	Helpap, 1995; Sesterhenn et al, 1996
PNA		+			+		←	←	←	Myers and Grizzle, 1997; Drachenberg and Papadimitriou, 1995

Marker							Reference
AR	−	+	−	+	−	+/−	Leav et al, 1996
ACT	(−)	(+)	(−)	(+)	(−)	+	Myers and Grizzle, 1997
FASE	+	+	+	+	↑	↑	Myers and Grizzle, 1997
hK2	+	+	+	+	↑	↑	Myers and Grizzle, 1997
LNGFR	+	+	+	+	→	→	Perez et al, 1997
GP A80	(+)	(+)	(+)	(+)	↑	↑	Gould et al, 1996
CK5	+	−	+	−	+		Yang et al, 1997
CK8	+	+	+	+	+	+	Yang et al, 1997
CK14	+	−	+	−	−		Yang et al, 1997
CK19	(+)	(+)	(+)	(+)	+		Yang et al, 1997
NE			+		+	+	di Sant Agnese, 1992; Iwamura et al, 1995
nm23-H1	+	+	+	+	↑	↑	Myers and Grizzle, 1997
MET	+	−	+	−	↑	↑	Myers and Grizzle, 1997
TAG72	+	+	+	+	↑	↑	Brenner et al, 1995
TGFA	+	+	+	+	↑	↑	Robertson et al, 1994; Myers et al, 1995

[a]BC= basal cells; NS=not specified; LC=luminal cells; Ki-67=proliferation marker; PCNA=proliferative cell nuclear antigen; EGFR=epidermal growth factor receptor; ERBB2, ERBB3 proto-oncogenes in the ERBB family; BCL2=gene involved in regulation of apoptosis; AB=apoptotic bodies; IGFBP2, IGFBP3=insulin like growth factor binding proteins 2 and 3; AgNOR=silver stained nucleolar organizing regions; PNA=peanut agglutinin lectin; ACT=antichymotrypsin; FASE=fatty acid synthetase; hK2=human kallekrein 2; LNGFR=low affinity nerve growth factor receptor; GP A80=glycoprotein A80; CK5,8,14,19=cytokeratins 5,8,14,19; NE=neuroendocrine differentiation; nm23-H1=metastasis associated gene; MET=metastasis associated gene; TAG72=tumour associated glycoprotein72; TGFA=transforming growth factor alpha

the peripheral zone, and its total volume is larger than that of invasive cancer as long as this is small. The recognition of low grade PIN as a precursor has to await further molecular genetic analysis, but it is clear that low grade invasive carcinomas also need a precursor to complete the tumour biological picture. The transforming events, inductive or functional mutations and secondary functional epigenetic ones, lead to dysregulation of three hypothetical sets of genes responsible for control of (a) growth and programmed cell death, (b) "social behaviour" and (c) cell differentiation. At a certain point of disharmony of regulation the prerequisites for malignant behaviour exist. The probability for this seems related to the degree of genetic derangement as well as to structural and functional derangement (malignancy grade). It can be anticipated that sets of markers for the events may be identified and organized (by neuronal network techniques?) to prognostically even more useful tools than those identified so far. The possibility that precancer lesions of the prostate may be reversible by hormonal manipulation is intriguing, and the possible contribution of angiogenesis to precancer→cancer progression needs to be further investigated.

CLINICAL IMPLICATIONS

The acceptance of high grade PIN as a premalignant lesion and its association with concomitant invasive carcinoma necessitates a protocol for its management when found in core biopsy material or in transurethral resectates from the prostate. Low grade PIN, however, is not per se considered of clinical importance, since there is no proof of its association with invasive cancer.

Only patients suitable for curative treatment of a prostate cancer should undergo further investigation of a PIN biopsy finding (Fig. 4).

In patients with high grade PIN on prostate biopsy, there is a significant risk of a co-existing invasive carcinoma—24–73% on repeat biopsy (Brawer *et al*, 1991; Weinstein and Epstein, 1993; Bostwick *et al*, 1995; Davidson *et al*, 1995). However, this does not justify radical treatment for prostate cancer on a PIN biopsy finding alone, since the incidence of cancer on repeat biopsy is still significantly less than 100%.

The original clinical finding that prompted a prostate biopsy should be taken into account.

Hence a palpable nodule on digital rectal examination and high grade PIN in the prostate biopsy are strongly associated with a cancer finding on repeat biopsy. In one published study 100% of the repeat biopsies after an initial finding of high grade PIN and 18% in the low grade PIN cases were positive (Brawer *et al*, 1991), Langer *et al* (1996) examined 1275 consecutive patients undergoing prostate needle biopsies. 61 of these were originally identified with PIN without concurrent carcinoma. Of the 61, 53 had repeat biopsies. This yielded carcinoma in 15, PIN without carcinoma in 8 and benign tissue in 30. Further analysis of the relationships between original findings and site specific findings of the second round of needle core biopsies led the authors to the fol-

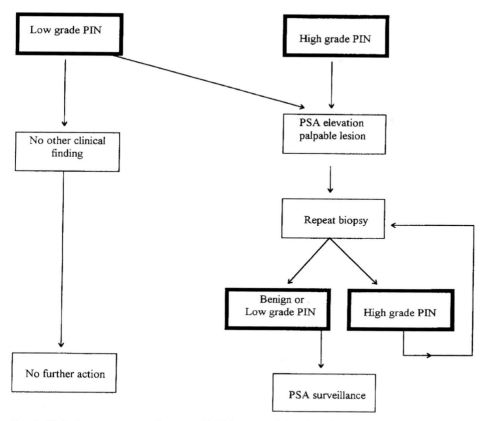

Fig. 4. Clinical management of cases with PIN on core biopsies of the prostate

lowing conclusions: repeat biopsies of patients with PIN should include random biopsies as well as biopsy of transrectal ultrasound abnormalities and of previous sites of PIN. We recommend the following strategy when PIN is diagnosed on a prostate biopsy (Fig. 5): high grade PIN found in a prostate biopsy should prompt rebiopsy; low grade PIN should cause further action only in cases where other cancer suspicious findings co-exist.

FUTURE RESEARCH

Although evidence is mounting for a relationship between PIN and invasive cancer, many questions remain.

The unique range of age distribution of PIN, latent and clinically diagnosed carcinoma demands better understanding of triggering events. What is the precise role of hormonal dysregulation for tumour progression? Is angiogenesis involved early? What is the contribution of other stromal components? What about viral oncogenesis in the prostate?

The existence of low grade invasive carcinoma raises the possibility that only high grade PIN may be a precursor. Further molecular analysis of lower grade lesions may reveal a closer association to invasiveness.

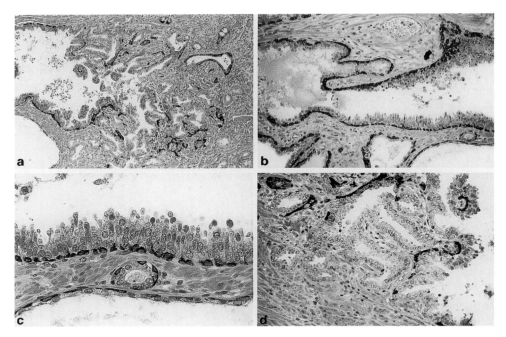

Fig. 5. Immunohistochemical stainings of basal cells illustrating the gradual separation and loss of basalcells as invasion occurs: (a) overview of portion of acinus with transition to invasive cancer; (b) focal separation of basal cells; (c) flat high grade PIN; (d) absence of basal cells in area of imminent invasion

A more detailed three dimensional assessment of the transition from PIN to invasive cancer, combined with molecular analysis of microdissected small numbers of cells or individual cells, may throw further light on progression events. Also the intriguing possibility that changes of the microvessel organization adjacent to PIN lesions may precede or go along with invasion should be investigated further.

The indications that PIN is sensitive to hormonal manipulation demand further study. The canine model of progression offers a promising approach in this respect (Waters and Bostwick, 1997).

As stated by Lalani *et al* (1997), current research in prostate cancer demands greater input from pathologists, with a requirement for improved morphological assessment, classification and grading of neoplasia. Lalani *et al* advocate optimal preservation of collected material and establishment of tissue banks to facilitate molecular analysis. Microdissection will help to get pure tumour DNA and mRNA, which can be further amplified by reverse transcriptase PCR. Experts in morphological analysis are essential members of the teams, which also include basic scientists and translational researchers. Finally, clinicians with a devoted interest in fundamental tumour biological research complete the future successful teams.

SUMMARY

The evolution of the malignant phenotype requires a set of genetic and epigenetic changes in sets of genes responsible for regulation of normal growth and cell death, of "social behaviour" and differentiation. The sum of these changes, not only the sequence, determines the malignancy as well as its grade. The probability of invasiveness shows a remarkable relationship to morphological changes, which in turn prove to be accompanied by a multitude of discrete molecular perturbations. Some of these can be characterized as functional, others as inductive with respect to their participation in the process. Since only the functional changes regulate malignant behaviour per se, it is an important task for future research to assemble a set of such changes, find markers for them and combine morphological and molecular indicators to achieve prognostically optimal scores. It should be emphasized, though, that rational use of such scores using biopsy samples as a source of information cannot be defined until biopsy strategies have been standardized and optimized.

References

Alcaraz A, Takahashi S, Brown JA et al (1994) Aneuploidy and aneusomy of chromosome 7 detected by fluorescence in situ hybridization are markers of poor prognosis in prostate cancer. *Cancer Research* **54** 3998–4002

Alers JC, Krijtenburg PJ, Vissers KJ, Bosman FT, van der Kwast TH and van Dekken H (1995) Interphase cytogenetics of prostatic adenocarcinoma and precursor lesions analysis of 25 radical prostatectomies and 17 adjacent prostatic intraepithelial neoplasias. *Genes, Chromosomes and Cancer* **12** 241–250

Algaba F, Trias l, Lopez L, Rodriguez-Vailejo JM and Gonzales-Esteban J (1995) Neuroendocrine cells in peripheral prostatic zone age, prostatic intraepithelial neoplasia and latent cancer-related changes. *European Urology* **27** 329–333

Allam CK, Bostwick DG, Hayes JA et al (1996) Interobserver variability in the diagnosis of high grade prostatic intraepithelial neoplasia and adenocarcinoma. *Modern Pathology* **6** 742–751 **(Supplement 71A)**

Amin MB, Ro JY and Ayala AG (1993a) Putative precursor lesions of prostatic adenocarcinoma: fact or fiction? *Modern Pathology* **6** 476–483

Amin MB, Schultz DS, Zarbo RJ, Kubus J and Shaheen C (1993b) Computerized static DNA ploidy analysis of prostatic intraepithelial neoplasia. *Archives of Pathology and Laboratory Medicine* **117** 794–798

Bandyk MG, Zhao L, Troncosos P et al (1994) Trisomy 7: a potential cytogenetic marker of human prostate cancer progression. *Genes, Chromosomes and Cancer* **9** 19–27

Baretton GB, Vogt T, Blasenbreu S and Lohrs U (1994) Comparison of DNA ploidy in prostatic intraepithelial neoplasia and invasive carcinoma of the prostate: an image cytometric study. *Human Pathology* **25** 506–513

Bartels PH, Thompson D, Bartels HG, Montironi R, Scarpelli M and Hamilton PW (1995a) Machine vision based histometry of premalignant and malignant prostatic lesions. *Pathology Research and Practice* **191** 935–944

Bartels PH, Thompson D, Montironi R, Hamilton PW and Scarpelli M (1995b) Diagnostic decision support for prostate lesions. *Pathology Research and Practice* **191** 945–957

Bastacky SI, Wojno KJ, Walsh PC, Carmichael MJ and Epstein JI (1995) Pathological features of hereditary prostate cancer. *Journal of Urology* **153** 987–992

Berges RR, Vukanovic J, Epstein JI *et al* (1995) Implication of cell kinetic changes during the progression of human prostate cancer. *Clinical Cancer Research* **1** 473

Berner A, Danielsen HE, Pettersen EO, Fossa SD, Reith A and Nesland JM (1993) DNA distribution in the prostate. Normal gland, benign and premalignant lesions, and subsequent adenocarcinomas. *Analytical and Quantitative Cytology and Histology* **15** 247–252

Bigler SA, Deering RE and Brawer MK (1993) Comparison of microscopic vascularity in benign and malignant prostate tissue. *Human Pathology* **24** 220–226

Bishop DT and Skolnick MH (1984) Genetic epidemiology of cancer in Utah genealogies: a prelude to the molecular genetics of common cancers. *Journal of Cellular Physiology* **3** **(Supplement)** 63–67

Boag AH and Young ID (1993) Immunohistochemical analysis of type IV collagenase expression in prostatic hyperplasia and adenocarcinoma. *Modern Pathology* **6** 65–68

Boag AH and Young ID (1994) Increased expression of the 72-kd type IV collagenase in prostatic adenocarcinoma. Demonstration by immunohistochemistry and in situ hybridization. *American Journal of Pathology* **144** 585–591

Bonkhoff H (1996) Role of the basal cells in the premalignant changes of the human prostate: a stemcell concept for the development of cancer. *European Urology* **30** 201–205

Bonkhoff H, Stein U, Walter C and Remberger K (1995) Differential expression of the pS2 protein in the human prostate and prostate cancer association with premalignant changes and neuroendocrine differentiation. *Human Pathology* **26** 824–828

Bookstein R, Rio P, Madreperla SA *et al* (1990) Promoter deletion and loss of retinoblastoma gene expression in human prostate carcinoma. *Proceedings of the National Academy of Sciences of the USA* **87** 7762–7766

Bookstein R, MacGrogan D, Hilsenbeck SG, Sharkey F and Allred DC (1993) p53 is mutated in a subset of advanced-stage prostate cancers. *Cancer Research* **53** 3369–3373

Bostwick DG (1988) Premalignant lesions of the prostate. *Seminars in Diagnostic Pathology* **5** 240–253

Bostwick DG (1994) c-erbB-2 oncogene expression in prostatic intraepithelial neoplasia: mounting evidence for a precursor role. *Journal of the National Cancer Institute* **86** 1108–1110

Bostwick DG (1995) High grade prostatic intraepithelial neoplasia: the most likely precursor of prostate cancer. *Cancer* **75** 1823–1836

Bostwick DG and Brawer MK (1987) Prostatic intraepithelial neoplasia and early invasion in prostate cancer. *Cancer* **59** 788–794

Bostwick DG, Cooner WH, Denis L, Jones GW, Scardino PT and Murphy GP (1992) The association of benign prostatic hyperplasia and cancer of the prostate. *Cancer* **70** **(Supplement 1)** 291–301

Bostwick DG, Amin MB, Dundore P, Marsh W and Shultz DS (1993) Architectural patterns of high grade prostatic intraepithelial neoplasia (PIN). *Human Pathology* **42** 298–310

Bostwick DG, Burke HB, Wheeler TM *et al* (1994a) The most promising surrogate endpoint biomarkers for screening candidate chemopreventive compounds for prostatic adenocarcinoma in short-term phase II clinical trials. *Journal of Cellular Biochemistry* **19** **(Supplement)** 283–289

Bostwick DG, Dousa MK, Crawford BG and Wollan PC (1994b) Neuroendocrine differentiation in prostatic intraepithelial neoplasia and adenocarcinoma. *American Journal of Surgical Pathology* **18** 1240–1246

Bostwick DG, Quian J and Frankel K (1995) The incidence of high grade prostatic intraepithelial neoplasia in needle biopsies. *Journal of Urology* **154** 1791–1794

Bova GS, Carter BS, Bussemakers MJG *et al* (1993) Homozygous deletion and frequent allelic loss of chromosome 8p22 loci in human prostate cancer. *Cancer Research* **53** 3869–3873

Braun MM, Partin AW, Page WF and Walsh PC (1995) Prostate cancer concordance rates among World War II veteran twins suggest hereditary influences. *Journal of Urology* **153** **(Supplement)** 504A

Brawer MK, Nagle MD, Bigler SA, Lange PH and Sohlberg OE (1991) Significance of prostatic intraepithelial neoplasia on prostate needle biopsy. *Urology* **38** 103–107

Brenner PC, Rettig WJ, Sanz-Moncasi MP *et al* (1995) TAG-72 expression in primary, metastatic and hormonally treated prostate cancer as defined by monoclonal antibody CC49. *Journal of Urology* **153** 1575–1579

Brooks JD, Bova GS and Isaacs WB (1995) Allelic loss of the retinoblastoma gene in primary human prostatic adenocarcinoma. *Prostate* **26** 35–39

Brothman AR, Peehl DM, Patel AM and McNeal JE (1990) Frequency and pattern of karyotypic abnormalities in human prostate cancer. *Cancer Research* **50** 3795–3803

Brown JA, Alcaraz A, Takahashi S, Persons DL, Lieber MM and Jenkins RB (1994) Chromosomal aneusomies detected by fluorescence in situ hybridization analysis in clinically localized prostate carcinoma. *Journal of Urology* **152** 1157–1162

Cannon L, Bishop DT, Skolnick M, Hunt S, Lyon JL and Smart CR (1982) Genetic epidemiology of prostate cancer in the Utah mormon genealogy. *Cancer Surveys* **1** 48–49

Carter BS, Beaty TH, Steinberg GD, Childs B and Walsh PC (1990a) Mendelian inheritance of familial prostate cancer. *Proceedings of the National Academy of Sciences of the USA* **89** 3367–3371

Carter BS, Epstein JI and Isaacs WB (1990b) Ras gene mutations in human prostate cancer. *Cancer Research* **50** 6830–6832

Carter BS, Ewing CM, Ward WS *et al* (1990c) Allelic loss of chromosome 16q and 10q in human prostate cancer. *Proceedings of the National Academy of Sciences of the USA* **87** 8751–8752

Carter BS, Bova GS, Beaty TH *et al* (1993a) Hereditary prostate cancer epidemiologic and clinical features. *Journal of Urology* **150** 797–802

Carter HB, Piantadosi S and Isaacs JT (1993b) Clinical evidence for and implications of the multistep development of prostate cancer. *Journal Urology* **143** 742–746

Cheng L, Shan A, Qian J *et al* (1998) Genetic heterogeneity in prostatic intraepithelial neoplasia and carcinoma: United States and Canadian Academy of Pathology annual meeting, Boston, Massachusetts, February 28–March 6 **444** 78A [Abstract]

Crissman JD, Sakr WA, Hussein ME *et al* (1993) DNA quantitation of intraepithelial neoplasia and invasive carcinoma of the prostate. *Prostate* **22** 155–162

Davidson D, Bostwick DG, Qian J *et al* (1995) Prostatic intraepithelial neoplasia is a risk factor for adenocarcinoma: predictive accuracy in needle biopsies. *Journal of Urology* **154** 1295–1299

de la Torre M, Hæggman M, Brændstedt S and Busch C (1993) Prostatic intraepithelial neoplasia (PIN) and invasive adenocarcinoma in total prostatectomy specimens. *British Journal of Urology* **72** 207–213

Deschenes J and Weidner N (1990) Nucleolar organiser regions (NOR) in hyperplastic and neoplastic prostate disease. *American Journal of Surgical Pathology* **14** 1148–1155

di Sant' Agnese PA (1992) Neuroendocrine differentiation in carcinoma of the prostate: diagnostic, prognostic and therapeutic implications. *Cancer* **70** 254–268

Dong JT, Isaacs WB and Isaacs JT (1997) Molecular advances in prostate cancer. *Current Opinion in Oncology* **9** 101–107

Drachenberg CB and Papadimitriou JC (1995) Aberrant pattern of lectin binding in low and high grade prostatic intraepithelial neoplasia. *Cancer* **75** 2539–2544

Drago JR, Mostofi FK and Lee F (1989) Introductory remarks and workshop summary. *Urology* **34 (Supplement)** 2–3

Effert PJ, McCoy RH, Walther PJ *et al* (1993) p53 gene alterations in human prostate carcinoma. *Journal of Urology* **150** 257–261

Emmert-Buck MR, Vocke CD, Pozzatti RO *et al* (1995) Allelic loss on chromosome 8p12-21 in microdissected prostatic intraepithelial neoplasia (PIN). *Cancer Research* **55** 2959–2962

Epstein JI, Cho KR and Quinn BD (1990) Relationship of severe dysplasia to stage A (incidental) adenocarcinoma of the prostate. *Cancer* **65** 2321–2327

Epstein JI, Grignon DJ, Humphrey PA *et al* (1995) Interobserver reproducibility in the diagnosis of prostatic intraepithelial neoplasia. *American Journal of Surgical Pathology* **19** 873–886

Ewing CM, Ru N and Morton RA (1995) Chromosome 5 suppresses tumourigenicity of PC-3 prostate cancer cells: correlation with re-expression of alpha-catenin and restoration of E-cadherin function. *Cancer Research* **55** 4813–4817

Ferguson J, Zincke H, Ellison E, Bergstrahi E and Bostwick DG (1994) Decrease of prostatic intraepithelial neoplasia (PIN) following androgen deprivation therapy in patients with stage T3 carcinoma treated by radical prostatectomy. *Urology* **44** 91–95

Giri DK, Wadhawa SN, Upadaya SN *et al* (1993) Expression of neu/her-2 oncoprotein (p185neu) in prostate tumors: an immunohistochemical study. *Prostate* **23** 329–336

Giroldi LA and Schalken JA (1993) Decreased expression of the intercellular adhesion molecule E-cadherin in prostate cancer: biological significance and clinical implications. *Cancer Metastasis Reviews* **12** 29–37

Giroldi LA, Bringuier PP and Schalken JA (1994–95) Defective E-cadherin function in urological cancers: clinical implications and molecular mechanisms. *Invasion Metastasis* **14** 71–81

Goldgar DE, Easton DF, Cannon-Albright LA and Skolnick MH (1994) Systematic population-based assessment of cancer risk in first-degree relatives of cancer probands. *Journal of the National Cancer Institute* **86** 1600–1608

Gould VE, Doljanskaia V, Gooch G and Bostwick DG (1996) Immunolocalization of glycoprotein A-80 in prostatic carcinoma and prostatic intraepithelial neoplasia. *Human Pathology* **27** 547–552

Gronberg H, Damber L and Damber JE (1994) Studies of genetic factors in prostate cancer in a twin population. *Journal of Urology* **152** 1484–1489

Gronberg H, Damber L, Damber JE and Iselius L (1997) Segregation analysis of prostate cancer in Sweden: support for dominant inheritance. *American Journal of Epidemiology* **146** 552–557

Gunthert U, Stauder R, Mayer B, Terpe H-J, Finke L and Friedrichs K (1995) Are CD44 variant isoforms involved in human tumour progression? *Cancer Surveys* **24** 19–42

Hamdy FC, Fadion EJ, Cottam D *et al* (1994) Matrix metalloproteinase expression in primary human prostatic adenocarcinoma and benign prostatic hyperplasia. *British Journal of Cancer* **69** 177–182

Hau J, Yang Y, McDaniel KM, Dalkin BL, Cress A and Nagle RB (1996) Differential expression of laminin 5 by human malignant and normal prostate. *American Journal of Pathology* **149** 1341–1349

Hedrick L and Epstein JI (1989) Use of Keratin 903 as an adjunct in the diagnosis of prostate carcinoma. *American Journal of Surgical Pathology* **113** 389–396

Hellstrom M, Haggman M, Brandstedt S *et al* (1993) Histopathological changes in andogen-deprived localized prostatic cancer: a study in total prostatectomy specimens. *European Urology* **24** 461–465

Helpap B (1988) Observations on the number, size and location of nucleoli in hyperplastic and neoplastic prostatic disease. *Histopathology* **13** 203–211

Helpap B (1995) Cell kinetic studies on prostatic intraepithelial neoplasia (PIN) and atypical adenomatous hyperplasia (AAH) of the prostate. *Pathology Research and Practice* **191** 904–907

Helpap B and Riede C (1995) Nucleolar and AgNOR-analysis of prostatic intraepithelial neoplasia (PIN), atypical adenomatous hyperplasia (AAH) and prostatic carcinoma. *Pathology Research and Practice* **191** 381–390

Hsieh JT, Luo W, Song W *et al* (1995) Tumour suppressive role of an androgen-regulated epithelial cell adhesion molecule (C-CAM) in prostate carcinoma cell revealed by sense and antisense approaches. *Cancer Research* **55** 190–197

Humphrey PA and Swanson PE (1995) Immunoreactive p53 protein in high-grade prostatic intraepithelial neoplasia. *Pathology Research and Practice* **191** 881–887

Ibrahim GK, Kerns BM, MacDonald JA *et al* (1993) Differential immunoreactivity of epidermal growth factor receptor in benign, dysplastic and malignant prostatic tissues. *Journal of Urology* **149** 170–173

Iwamura M, Gershagen S, Lapets O *et al* (1995) Immunohistochemical localization of parathyroid hormone related protein in prostatic intraepithelial neoplasia. *Human Pathology* **26** 797–801

Kanthoff PW, Febbo PG, Giovannucci E *et al* (1997) A polymorphism of the α–reductase gene and its association with prostate cancer: a case control analysis. *Cancer Epidemiology, Biomarkers and Prevention* **6** 189–192

Kastendieck H (1980) Correlations between atypical primary hyperplasia and carcinoma of the prostate. *Pathology Research and Practice* **169** 366–387

Kastendieck H and Helpap B (1989) Prostatic "dysplasia/atypical hyperplasia". Terminology, histopathology, pathobiology, and significance. *Urology* **(Supplement)** **34** 28–42

Kleinerman DI, Troncoso P, Sue-Hwa L *et al* (1995) Consistent expression of an epithelial cell adhesion molecule (CAM) during human prostate development and loss of expression in prostate cancer: implication as a tumor suppressor. *Cancer Research* **55** 1215–1220

Knox JD, Crew AE, Clark V *et al* (1994) Differential expression of extracellular matrix molecules and the alpha-6-integrins in the normal and neoplastic prostate. *American Journal of Pathology* **145** 167–174

Kovi J, Mostofi FK, Heshmat MY and Enterline JP (1988) Large acinar atypical hyperplasia and carcinoma of the prostate. *Cancer* **61** 555–561

Kubota Y, Shuin T, Fujinami K *et al* (1995) Tumor suppressor gene p53 mutations in human prostate cancer. *Prostate* **27** 18–24

Kuczyk M, Serth J, Denil J, Hofner K, Allhoff E and Jonas U (1994) Cathepsin D expression and the possible role of lysosomal proteases as a prognostic factor in prostate cancer. *Journal of Urology* **151** [Abstract 286]

Kuhn EJ, Kurnot RA, Sesterhenn IA *et al* (1993) Expression of the c-erbB-2 (HER2/neu) onco-protein in human prostatic carcinoma. *Journal of Urology* **150** 1427–1433

Lalani E-N, Stubbs A and Stamp GWH (1997) Prostate cancer the interface between pathology and basic scientific research. *Seminars in Cancer Biology* **8** 53–59

Langer JE, Rovner ES, Coleman BG *et al* (1996) Strategy for repeat biopsy of patients with pro-static intraepithelial neoplasia detected by prostate needle biopsy. *Journal of Urology* **155** 228–231

Langston AA, Stanford JL, Wicklund KG, Thompson JD, Blazej RG and Ostrander EA (1996) Germ-line mutations in selected men with prostate cancer. *American Journal of Human Genetics* **58** 885–888

Leav I, McNeal JE, Kwan PW, Komminoth P and Merk FB (1996) Androgen receptor expression in prostatic dysplasia (prostatic intraepithelial neoplasia) in the human prostate: an immuno-histochemical and in situ hybridization study. *Prostate* **29** 137–145

Lowe FC, Hillel K, Thiel R, Chen R and Luderer AA (1996) Follow-up of high grade prostatic intraepithelial neoplasia: clinical implications. *Journal of Urology* **155** [Abstract 605]

McIndoe RA, Stanford JL, Gibbs M *et al* (1997) Linkage analysis of 49 high-risk families does not support a common familial prostate cancer-susceptibility gene at 1q24-25. *American Journal of Human Genetics* **61** 347–353

McNeal JE and Bostwick DG (1986) Intraductal dysplasia: a premalignant lesion of the prostate. *Human Pathology* **17** 64–71

McNeal JE, Leav I, Alroy J and Skutellsky E (1988a) Differential lectin staining of the central and peripheral zones of the prostate and alterations in dysplasia. *American Journal of Clinical Pathology* **89** 41–48

McNeal JE, Alroy J, Leav I, Redwine EA, Freiha FS and Stamey TA (1988b) Immunohistochemical evidence for impaired cell differentiation in the premalignant phase of prostate carcinogenesis. *American Journal of Clinical Pathology* **90** 23–32

McNeal JE, Villers A, Redwine EA, Freiha FS and Stamey TA (1991) Microcarcinoma of the prostate: its association with duct-acinar dysplasia. *Human Pathology* **22** 644–652

Macoska JA, Micale MA, Sakr WA, Benson PD and Wolman SR (1993) Extensive genetic alter-ations in prostate cancer revealed by dual PCR and FISH analysis. *Genes, Chromosomes and Cancer* **8** 88–97

Macoska JA, Trybus TM, Sakr WA *et al* (1994) Fluorescence in situ hybridization analysis of 8p allelic loss and chromosome 8 instability in human prostate cancer. *Cancer Research* **54** 3824–3830

Macoska JA, Trybus TM, Benson PD *et al* (1995) Evidence for three tumor suppressor gene loci on chromosome 8p in human prostate cancer. *Cancer Research* **55** 5390–5395

Makar R, Mason A, Kittelson JM, Bowden GT, Cress AE and Nagle RB (1994) Immunohistochemical analysis of cathepsin D in prostate carcinoma. *Modern Pathology* **7** 747–751

Maygarden SJ (1994) Applications of immunohistochemistry to the diagnosis and prognostication of prostate carcinoma and prostatic intraepithelial neoplasia. *Pathology Annual* **29** 303–320

Maygarden SJ, Strom S and Ware JL (1992) Localization of epidermal growth factor receptor by immunohistochemical methods in human prostatic carcinoma, prostatic intraepithelial neoplasia, and benign hyperplasia. *Archives of Pathology and Laboratory Medicine* **116** 269–273

Meilon K, Thompson S, Charlton RG *et al* (1992) p53, c-erbB-2 and the epidermal growth factor receptor in the benign and malignant prostate. *Journal of Urology* **147** 496–499

Miller A and Seljelid R (1971) Cellular dysplasia in the prostate. *Scandinavian Journal of Urology and Nephrology* **5** 17–21

Min KW, Jin J-K, Blank J and Hemstreet G (1990) AGNOR in the human prostatic gland. *American Journal of Clinical Pathology* **95** 508–512

Mirchandani D, Zheng J, Miller GJ *et al* (1995) Heterogeneity in intratumor distribution of p53 mutations in human prostate cancer. *American Journal of Pathology* **47** 92–101

Montironi R, Scarpelli M, Sisti S, Braccisch A and Mariuzzi GM (1990) Quantitative analysis of prostatic intra-epithelial neoplasia on tissue sections. *Analytical and Quantitative Cytology and Histology* **12** 366–372

Montironi RM, Scarpelli M, Galuzzi CM and Diamanti L (1992) Aneuploidy and nuclear features of prostatic intraepithelial neoplasia (PIN). *Journal of Cellular Biochemistry* **Supplement 16H** 47–53

Montironi R, Magi Gailuzzi C, Diamanti L *et al* (1993a) Prostatic intra-epithelial neoplasia: qualitative and quantitative analyses of the blood capillary architecture on thin tissue sections. *Pathology Research and Practice* **189** 542–548

Montironi R, Magi-Galluzzi C, Diamanti L *et al* (1993b) Prostatic intra-epithelial neoplasia: expression and location of proliferating cell nuclear antigen (PCNA) in epithelial, endothelial and stromal nuclei. *Virchows Archiv A, Pathological Anatomy and Histopathology* **422** 185–192

Montironi R, Magi Galiuzzi C, Scarpelli M, Giannulis I and Diamanti L (1993c) Occurrence of cell death (apoptosis) in prostatic intra-epithelial neoplasia. *Virchows Archiv A, Pathological Anatomy and Histopathology* **423** 351–357

Montironi R, Bartels PH, Thompson D, Bartels HG, Scarpelli M and Hamilton PW (1994a) Prostatic intraepithelial neoplasia: development of a Bayesian Belief Network for diagnosis and grading. *Analytical and Quantitative Cytology and Histology* **16** 101–112

Montironi R, Magi-Gailuzzi C, Muzzonigro G, Prete E, Polito M and Fabris G (1994b) Effects of combination endocrine treatment on normal prostate, prostatic intraepithelial neoplasia, and prostatic adenocarcinoma. *Journal of Clinical Pathology* **47** 906–913

Montironi R, Bartels PH, Thompson D, Bartels HG, Scarpelli M and Hamilton PW (1995a) Prostatic intraepithelial neoplasia (PIN): performance of Bayesian Belief Network for diagnosis and grading. *Journal of Pathology* **177** 153–162

Montironi R, Bartels PH, Thompson D, Bartels HG and Scarpelli M (1995b) Prostatic intraepithelial neoplasia: quantitation of the basal cell layer with machine vision system. *Pathology Research and Practice* **191** 917–923

Montone KT and Tomaszewski JE (1993) In situ hybridization for epidermal growth factor receptor (EGFR) external domain transcripts in prostatic adenocarcinoma. *Journal of Clinical and Laboratory Analysis* **7** 188–195

Morton RA, Ewing CM, Nagafuchi A, Tsukita S and Isaacs WB (1993) Reduction of E-cadherin levels and deletion of the alpha-catenin gene in human prostate cancer cells. *Cancer Research* **53** 3585–3590

Mostofi FK (1984) Precancerous lesions of the prostate, In Carter RL (ed). *Precancerous States*, pp 304–316, Oxford University Press, New York

Mostofi FK, Sesterhenn IA and Davis CJ (1989) Malignant change in hyperplastic prostate glands: the

AFIP experience. *Urology* **34** 49–51

Murant SJ, Handley J, Stower M, Reid N, Cussenot O and Maitland NJ (1997) Co-ordinated changes in expression of cell adhesion molecules in prostate cancer. *European Journal of Cancer* **33** 263–271

Myers RB and Grizzle WE (1997) Changes in biomarker expression in the development of prostatic adenocarcinoma. *Biotechnology and Histochemistry* **72** 86–95

Myers RB, Kudlow JE and Grizzle WE (1993) Expression of transforming growth factor-alpha, epidermal growth factor and the epidermal growth factor receptor in adenocarcinoma of the prostate and benign prostatic hyperplasia. *Modern Pathology* **6** 733–737

Myers RB, Oelschlager D, Srivastava S and Grizzle WE (1994a) Accumulation of the p53 protein occurs more frequently in metastatic than in localized prostatic adenocarcinomas. *Prostate* **25** 243–248

Myers RB, Srivastava S, Oelschlager DK and Grizzle WE (1994b) Expression of p160erbB-3 and p185erbB-2 in prostatic intraepithelial neoplasia and prostatic adenocarcinoma. *Journal of the National Cancer Institute* **86** 1140–1145

Myers RB, Lampejo O, Herrera GA *et al* (1995) TGF-alpha expression is a relatively late event in the progression of prostatic adenocarcinoma. *Journal of Urology Pathology* **3** 195–204

Nagle RB, Brawer MK, Kittelson J and Clark V (1991) Phenotypic relationships of prostatic intraepithelial neoplasia to invasive prostatic carcinoma. *American Journal of Pathology* **138** 119–128

Nagle RB, Hao J, Know JD, Dalkin BL, Clark V and Cress AE (1995) Expression of hemidesmosomal and extracellular matrix proteins by normal and malignant human prostate tissue. *American Journal of Pathology* **146** 1498–1507

O'Malley F, Grignon D, Keeney M, Kerkvliet N and McLean C (1991) DNA flow-cytometric studies of prostatic intraepithelial neoplasia. *Modern Pathology* **4** [Abstract 50]

Oyasu R, Bahnson RR, Nowels K and Garnett JE (1986) Cytological atypia in the prostate gland: frequency, distribution and possible relevance to carcinoma. *Journal of Urology* **135** 959–962

Perez M, Regan T, Pflug B, Lynch J, and Djakiew D 1997. Loss of low affinity nerve growth factor receptor during malignant transformation of the human prostate. *Prostate* **30** 274–279

Petein M, Michel P, Van Velthoven R *et al* (1991) Morphonuclear relationship between prostatic intraepithelial neoplasia and cancers as assessed by digital cell image analysis. *American Journal of Clinical Pathology* **96** 628–634

Qian J and Bostwick DG (1995) The extent and zonal location of prostatic intraepithelial neoplasia and atypical adenomatous hyperplasia: Relationship with carcinoma in radical prostatectomy specimens. *Pathology Research and Practice* **191** 860–867

Qian J, Bostwick DG, Takahashi S *et al* (1995) Chromosomal anomalies in prostatic intraepithelial neoplasia and carcinoma detected by fluorescence in situ hybridization. *Cancer Research* **55** 5408–5414

Qian J, Wollan P and Bostwick DG (1997) Extent and multicentricity of high grade prostatic intraepithelial neoplasia in clinically localized prostatic adenocarcinoma. *Human Pathology* **28** 143–148

Quinn BD, Cho KR and Epstein JI (1990) Relationship of severe dysplasia to stage B adenocarcinoma of prostate. *Cancer* **65** 2328–2337

Robertson CN, Roberson KM, Herzberg AJ, Kerns BJM, Dodges RK and Pauison DF (1994) Differential immunoreactivity of transforming growth factor alpha in benign, dysplastic and malignant prostatic tissues. *Surgical Oncology* **3** 237–242

Sakr WA, Haas GP, Drozdowicz SM *et al* (1992) Nuclear DNA content of prostatic carcinoma and intraepithelial neoplasia (PIN) in young males. An image analysis study. *Modern Pathology* **5** [Abstract 58]

Sakr WA, Haas GP, Cassin BF, Pontes JE and Crissman JD (1993a) The frequency of carcinoma and intraepithelial neoplasia of the prostate in young male patients. *Journal of Urology* **150** 379–385

Sakr WA, Sarkar FH, Sreepathi P, Drozdowicz S and Crissman JD (1993b) Measurement of cellular proliferation in human prostate by AGNOR, PCNA and SPF. *Prostate* **22** 147–154

Sakr WA, Grignon DJ, Crissman JD *et al* (1994) High grade prostatic intraepithelial neoplasia (HGPIN) and prostatic adenocarcinoma between the ages of 20-69: an autopsy study of 249 cases. *In Vivo* **8** 439–443

Salem CE, Tomasic NA, Elmajian DA *et al* (1997) p53 protein and gene alterations in pathological stage C prostate carcinoma. *Journal of Urology* **158** 510–514

Sarkar FH, Sakr W, Li YW *et al* (1992) Analysis of retinoblastoma (RB) gene deletion in human prostatic carcinomas. *Prostate* **21** 145–152

Sesterhenn IA, Becker RL, Avallone FA, Mostofi FK, Lin TE and Davis CJ (1991) Image analysis of nucleoli and nucleolar organiser regions in prostatic hyperplasia, intraepithelial neoplasia, and prostatic carcinoma. *Journal of Urogenital Pathology* **1** 61–74

Shah IA, Schlageter MO, Stinnett P and Lechago J (1991) Cytokeratin immunohistochemistry as a diagnostic tool for distinguishing malignant from benign epithelial lesions of the prostate. *Modern Pathology* **4** 220–224

Sheng S, Carey J, Seftor EA *et al* (1996) Maspin acts at the cell membrane to inhibit invasion and motility of mammary and prostatic cancer cells. *Proceedings of the National Academy of Sciences of the USA* **93** 11669–11674

Sikes RA and Chung LWK (1992) Acquisition of a tumorigenic phenotype by a rat ventral prostate epithelial cell line expressing a transfected activated neu oncogene. *Cancer Research* **52** 3174–3178

Sinha AA, Wilson LU, Gleason DF, Reddy PK, Sameni M and Sloane BF (1995) Immunohistochemical localization of cathepsin B in neoplastic human prostate. *Prostate* **26** 171–178

Smith JR, Freije D, Carpten JD *et al* (1996) Major susceptibility locus for prostate cancer on chromosome 1 suggested by a genome-wide search. *Science* **274** 1371–1374

Stattin P, Damber JE, Karlberg L, Nordgren H and Bergh A (1996) Bcl-2 immunoreactivity in prostate tumorigenesis in relation to prostatic intraepithelial neoplasia, grade, hormonal status, metastatic growth and survival. *Urological Research* **24** 257–264

Stearns ME and Stearns M (1993) Autocrine factors, type IV collagenase secretion and prostatic cancer cell invasion. *Cancer Metastasis Reviews* **12** 39–52

Takahashi S, Qian J, Brown JA *et al* (1994) Potential markers of prostate cancer aggressiveness detected by fluorescence in situ hybridization. *Cancer Research* **54** 3574–3579

Tennant MK, Trasher JB, Twomey PA, Birnbaum RS, and Plymate SR (1996) Insulin-like growth factor-binding protein (IGFB)-4, -5 and 6 in the benign and malignant human prostate: IGFB-5 messenger ribonucleic acid localization differs from IGFB-5 protein localization. *Journal of Clinical Endocrinology and Metabolism* **81** 3783–3792

Troncoso P, Babaian RJ, Ro JY, Grignon DJ, Eschenbach AC and Ayala AG (1989) Prostatic intraepithelial neoplasia and invasive prostatic adenocarcinoma in cystoprostatectomy specimens. *Urology* **34** (**Supplement**) 52–56

Turkeri LN, Sakr WA, Wykes SM, Grignon DJ, Pontes JE and Macoska JA (1994) Comparative analysis of epidermal growth factor receptor gene expression and protein product in benign, premalignant and malignant prostate tissue. *Prostate* **25** 199–205

Ware JL (1993) Growth factors and their receptors as determinants in the proliferation and metastasis of human prostate cancer. *Cancer Metastasis Reviews* **12** 287–301

Waters DJ and Bostwick DG (1997) The canine prostate is a spontaneous model of intraepithelial neoplasia and prostate cancer progression. *Anticancer Research* **17** 1467–1470

Weinberg DS and Weidner N (1993) Concordance of DNA content between prostatic intraepithelial neoplasia and concomitant carcinoma evidence that prostatic intraepithelial neoplasia is a precursor of invasive prostatic carcinoma. *Archives of Pathology and Laboratory Medicine* **117** 1132–1137

Weinstein MH and Epstein JI (1993) Significance of high grade prostatic intraepithelial neoplasia on needle biopsy. *Human Pathology* **24** 624–629

Woolf CM (1960) An investigation of the familial aspects of carcinoma of the prostate. *Cancer* **13** 739

Zenkiusen JC, Thompson JC, Troncoso P, Kagan J and Cont CJ (1994) Loss of heterozygosity in human primary prostatic carcinomas: a possible tumor suppressor gene at 7q3l.l. *Cancer Research* **54** 6870–6873

Zhau HE, Wan DS, Zhou J *et al* (1992) Expression of c-erbB-2/neu proto-oncogene in human prostatic cancer, tissues and cell lines. *Molecular Carcinogenesis* **5** 320–327

Zitzeisberger H, Szves S, Weier HU *et al* (1994) Numerical abnormalities of chromosome 7 in human prostate cancer detected by fluorescence in situ hybridization (FISH) on paraffin embedded tissue sections with centromere-specific DNA probes. *Journal of Pathology* **172** 325–335

Zou Z, Anisowicz A, Hendrix MJC *et al* (1994) Maspin, a serpin with tumour suppressing activity in human mammary epithelial cells. *Science* **263** 526–529

The authors are responsible for the accuracy of the references.

The Dynamics of Early Intestinal Tumour Proliferation: To Be or Not to Be

DARRYL SHIBATA

University of Southern California, School of Medicine, Los Angeles, CA 90033

INTRODUCTION

Colorectal cancer is one of the most well characterized examples of multistep tumour progression. A number of loci frequently mutated in colorectal cancer have been identified and associated with specific phases of the adenoma–carcinoma sequence. This chapter will not stress the genetic barriers to colorectal cancer (recently reviewed by Kinzler and Vogelstein, 1996) but instead focuses on the dynamics of multistep tumour progression. Compared to the detailed dissections of the altered genotypes and abnormal intracellular pathways in cancer, little is known about the consequent dynamic phenotype of "uncontrolled proliferation". An ultimate description of multistep progression would include both mutational and proliferation patterns. Since multiple mutations are necessary for malignant transformation, there are likely to be different types or degrees of uncontrolled proliferation. What proliferation patterns allow a single cell to progress eventually to cancer?

Cancer Surveys Volume 32: *Precancer: Biology, Importance and Possible Prevention*
© 1998 Imperial Cancer Research Fund. 0-87969-540-4/98. $5.00 + .00

HEREDITARY NON-POLYPOSIS COLORECTAL CANCER: A MODEL SYSTEM OF TUMOUR EVOLUTION

Hereditary non-polyposis colorectal cancer (HNPCC, also known as Lynch syndrome) is one of the most common forms of hereditary colon cancer (Lynch *et al*, 1996). Approximately 5% of all colorectal cancers occur in HNPCC families. Heterozygous germline mutations in DNA mismatch repair (MMR) genes are responsible for its autosomal dominant inheritance. The most common germline mutations are in *hMLH1* and *hMSH2*, with a few families with *hPMS2* and *hPMS1* mutations (Kinzler and Vogelstein, 1996).

Microsatellite Instability

A hallmark characteristic of HNPCC tumours is genomic instability defined by the ubiquitous presence of somatic mutations in the majority of microsatellite (MS) loci (Aaltonen *et al*, 1993; Ionov *et al*, 1993; Thibodeau *et al*, 1993). MS loci are simple repeat (mono- to tetranucleotide) sequences predominantly present in non-coding genomic regions. For example, dinucleotide repeats are typically defined as $(CA)_N$ with N between 10 and 30. There are thousands of MS loci and their roles are unknown. Different sized alleles are likely to have little selective value since MS loci are highly polymorphic in human populations (Weber, 1990).

Frameshifts in MS loci predominantly occur through slippage during DNA replication (Strand *et al*, 1993; Streisinger *et al*, 1966). Lack of subsequent DNA MMR results in novel alleles with different numbers of repeat units. Therefore, the majority of MS loci in HNPCC tumours exhibit alleles larger or smaller than germline since HNPCC tumour cells have lost or mutated the normal repair allele and are MMR deficient (Aaltonen *et al*, 1994; Kinzler and Vogelstein, 1996).

A Long Journey

When does cancer initiate? Although certain alterations may occur very early in life, for most HNPCC individuals, the first critical event can be traced before conception. In Finland, many individuals have the same *hMLH1* germline mutation traced back as far as 1505 to ancestors near the town of Jyvaskyla (Nystrom-Lahti *et al*, 1994). Therefore, a contemporary colorectal tumour arising in this extended HNPCC family can trace its origins way back to the 14th century.

How did this 14th century mutation eventually transform 20th century intestinal cells?

Genetic events are linked through time by their accumulation and transmission on single genomes. The mutant *hMLH1* locus is not the only "message" transmitted to the 20th century. Phylogenetic analysis of other loci can unravel other legacies recorded in the human genome (von Haeseler *et al*, 1996). For example, polymorphisms in contemporary populations scattered throughout the world reveal a likely human origin "out-of-Africa" about 100 000 to 200 000 years ago (Cavalli-Sforza *et al*, 1993; Ayala, 1995; Goldstein *et al*, 1995; von Haeseler *et al*, 1996). Tumour genomes should also record similar information about tumour dynamics, ages and origins (Shibata *et al*, 1996; Shibata, 1997). Of note, phylogenetic information or messages are not immutable relics but rather dynamic loci that are expected to mutate with division. An approach to extract some of this information recorded by MS loci in HNPCC tumours follows in later sections.

Affected HNPCC individuals are phenotypically normal and appear to have no selective advantage or disadvantage with the usual 50:50 ratio of affected siblings characteristic of autosomal dominant inheritance. Germline transmission is random. The 14th century germline *hMLH1* mutation could have disappeared long ago either due to the lack of offspring or by random failure of transmission to offspring. In fact, with the random process of human procreation, most polymorphisms do not become "fixed" in the population but are eliminated by chance (Ayala, 1995). Robert Malthus indirectly observed this phenomenon by noting that most last names in small medieval English towns tend to die out.

Although germline transmission is random, the actual dynamics have been completely documented with Finnish pedigrees extending from the 14th into the 20th century (Nystrom-Lahti *et al*, 1994). However, the contemporary period between conception and clinical presentation of a colon tumour represents a void. How did one intestinal cell become transformed?

TISSUE DYNAMICS

The dynamics of multistep tumour progression are often implied from static morphological phenotypes. A low stage tumour is an "early" lesion. A focus of cancer within an adenoma is evidence of "recent" transformation. Although these impressions are logical, objective evidence is lacking as morphology is dogmatic. Better understanding of the underlying proliferation patterns responsible for tissue construction could validate these morphological impressions.

Normal Intestinal Dynamics

Transformation occurs from the background of normal intestinal development and regeneration. The murine intestine will be discussed since it has been extensively studied with techniques generally impractical in humans (Griffiths *et al*, 1988; Winton *et al*, 1988). Chimaeric studies reveal that relatively large patches (hundreds of crypts) of intestinal epithelium develop from single cells (Ponder *et al*, 1985). At the junctions between patches, crypts are initially polyclonal at birth with contributions from both adjacent patches. Therefore, initially crypts are maintained by a number of stem cells. However, by two weeks of age, the crypts at the patch junctions become monoclonal with all cells from either one of the patches, allowing the conclusion that crypts are derived from a single cell or a very small number of cells. This process of elimination to a single crypt progenitor is called purification (Schmidt *et al*, 1988).

After development, the normal crypt structure is maintained by a small number of functional stem cells (Potten and Loeffler, 1990; Gordon *et al*, 1992). Approximately 6–20 of such stem cells are present near the base of each crypt. A proliferative zone of approximately 150 cells is present in the lower crypt. These non-stem cells divide approximately 4–6 times before terminal differentiation. Most of these cells die within a week as they migrate towards the lumen.

This intestinal crypt structural hierarchy provides inherent protection against neoplasia since the number of immortal cells is relatively small, and most crypt cells are terminally differentiated and actively migrating towards the lumen (Cairns, 1975). The majority of crypt divisions occur in non-stem cells. Mutations acquired in non-stem cells will be rapidly lost through death. It appears to be very difficult for non-stem cells to acquire sufficient numbers of mutations to persist. Expression of transgenes (*Ras, TP53, SV40 TAg*) in differentiated enterocytes but not stem cells alters phenotype but does not lead to neoplasia (Kim *et al*, 1993).

Therefore, crypt stem cells are the most likely progenitors of colorectal cancer (Cairns, 1975). This progenitor faces numerous challenges since it must divide to accumulate sufficient numbers of oncogenic mutations and yet persist for decades. Intestinal epithelium is mitotically active with divisions balanced by death. Every division provides opportunities for either renewal, loss or growth. The division of crypt stem cells is a complex subject (Potten and Loeffler, 1990; Morrison *et al*, 1997). Since stem cells are difficult to identify and study directly, indirect measurements of their behaviour are necessary. Sophisticated mathematical models and simulations can account for many of the observations, but much remains unknown.

Crypt stem cells most often divide to produce one stem cell daughter and one daughter destined to die. This form of renewal allows persistence with unlimited divisions and is called asymmetrical division (Fig. 1). The mechanisms responsible for asymmetrical division are unknown. Stem cells also appear occasionally to divide symmetrically (Winton and Ponder, 1990; Loeffler *et al*, 1993; Bjerknes, 1994). In symmetrical division, both daughters either survive or die (Fig. 1). For homoeostasis, whenever both daughter cells survive, both daughters of another division must die. Symmetrical division is needed to replace stem cells lost normally or through disease. The proportion of symmetrical versus asymmetrical stem cell divisions is uncertain in normal intestines. Superficially, the number of stem cells can remain constant with any combination of asymmetrical or symmetrical divisions. However, kinetic observations of murine intestines are consistent with predominantly asymmetrical divisions since polyclonal crypts induced by mutagens only slowly become monoclonal (Winton and Ponder, 1990; Loeffler *et al*, 1993; Bjerknes, 1994). Asymmetrical

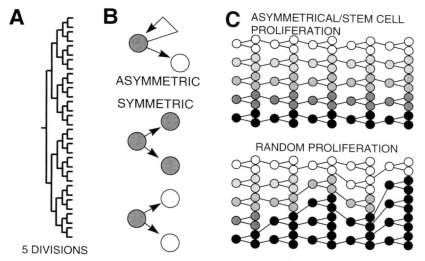

Fig. 1. (A) Binary branching of cell division. A single cell dividing five times could follow 32 different paths. Such exact tumour descriptions are desirable but impractical for large numbers of cells and divisions. (B) Diagrams of asymmetrical and symmetric divisions. Open circles represent cells destined to die. (C) Division patterns in stable populations. In asymmetrical division, survival of every lineage is assured. Therefore, mutations accumulate. In random proliferation (symmetrical or asymmetrical division) lineages terminate at random. Therefore, many mutations are eliminated by death. Superficially it is difficult to distinguish between random proliferation and selection since the consequences are similar—a reduction in diversity

stem cell division appears to occur more than 80% of the time (Loeffler *et al*, 1993).

Tumour Dynamics

Although the majority of human tumours appear to have defects in cell cycle regulation (Strauss *et al*, 1995), the consequent phenotype is usually described simply as "increased proliferation". Tumours may be stable, shrink or grow depending on the balance between proliferation and death. For tumours stable in size, cell division must equal cell death. Older kinetic studies of human tumours reveal that more than 90% of tumour cells must die since mitotic rates greatly exceed growth rates (Steele, 1967, 1977). Death rates rather than mitotic rates control tumour sizes (Steele, 1977). A recent radiographic study revealed that most colorectal adenomas are stable in size (Otchy *et al*, 1996).

A balance between division and death can occur with an almost infinite number of proliferation combinations (asymmetrical and symmetrical divisions). The ultimate description of tumour dynamics would reconstruct the pedigrees of every tumour cell. The time, phenotype, genotype and physical location would be recorded for each branch point. However, such precise descriptions of proliferation are extremely difficult since branching leads to exponential numbers of possible pathways (Fig. 1A). An alternative dynamic description is the average behaviour of cells. Do certain types of cells exhibit characteristic proliferation patterns?

To Be or Not to Be

Proliferation is a binary process (Fig. 1A). One cell divides to yield two cells. With asymmetrical division, one daughter cell persists and the other one eventually dies. The fate of each daughter is likely to be predetermined by inherent mechanisms that are only poorly understood. Stem cells characteristically undergo asymmetrical division.

In contrast, divisions of established cell lines yield two potentially immortal daughters. The frequent inactivation of cell cycle control loci in human tumours (Strauss *et al*, 1995) may be responsible for the relentless cycles of division and death observed in tumours (Steele, 1977). Cell lines have lost the ability to determine the inherent fate of their progeny. Instead, external forces decide life or death. Exponential growth occurs in the proper environment. Under limiting conditions, cell lines can have both symmetrical (both daughters die or survive) or asymmetrical division. Survival or death poses a dilemma since the daughters are almost completely identical and adjacent. Given this similarity, death under steady state conditions is likely to be random. Since death prevents further proliferation, random death is equivalent to random proliferation.

Therefore, two tumours stable in size may be superficially identical but markedly different in terms of dynamic regulation. With asymmetrical division, population size regulation is inherent whereas with random death, size regulation is likely to be due to environmental limitations. If one could mark and follow individual cells, one could distinguish between random death/proliferation and asymmetrical division (Fig. 1C).

MICROSATELLITE LOCI AS MOLECULAR TUMOUR CLOCKS

MS loci in cells deficient in MMR are potentially such markers or molecular clocks since they will become polymorphic after relatively few divisions. Heterozygous HNPCC cells are repair proficient and do not accumulate significant numbers of somatic MS mutations. Loss of the normal repair allele essentially "starts" the molecular clock and theoretically the bulk of mutations can be traced to this initiating event.

The Approach: Reconstructing the Past

The somatic MS mutations characteristic of MMR deficiency are initially rare since mutation rates, although absolutely high (up to 0.01 mutations per division) are still relatively low. At a 1% mutation rate, about 70 divisions are needed for a 50% probability of a single mutation (Li *et al*, 1996). Probabilities must be used since mutations are not accumulated with mechanical clock like reliability but rather like the stochastic process of radioactive decay.

Interpretation of the complex MS distributions of mutator phenotype tumours requires extensive mathematical or computer analysis. Phylogenetic reconstruction of historical division patterns recorded by MS loci depends on models that describe how cells divide, die and acquire mutations. Model building requires numerous assumptions that may be not strictly correct or difficult to prove. Models cannot prove mechanisms and are at best consistent with experimental data. Nevertheless, models are invaluable since they clearly project the results expected with specific assumptions.

Models of MS loci may be mathematical (Goldstein *et al*, 1995; Shibata *et al*, 1996) or simulated on computers (Tsao *et al*, 1997). Simulations will be discussed here since very complex models can be formulated by a few basic rules illustrated in Table 1. Potential flaws or weaknesses can be identified (and corrected) since the rules are relatively easy to understand (compared to mathe-

TABLE 1. Simulation of cell dynamics

RULES:

1. One cell divides to yield two cells
2. Number of cells remains constant
3. Cell loss is either asymmetrical (one daughter from each division dies) or at random (cells are eliminated at random from the entire population)
4. Equal numbers of divisions between cells
5. Constant mutation rates
6. Stepwise mutation (single repeat unit additions or deletions)

RATIONALE:

1. Known to occur
2. Approximately true in most tumours since macroscopic tumour growth is slow
3. Model assumptions
4. Unlikely to be strictly true but similar numbers of divisions are likely since the cells are clonally related (especially in small tumour dots)
5. MS mutations in cells deficient in MMR probably occur almost exclusively by slippage of DNA polymerase during replication. Therefore, the number of mutations is likely to be directly proportional to the number of divisions. In HNPCC patients, loss of the normal repair allele appears to occur early in tumour progression (Shibata *et al*, 1994) and results in cells completely repair deficient by standard assays (Parsons *et al*, 1993). Significant changes in MS mutation rates after loss of DNA MMR therefore appear unlikely. A recent study illustrated a conditional mutator phenotype with increased frequencies of mutation in two ovarian cell lines under growth limitations (Richards *et al*, 1997). These experiments illustrate possible pitfalls in using MS loci as molecular clocks. However, evidence of increased mutation rates in stable xenografts of mutator colorectal cell lines has not been observed (unpublished data).
6. Most MS mutations between cell and human generations are changes of a single repeat unit, with both additions and deletions observed (Weber and Wong, 1993; Bhattacharyya *et al*, 1994; Shibata *et al*, 1994).

matical descriptions). The simulation is essentially a large spreadsheet in which MS genotypes are stored electronically in database cells instead of in the DNA of cells. Each electronic cell and its MS allele undergo analysis every division cycle based on the rules. Similar to but cheaper and faster than laboratory experiments, the rules can be modified to explore their influence on the accumulation of mutations. The current simulation (Tsao *et al*, 1997) runs on Pentium based computers and fits on a single 1.4 MB diskette. The stepwise nature of MS mutations (both single repeat unit addition or deletions) complicates analysis since time cannot be determined by absolute repeat unit differences between tumour and germline. Instead, after an initial clonal expansion, MS loci are expected to become polymorphic (Fig. 2). The MS diversity or spread of the distribution, defined mathematically as variance, reflects the number of divisions since the last clonal expansion. With asymmetrical division, median variance is directly proportional to the number of divisions (Shibata *et al*, 1996).

Simulations and Experimental Reality

Simulations are often criticized as having little to do with biological realities. It seems unwise to simulate an entire tumour unless more is known about its dynamics. Do tumours arise gradually or in stages? Is growth uniform? How similar are different parts of a tumour? If dynamic tumour heterogeneity exists, descriptions of average tumour behaviour may have little meaning.

The large number of cells present even in small tumours also represents enormous computational burdens. Therefore, we have chosen an approach that simplifies both the simulations and the experimental analysis. This strategy describes the dynamics of topographically defined small contiguous cell groups or tumour dots isolated by microdissection. Tumours are physical representations of large phylogenetic trees rooted in a common progenitor. Compared to the entire tumour, the 200–400 cells present within each small region should have more immediate ancestors and therefore are more likely to have similar genotypes and phenotypes. Progeny are likely to remain neighbours as topographical heterogeneity is observed in adenomas (Shibata *et al*, 1993; Borland *et al*, 1995). Significant mixing of cells may not occur since detachment from basement membranes is likely to result in death or anoikis (Frisch and Francis, 1994).

The DNA isolated from each small tumour dot can be analysed by dilution prior to polymerase chain reaction (PCR). Assuming the ability to amplify single molecules, each PCR product essentially represents a single allele if 50–66% of the reactions yield products. Another experimental simplification is the use of MS loci on the X chromosome and male patients. The frequency distributions (size of each MS allele v. number of each allele) represent the population of tumour cells present within each dot. These frequency distributions are compared between different dots randomly isolated throughout the tumour.

A

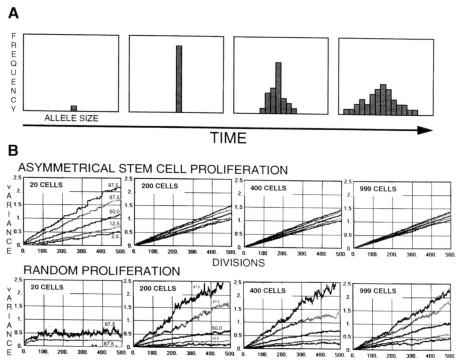

Fig. 2. (A) Schematic of the increased MS diversity or variance expected with division. A clonal expansion initially has limited diversity. However, with further division, greater diversity is expected. The number of elapsed divisions can be estimated from the extent of the MS diversity. (B) Computer simulations of the variance expected with different types and numbers of divisions. The mutation rate is 0.0025 mutations per division. With asymmetrical division, variance increases linearly with division. With small numbers of immortal cells, outcomes are more variable due to the stochastic nature of mutation. Therefore, outcomes are best expressed with confidence intervals (75 and 95%) and median variances. With larger numbers of cells, stochastic variation is decreased. A different pattern is seen with random proliferation. In this case, variance is limited with small numbers of immortal cells (<400 cells). Mutations which contribute to the variances are frequently lost by death with random proliferation. Therefore, analysis of small microdissected cell groups should be able to distinguish between asymmetric and random proliferation after about 400 divisions. Median MS variances greater than 1.0 would indicate asymmetrical division whereas MS variances less than 1.0 are consistent with either young tumours with asymmetrical division or tumours with random proliferation. The MS variances in normal murine intestines match the 20 cell asymmetrical simulations (Tsao et al, 1997). The MS variances in xenografts composed of mutator phenotype colorectal cancer cell lines match the 200–400 cell random proliferation simulations (unpublished data)

Simulations of relatively small numbers of cells are easily performed and are illustrated in Fig. 2B. With asymmetrical division, MS diversity or variance increases with division. With random death, MS diversity reaches a limit and it is difficult to exceed median variances greater than 1.0 at reasonable mutation rates (<1%) with small populations (<400 cells). This is because with asymmetrical division, lineages and all associated mutations persist (Fig. 1C). With random death, lineages terminate and rarer mutations, which contribute to diversity, are frequently lost through death as there is less than a 1% chance of acquiring a mutation but a 25% chance of elimination.

Another interesting phenomenon is the effect of stochastic mutation. Although most experiments are designed to provide unequivocal and reproducible measurements, stochastic processes are expected to yield many different outcomes. For example, coin flips will yield on average equal numbers of heads and tails. However, a series of four coin flips will sometimes yield zero, one, two, three or four heads. Similarly, stochastic mutation is expected to yield variable outcomes that are reflected in the simulations of Fig. 2B as confidence intervals. Smaller numbers of immortal cells have greater stochastic variation. Although increasing the number of measured cells should reduce stochastic variation, biologically relevant information may be lost. As noted above, crypts are composed of relatively small numbers of immortal stem cells and the stochastic variation expected with such a system is not experimental noise but rather biological information. Unfortunately, multiple measurements are necessary to extract this type of information.

Experimental Models of Asymmetrical and Random Proliferation

MS molecular tumour clocks and their associated theoretical models can be validated with experimental models.

Transgenic Mice

An experimental model of asymmetrical stem cell division is the normal intestine of mice deficient in DNA MMR (Tsao *et al*, 1997). Mice with homozygous knockouts of the MMR locus *Pms2* develop normally and have increased frequencies of lymphomas but not intestinal tumours. Experimental data (Tsao *et al*, 1997) are consistent with the intestinal dynamics inferred by other techniques. MS mutations progressively accumulate with age in *Pms2–/–* mice with a pattern consistent with the simulations of asymmetric divisions with 20 or fewer immortal stem cells (Fig. 2B). The scatter of the variances from multiple dots (each with 200–400 cells) located throughout the intestines reflects the stochastic nature of mutation. Note that the number of immortal stem cells consistent with the data (20 or fewer) is less than the number of analysed alleles (typically 40–80 alleles per dot). However, it is unnecessary directly to isolate, identify and analyse only the stem cells because the genotypes of the non-stem cells will reflect the genotypes of their stem cells since only a few divisions are likely to intervene (Tsao *et al*, 1997). For normal mucosa, only four to six divisions precede stem cell division (Potten and Loeffler, 1990).

Mice deficient in other repair loci (*Mlh1*, *Msh2*, etc) are available. Other organs, development and disease processes could be examined with MS clocks since all cells are repair deficient. Additional genetic manipulations such as crosses with mice mutated in other pertinent loci, or exposures to different environments, offer opportunities to examine their effects on tissue dynamics as reflected by the accumulations of MS mutations.

Xenografts of MMR Deficient Cell Lines

An experimental model of cells likely to undergo division with random death are xenografts derived from single clones of mutator phenotype colorectal cancer cell lines. Xenografts isolated at specific time points after injection offer serial observations of their tumour dynamics. Every daughter cell is potentially immortal and xenografts, despite being mitotically active, do not grow exponentially after reaching macroscopic sizes. Therefore, most progeny must die in xenografts. Median MS diversity or variance increases initially in small xenograft populations, but then does not subsequently further increase with xenograft age, which is consistent with the simulations of random death (with 200–400 cells) illustrated in Fig. 2B (data not shown).

ADENOMAS: WHEN DOES THE TRANSITION TO RANDOM PROLIFERATION OCCUR?

The dynamic behaviour of normal intestinal mucosa (asymmetrical stem cell division) can be distinguished from fully transformed carcinoma cell lines (random death) by both simulations and experimental data. The differences become apparent only after a large number of divisions (about 400) as median MS variances exceed 1.0 with stem cell division but remain below 1.0 with random death (with mutation rates below 1%). When in the course of human colorectal tumour progression does the transition from asymmetrical stem cell division to random proliferation occur?

Examination of human adenomas may provide the necessary information. Examples are two metachronous HNPCC adenomas (Fig. 3). Metachronous tumours are common in HNPCC patients and provide unique opportunities to examine independent tumours evolving from identical genetic and similar environmental backgrounds. The MS alterations of both polyps have arisen within two years since they were obtained during biennial surveillance colonoscopy. Despite identical germline points of initiation, the distributions are different in the two polyps, likely reflecting their independent origins and differences in their relative ages since they could have arisen at any time between the biennial surveillance intervals.

Adenoma-A appears to be a relatively recent clonal expansion. Each small tumour dot contains a population of MS alleles consistent with a number of divisions and deaths since clonal expansion. The information from both loci appears consistent. It is uncertain if the polyp is a new clonal expansion with asymmetrical division or an old polyp with random proliferation since the median variances are less than 1.0 and both are possible with the models of Fig. 2B. Assuming asymmetrical division, fewer than 400 divisions have occurred since clonal expansion. The MS genotype of the progenitor cell of the last clonal expansion is likely to be +4 (units relative to germline) for DXS556 and +3 for DXS418 since this is the most common genotype present throughout the tumour.

Adenoma-B is larger and more complex. The MS distributions are more diverse than in Adenoma-A. The median MS variances exceed 1.0, which is inconsistent with a model of random proliferation but consistent with more than 400 asymmetric divisions. There appear to be no consistent regional vari-

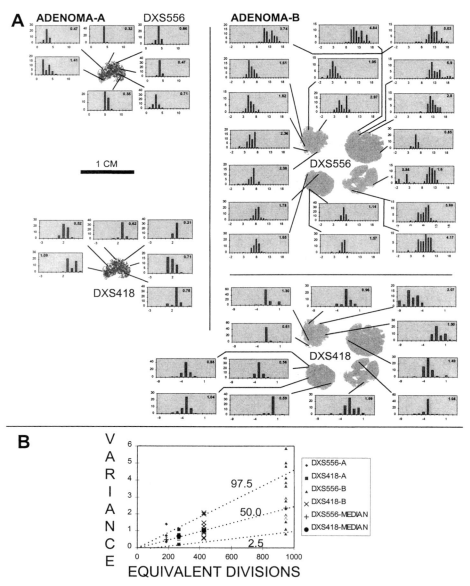

Fig. 3. (See facing page for legend)

ance differences, suggesting a similar age for the entire adenoma. However, heterogeneity with respect to the modes of the MS distributions is present, with some distributions lacking overlap with others. The MS genotype of the progenitor cell for the last clonal expansion is more difficult to discern as wider distributions of alleles are present throughout the adenoma. For DXS556, the modes of the distributions range from +3 to +12. For DXS418, the modes of the distributions range from −7 to germline. Simulations demonstrate that MS modes will vary from each other with time, although the modal differences are typically more like those seen in Adenoma-A and not the extreme differences seen in Adenoma-B. Another possibility, discussed later, is a multiclonal origin of tumours.

Considerable variation in the variances is noted in both adenomas. According to the simulations (Fig. 2B), the number of immortal cells affects this variation with small numbers of stem cells leading to greater stochastic fluctuation. For normal murine intestinal mucosa, the data are consistent with 20 or fewer stem cells within each 200–400 cell dot (Tsao *et al*, 1997), as expected with current models of intestinal renewal (Potten and Loeffler, 1990; Gordon *et al*, 1992). A similar number (<20 adenoma stem cells) also appear to be present in human adenomas (Fig. 3B). Therefore, the human adenoma data are consistent with both asymmetrical division and a small proportion of immortal adenoma stem cells. The majority of adenoma cells appear not to contribute future progeny and are effectively terminally differentiated. Note that although the analysis suggests that the dynamics of adenomas and normal mucosa are similar, it does not identify the location of the adenoma stem cells. The adenoma

Fig. 3. (A) Topographical locations of the MS frequency distributions of the metachronous HNPCC Adenomas A and B. Findings are consistent with asymmetrical proliferation. The frequency of each allele, their relative sizes and the variance of each distribution are given. Germline ((CA)$_{20}$ for DXS556 and (CA)$_{22}$ for DXS418) is noted as "0" with relative repeat unit additions and deletions given on the horizontal axis. The MS distributions for Adenoma-A are relatively homogeneous compared to Adenoma-B. In Adenoma-B some portions of the adenoma have apparent bimodal distributions and others lack overlap between each other. The distinct populations seen in Adenoma-B imply both topographical and time isolation. Topographical isolation or the lack of mixing can be maintained by the crypt like branching structure of adenomas. Time isolation is required to generate the very different size distributions between regions. If the cells in Adenoma-B are related, divergence or their last common ancestor was ancient. In contrast, it is easy to see that the cells in Adenoma-A are related and their last common ancestor was much more recent. Both metachronous adenomas arose from the identical genetic background. (B) Plot of the variances obtained from the two adenomas. The data suggest a hierarchy—a small number of immortal adenoma stem cells maintain a larger number of differentiated adenoma cells. The confidence intervals from Fig. 2B for asymmetrical division with 20 stem cells are also plotted for reference. The scatter of the adenoma variances is wide and consistent with the pattern observed in normal murine intestines (asymmetrical division with <20 immortal stem cells). Note that although a single adenoma should have the same number of divisions for each locus, the mutation rates are likely to vary between individual MS loci. These different mutation rates can be normalized by using "equivalent" divisions (product of relative mutation rate and cell division). For example, DXS556 is likely to have a higher mutation rate than DXS418 in Adenoma-B. Mutation rates appear generally to increase with the number of MS repeat units

stem cells may be in aberrant locations. Therefore, the topographically disorganized patterns of division observed in adenomas (see, for instance, El-Deiry *et al*, 1995 and Polyak *et al*, 1996) may reflect abnormalities in location but not in the underlying asymmetrical proliferation.

In summary, for some HNPCC adenomas, "initiation" can be traced to a mutation acquired before the 14th century, passed at random between generations into the 20th century. After conception, a single cell populated a relatively large patch of colonic epithelium. The ultimate progenitor was a stem cell that survived the ordeal of purification and persisted for decades near the base of a single crypt, preserving its genome through predominantly asymmetrical divisions. At some point in time, the normal "caretaker" repair allele was inactivated and the cell became MMR deficient. With an increased mutation rate, the MMR deficient cell accelerated its accumulation of somatic mutations in coding and MS loci, eventually transforming the normal stem cell to an adenoma stem cell. Loss of a gatekeeper function led to net proliferation or symmetrical expansion (both daughter cells survive) and adenoma formation. However, despite gatekeeper and caretaker deficits (Kinzler and Vogelstein, 1997), asymmetrical division can remain the predominant pattern of division in adenomas. Loss of intrinsic stem cell behaviour may not occur early in colorectal cancer progression.

STEM CELL ADENOMA: IMPLICATIONS OF A HIERARCHY

A stem cell adenoma model is consistent with many adenoma characteristics. Asymmetrical division can account for the persistence of adenomas for years without apparent progression (Koretz, 1993). The small proportion of immortal stem cells may be responsible for the low to absent telomerase activity in adenomas (Chadeneau *et al*, 1995). The relatively small number of immortal cells may also account for the relatively infrequent conversion of adenomas to cancers (Koretz, 1993).

A stem cell adenoma also imposes a natural structural hierarchy. Adenoma stem cells may be inconspicuous with the polyp phenotype dependent on the abnormal expression of genes not expressed in stem cells. In normal intestines, different genes are expressed as cells differentiate with luminal migration (Potten and Loeffler, 1990; Gordon *et al*, 1992). Therefore, some somatic mutations may be differentially expressed or have different consequences in adenoma stem cells compared to differentiated cells. For example, a mutation delaying death may lead to greater numbers of differentiated adenoma cells and a larger polyp, but would have fewer consequences on the already immortal adenoma stem cell. A mutation altering cell cycle regulation may have different consequences depending on its expression in stem versus non-stem cells. This hierarchy may account for the regression of polyps by non-steroidal anti-inflammatory drugs (NSAID) but apparent persistence of the risk for subsequent cancer (Giardiello *et al*, 1993; Niv and Fraser, 1994; Thorson *et al*, 1994). NSAID may eliminate or reduce the differentiated, macroscopic component of adenomas but not the underlying potential stem cell progenitors to cancer. Polypectomy would remove both adenoma stem and non-stem cells and has been noted to decrease the risk of HNPCC cancers (Jarvinen *et al*, 1995). Recent studies of acute myelogenous leukaemia have also noted a hierarchy of more differentiated leukaemia cells maintained by small numbers of leukaemic stem cells (Bonnet and Dick, 1997).

FUTURE PREDICTIONS: HOW DIFFERENT IS TUMOUR PROGRESSION FROM SPECIES EVOLUTION?

The conversion from asymmetrical stem cell division to proliferation in which both daughter cells are potentially immortal may be a defining and characteristic feature of malignancy. Little is known about the regulation of asymmetrical division, but recognition of this critical dynamic transition may assist in identifying its critical factors.

Current models of colorectal cancer progression (Kinzler and Vogelstein, 1996) imply a linear process with sequential replacements by expansions with greater numbers of selective mutations. MS tumour clocks provide another opportunity to examine this pathway rigorously. The deeply branching pathways associated with episodic or punctated evolution of species (Gould and Eldredge, 1993) are alternative models of tumour progression. Adenomas and carcinomas must coexist for some period of time. The last common ancestor between cancers and their adenomas are presumed to be quite recent. However, gradual or phyletic transitions between species rarely occur. For example, it is highly unlikely that a monkey will eventually evolve into a human. However, we shared over 90% sequence similarities, with certain genomic stretches highly conserved between humans and primates. According to reasoning commonly applied to adenoma–carcinoma progression, the presence of the same sequences in monkeys and humans implies that humans evolved from monkeys (or vice versa). Of course the key elements here are the specific sequences used for comparison and the time of divergence between species. Comparing sequences between different entities is fraught with ambiguities unless the frequencies of expected polymorphisms are well defined. Sequences which only rarely acquire mutations (slow molecular clocks) are not expected to be different and divergence may be relatively recent or distant. Depending on the mutation rate, the time frame of different types of molecular tumour clocks may be years to decades. For example, if the mutation rate for a base substitution is 0.0001, about 7000 divisions (19 years if a cell divides every day) must occur for a 50% probability of mutation (Li *et al*, 1996). MS sequences in MMR deficient tumours have extremely high mutation rates (up to 0.01) and therefore can more easily distinguish between recent events.

A key test for the evolution of cancers directly from adenomas is the degree of similarity between their MS distributions (Fig. 4A). If cancers directly evolve

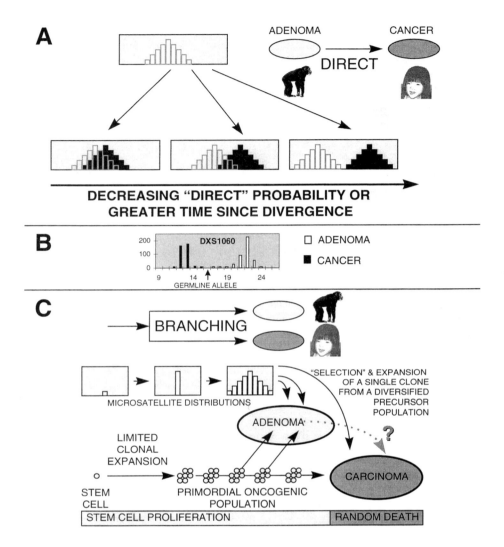

Fig. 4. (A) The current direct model of colorectal cancer. If cancers directly arise from adenomas, then their MS distributions should be similar. Differences between the MS distributions imply either completely independent origins or a long time since divergence. (B) MS distribution data from an adenoma and directly adjacent HNPCC carcinoma. Multiple adenoma and carcinoma regions were sampled. Although the distributions are relatively uniform within the adenoma and carcinoma, there is a complete lack of overlap between the two distributions. (C) A branching model of tumour progression. It is the same as direct models of multistep tumour progression except that mutations are not accumulated in macroscopic precursors. Instead, mutations continue to accumulate in an underlying and persistent primordial oncogenic population. Adenomas or cancers arise directly from this primordial oncogenic population. Therefore, clonal expansions are related but can have very different MS distributions. In addition, multiple clones can expand simultaneously after the proper environmental triggers since occult oncogenic populations allow for parallel evolution. Evolution proceeding in occult progenitor populations allows significant mutations to accumulate throughout life and not just in the "compressed" interval of the last decades after polyps appear

from adenomas, their MS distributions should resemble their adenoma distributions. Note that MS loci lack selective value and serve merely as unbiased molecular markers of the populations. Differences between adenoma and carcinoma MS distributions imply either distinct origins or a number of divisions intervening since their last common ancestor. Rare examples of cancers directly adjacent to adenomas have been used as histological evidence to support the adenoma–carcinoma sequence. Examination of their MS distributions provide opportunities to test their genetic distances.

Evolution is characterized by diversity and dead ends. The dominant species of today were often occult members in the past. Most adenomas are physically dead ends as many more individuals die with polyps than of colorectal cancer (Koretz, 1993). Preliminary evidence suggests that some adenomas next to cancers are not their direct precursors (Fig. 4B). What mechanisms account for MS distributions that are virtually distinct between adenoma and adjacent cancer but relatively homogeneous within each tumour? The heterogeneous MS distributions of Adenoma-B (Fig. 3) also suggest that adenomas may arise from more than one immediate progenitor. Perhaps multiple, occult but genetically altered clones (which could reside in aberrant crypt foci; Heinen *et al*, 1996) require environmental changes to trigger their simultaneous expansion. Although completely independent origins for tumour populations are possible (Novelli *et al*, 1996), branching pathways to cancer (Fig. 4C) allow for differences between tumour regions but an ultimate clonal origin (Fearon *et al*, 1987). Somatic mutations in more stable loci acquired before divergence are the expected common link between branches. In more unstable MS loci, measurable differences are expected to arise if a large number of divisions intervene before clonal expansion. Since the differences between some tumour populations appear large (Fig. 4B), evolution is likely to occur (perhaps for decades) in occult tumour populations.

Branching evolution is consistent with current models of multistep tumourigenesis except that progression occurs in occult precursor populations and not directly through macroscopic lesions. With current adenoma–carcinoma models, progression is "compressed" since it occurs during the last decades of life after polyps appear. With occult progenitor populations, mutations can accumulate throughout life—adenomas and cancers represent terminal phases of evolution that allow for the deep phylogenetic roots or long branches postulated in Fig. 4C. This hypothesis suggests that some adenomas are genetic dead ends which nevertheless signal the underlying presence of unstable occult populations that retain the potential for further deadly evolution.

SUMMARY

New data and approaches bring novel perspectives and possibilities to old problems. The speculation of this chapter attempts to merge the puzzling MS data observed in human tumours (Figs. 3 and 4B) within a multistep tumour progression model. Clearly the current models are gross simplifications and other, more sophisticated models may better account for the distribution of MS alleles found in human tumours. The findings and the data are also limited to MMR deficient tumours, and studies in non-mutator phenotype tumours may be more difficult since fewer polymorphisms will arise during progression. The current model, however, precisely defines proliferation and clearly delineates two very distinct patterns. Further studies using MS loci in MMR deficient tumours will allow fairer tests of alternative pathways (Fig. 4C) to cancer. Evolution proceeding in occult progenitor populations allows mutations to accumulate throughout life and not just in the last decades after polyps appear.

Acknowledgements

The author thanks the collaborative efforts of Drs Reijo Salovaara, Heikki J Jarvinen, Jukka-Pekka Mecklin and Lauri Aaltonen in Finland, and support by grants from the Public Health Service (CA58704 and CA70858).

References

Aaltonen LA, Peltomaki P, Leach FS *et al* (1993) Clues to pathogenesis of familial colorectal cancer. *Science* **260** 812–816

Aaltonen LA, Peltomaki P, Mecklin JP *et al* (1994) Replication errors in benign and malignant tumors from hereditary nonpolyposis colorectal cancer patients. *Cancer Research* **54** 1545–1548

Ayala FJ (1995) The myth of Eve: molecular biology and human origins. *Science* **270** 1930–1936

Bhattacharyya NP, Skandalis A, Ganesh A, Groden J and Meuth M (1994) Mutator phenotypes human colorectal carcinoma cell lines. *Proceedings of the National Academy of Sciences of the USA* **91** 6319–6323

Bjerknes M (1994) Simple stochastic theory of stem cell differentiation is not simultaneously consistent with crypt extinction probability and the expansion of mutated clones. *Journal of Theoretical Biology* **168** 349–365

Bonnet D and Dick JE (1997) Human acute myeloid leukemia is organized as a hierarchy that originates from a primitive hematopoietic cell. *Nature Medicine* **3** 730–737

Borland CR, Sato J, Appelman HD, Bresalier RS and Feinberg AP (1995) Microallelotyping defines the sequence and tempo of allelic losses at tumor suppressor gene loci during colorectal cancer progression. *Nature Medicine* **1** 902–909

Cairns J (1975) Mutation selection and the natural history of cancer. *Nature* **255** 197–200

Cavalli-Sforza LL, Menozzi P and Piazza A (1993) Demic expansions and human evolution. *Science* **259** 639–646

Chadeneau C, Hay K, Hirte HW, Gallinger S and Bacchetti S (1995) Telomerase activity associated with acquisition of malignancy in human colorectal cancer. *Cancer Research* **55** 2533–2536

El-Deiry WS, Tokino T, Waldman T, *et al* (1995) Topological control of p21 (Waf1/Cip1) expression in normal and neoplastic tissues. *Cancer Research* **55** 2910–2919

Fearon ER, Hamilton SR and Vogelstein B (1987) Clonal analysis of human colorectal tumors. *Science* **238** 193–197

Frisch SM and Francis H (1994) Disruption of epithelial cell-matrix interactions induces apoptosis. *Journal of Cell Biology* **124** 619–626

Giardiello FM, Hamilton SR, Krush AJ *et al* (1993) Treatment of colonic and rectal adenomas with sulindac in familial polyposis adenomatous polyposis. *New England Journal of Medicine* **328** 1313–1316

Goldstein DB, Linares AR, Cavalli-Sforza LL and Feldman MW (1995) Genetic absolute dating based on microsatellites and the origin of modern humans. *Proceedings of the National Academy of Sciences of the USA* **92** 6723–6727

Gordon JI, Schmidt GH and Roth KA (1992) Studies of intestinal stem cells using normal, chimeric, and transgenic mice. *FASEB Journal* **6** 3039–3050

Gould SJ and Eldredge N (1993) Punctated equilibrium comes of age. *Nature* **366** 223–227

Griffiths DFR, Davies SJ, Williams D, Williams GT and Williams ED (1988) Demonstration of somatic mutation and colonic crypt clonality by X-linked enzyme histochemistry. *Nature* **333** 461–463

Heinen CD, Shivapurkar H, Tang Z, Groden J and Alabaster O (1996) Microsatellite instability in aberrant crypt foci from human colons. *Cancer Research* **56** 5339–5341

Ionov Y, Peinado MA, Malkhosyan S, Shibata D and Perucho M (1993) Ubiquitous somatic mutations in simple repeat sequences reveals a new mechanism for colorectal carcinogenesis. *Nature* **363** 558–561

Jarvinen HJ, Mecklin JP and Sistonen P (1995) Screening reduces colorectal cancer rate in families with hereditary nonpolyposis colorectal cancer. *Gastroenterology* **108** 4405–4411

Kim SH, Roth KA, Moser AR and Gordon JI (1993) Transgenic mouse models that explore the multistep hypothesis of intestinal neoplasia. *Journal of Cell Biology* **123** 877–893

Kinzler KW and Vogelstein B (1996) Lessons from hereditary colorectal cancer. *Cell* **87** 159–170

Kinzler KW and Vogelstein B (1997) Gatekeepers and caretakers. *Nature* **386** 761–763

Koretz RL (1993) Malignant polyps: are they sheep in wolves' clothing? *Annals of Internal Medicine* **118** 63–68

Li ZH, Aaltonen LA, Shu Q, Srivastava S, Grizzle WE and Shibata D (1996) Effects of mutation and growth rates on patterns of microsatellite instability. *American Journal of Pathology* **148** 1757–1761

Loeffler M, Birke A, Winton D and Potten C (1993) Somatic mutation, monoclonality and stochastic models of stem cell organization in the intestinal crypt. *Journal of Theoretical Biology* **160** 471–491

Lynch HT, Smyrk T and Lynch JF (1996) Overview of natural history, pathology, molecular genetics and management of HNPCC (Lynch syndrome). *International Journal of Cancer* **69** 38–43

Morrison SJ, Shah NM and Anderson DJ (1997) Regulatory mechanisms in stem cell biology. *Cell* **88** 287–298

Niv Y and Fraser GM (1994) Adenocarcinoma in the rectal segment in familial polyposis coli is not prevented by sulindac therapy. *Gastroenterology* **107** 854–857

Novelli MR, Williamson JA, Tomlinson IPM *et al* (1996) Polyclonal origin of colonic adenomas in an XO/XY patient with FAP. *Science* **272** 1187–1190

Nystrom-Lahti M, Sistonen P, Mecklin JP *et al* (1994) Close linkage to chromosome 3p and conservation of ancestral founding haplotype in hereditary nonpolyposis colorectal cancer families. *Proceedings of the National Academy of Sciences of the USA* **91** 6054–6058

Otchy DP, Ransohoff DF, Wolff BG, Waver A, Ilstrup D, Carlson H and Rademacher D (1996) Metachronous colon cancer in persons who have had a large adenomatous polyp. *American Journal of Gastroenterology* **91** 448–454

Parsons R, Li GM, Longley MJ, *et al* (1993) Hypermutability and mismatch repair deficiency in RER+ tumor cells. *Cell* **75** 1227–1236

Polyak K, Hamilton SR, Vogelstein B and Kinzler KW (1996) Early alteration of cell-cycle-regulated gene expression in colorectal neoplasia. *American Journal of Pathology* **149** 381–387

Ponder BAJ, Schmidt GH, Wilkinson MM, Wood M, Monk M and Reid A (1985) Derivation of mouse intestinal crypts from single progenitor cells. *Nature* **313** 689–691

Potten CS and Loeffler M (1990) Stem cells: attributes, cycles, spirals, pitfalls, and uncertainties. Lessons for and from the crypt. *Development* **110** 1001–1020

Richards B, Zhang H, Phear G and Meuth M (1997) Conditional mutator phenotypes in hMSH2-

deficient tumor cell lines. *Science* **277** 1523–1526

Schmidt GH, Winton DJ and Ponder BAJ (1988) Development of the pattern of cell renewal in the crypt-villus unit of chimaeric mouse small intestine. *Development* **103** 785–790

Shibata D (1997) Molecular tumor clocks and dynamic phenotype. *American Journal of Pathology* **151** 643–646

Shibata D, Schaeffer J, Li ZH, Capella G and Perucho M (1993) Genetic heterogeneity of the c-K-*ras* locus in colorectal adenomas but not adenocarcinomas. *Journal of the National Cancer Institute* **85** 1058–1063

Shibata D, Peinado MA, Ionov Y, Malkhosyan S and Perucho M (1994) Genomic instability in repeated sequences is an early somatic event in colorectal tumorigenesis that persists after transformation. *Nature Genetics* **6** 273–281

Shibata D, Navidi W, Salovaara R, Li ZH and Aaltonen LA (1996) Somatic microsatellite mutations as molecular tumor clocks. *Nature Medicine* **2** 676–681

Steele GG (1967) Cell loss as a factor in the growth rate of human tumors. *European Journal of Cancer* **3** 381–387

Steele GG (1977) *Growth Kinetics of Tumors,* pp 185–216, Clarendon, Oxford

Strand M, Prolla TA, Liskay RM and Petes TD (1993) Destabilization of tracts of simple repetitive DNA in yeast by mutations affecting DNA mismatch repair. *Nature* **365** 274–276

Strauss M, Lukas J and Bartek J (1995) Unrestricted cell cycling and cancer. *Nature Medicine* **1** 1245–1246

Streisinger G, Okada Y, Emrich J, Newton J, Tsugita A, Terzaghi E and Inouye M (1966) Frameshift mutations and the genetic code. *Cold Spring Harbor Symposia on Quantitative Biology* **31** 77–84

Thibodeau SN, Bren G and Schaid D (1993) Microsatellite instability in cancer of the proximal colon. *Science* **260** 816–819

Thorson AG, Lynch HT and Smyrk TC (1994) Rectal cancer in FAP patient after sulindac. *Lancet* **343** 180

Tsao JL, Davis SD, Baker SM, Liskay RM and Shibata D (1997) Intestinal stem cell divisions and genetic diversity: a computer and experimental analysis. *American Journal of Pathology* **151** 573–579

von Haeseler A, Sajantila A and Paabo S (1996) The genetic archaeology of the human genome. *Nature Genetics* **14** 135–140

Weber JL (1990) Informativeness of human (dC-dA)n.(dG-dT)n polymorphisms. *Genomics* **7** 524–530

Weber JL and Wong C (1993) Mutation of human short tandem repeats. *Human Molecular Genetics* **2** 1123–1128

Winton DJ, Blount MA and Ponder BAJ (1988) A clonal marker induced by mutation in mouse intestinal epithelium. *Nature* **333** 463–466

Winton DJ and Ponder BAJ (1990) Stem-cell organization in mouse small intestine. *Proceedings of the Royal Society of London B* **241** 13–18

The author is responsible for the accuracy of the references.

Precancer of the Human Cervix

J PONTÉN • ZHONGMIN GUO

Department of Genetics and Pathology, University of Uppsala, UAS, 751 85 Uppsala

INTRODUCTION

Cancer of the cervix is one of the common malignancies in women (Parkin *et al*, 1993). It has the epidemiological features of a sexually transmitted, very widely spread "endemic" disease, with human papillomavirus (HPV) as the important infectious agent (zur Hausen, 1977, 1987). Until the pioneering work of George Papanicolaou (Papanicolaou and Traut, 1943) not much was known about any lesions preceding clinical cancer. Vaginal cytology revolutionized the entire area. Dysplasia and cancer in situ (CIS) of the cervix are now the most widely studied human precancers. Outstanding questions are the precise aetiological and pathogenetic role of HPV and other factors and the determinants of progression to invasive cancer. An authoritative review exists (WHO, 1995).

PATHOLOGY

Conventionally dysplasia and CIS were defined in pure histological terms (see Burghardt, 1973), which took two main features into consideration: cellular atypia and degree of loss of differentiation. The elaborate original histological-

Cancer Surveys Volume 32: *Precancer: Biology, Importance and Possible Prevention*
© 1998 Imperial Cancer Research Fund. 0-87969-540-4/98. $5.00 + .00

ly based subdivisions have to a large extent been replaced by simplified schemes, either the cervical intraepithelial neoplasia (CIN) 1–3 scale (National Cancer Institute Workshop, 1989) or the low grade squamous intraepithelial lesion (LSIL)/high grade squamous intraepithelial lesion (HSIL) system. Although these are useful for practical purposes, they fail to deliver the rich information contained in tissue sections (Anderson *et al*, 1991). This chapter, with its tumour biological orientation, will therefore as much as possible draw from studies in which lesions have been studied in morphological detail and not only been cytologically defined. The fact that CIN 1 will by definition also contain lesions with cytological koilocytosis in the absence of any other atypia is a source of irreparable confusion (Crum and McLachlin, 1995).

Dysplasia and CIS have certain key features, which deserve attention as clues to understanding the disease.

First, sharp demarcation from surrounding normal epithelium and uniform morphology within the lesion suggest neoplastic expansion of cells "locked" in a fixed scheme of differentiation and expanding sideways at the expense of normal cells. This contrasts with hyperplasia, which probably involves a whole "field" of cells. The growth pattern suggests that precancers have taken their origin from a single cell (monoclonality) or a few cells (oligoclonality).

Second, there are large differences between individual lesions. Detailed examination has revealed apparently endless variations in the appearance of dysplasia (Burghardt, 1973). Three features are generally taken into account: (a) nuclear morphology, (b) pattern of disturbed differentiation and (c) intraepithelial disorder, namely differences between individual adjacent cells ("unicellular dyskeratosis"). Keen observation will for instance distinguish smooth uniform inhibition of differentiation across the entire height of the epithelium from abrupt resumption of differentiation at a certain level.

The degree of cellular atypia will generally correlate with lack of differentiation, but occasionally differentiation may seem to proceed normally in spite of very pronounced changes in shape and size of the nuclei.

Taken together, these features suggest sets of multiple genomic changes, the composition of which varies from lesion to lesion.

Third, no scheme for classification of dysplasia/CIS is satisfactory from a cell biological viewpoint. The conventional division into three grades of mild, moderate and severe dysplasia is an oversimplification, arbitrarily based on the relative thickness of poorly differentiated epithelial layers. For lack of a good alternative, and because most publications are founded on such a scheme, it will, however, be followed here.

Fourth, lesions are often multiple. The same cervix may contain two or more lesions, which occupy different areas and are separated by normal epithelium. There is a tendency towards a peripheral → central gradient in histological severity. Mild dysplasia lateral of the external os may for instance coexist with CIS at the transformation zone and endocervical invasive cancer (Burghardt and Ostor, 1983).

Salient but still unexplained morphological features of cervical precancer are shown in Fig. 1.

NATURAL HISTORY

The development of cervical cancer can be divided into two phases centred around the influence of HPV:

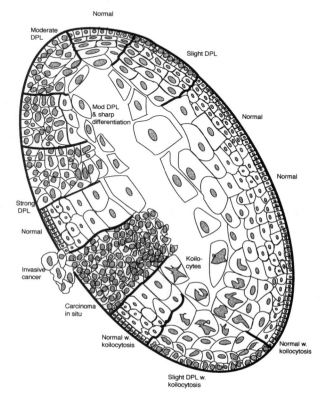

Fig. 1. Schematic representation of the salient features of cervical precancer and cancer. All precursors are shown with sharp lateral borders. Slight dysplasia (DPL) is depicted as a smooth transition from delicate cellular atypia mainly in the basal layer but with no significant atypia in spontaneously shed superficial cells. Moderate dysplasia is drawn as two variants, one with smooth transition from basal to superficial cells and the other with "sudden" differentiation along a horizontal line at about two-thirds of the total thickness of the epithelium. Differentiation should by definition be visible only in the top third of the epithelium. Strong dysplasia is illustrated by lack of differentiation in all but the most superficial layers. Carcinoma in situ should show no differentiation and moderate to severe cellular atypia. Illustrated is also the beginning of invasion, which typically is often accompanied by signs of differentiation, ie keratinization. With this exception invasive cancers tend to maintain a similarity with regard to atypia and differentiation pattern when compared with their precursors, which morphologically may range from moderate dysplasia to in situ cancer. Koilocytosis typically dominates in superficial squamous epithelium, in contrast to atypia associated with dysplasia, which will always be present in the basal epithelial layers. Slight dysplasia combined with koilocytosis is virtually impossible to single out with confidence as an entity, particularly if only cytological specimens are examined.

1. Infection by genital HPV
2. Development of morphological abnormalities.

Elucidation of the natural history of the disease has been hampered by the difficult propagation of HPV in vitro, few correlative morphological-virological studies, therapeutic intervention and lack of access to any robust method for in vitro cultivation of lesions under study. But in spite of these technical obstacles progress has been remarkable. We seem to be rapidly approaching a good understanding of a complex process.

INFECTION BY GENITAL HUMAN PAPILLOMAVIRUS (HPV)

Human Types of HPV

Many vertebrate species are carriers of their own kind of papillomavirus. Human papillomaviruses have never been found in non-humans. Close to 100 different types of HPV have been defined, and still no ceiling has been reached. By convention a new type is accepted when its gene sequence in L1 differs by over 10% from any previously known type. Subtypes have 2–10% divergence and variants less than 2% (van Ranst *et al*, 1993; Berard *et al*, 1994). One group of HPV has, because of its dominant target, been termed mucosal. It is within this group that the approximately 30 genital types are found.

The slow rate at which HPV has evolved, the relatively similar distribution of types in widely separated geographical locations and the small intratype diversity suggest that HPV evolved in extinct hominoid species in Africa before *Homo sapiens* emerged and migrated to other continents, carrying with it a spectrum of HPV types (Ong *et al*, 1993). This has given both host and virus ample time for mutual adaptation.

HPV types are noted for their tissue tropism and consequent association with a variety of site specific pathological lesions, many of which are neoplastic. However, these traits are not absolute—classical mucosal types such as HPV 16 have, for instance, been detected in precancer and cancer of the skin (Wieland and Pfister, 1997). HPV 16 is not only the best studied type but is also most prevalent in cervical cancer and precancer, where it has been found in about 50% of all HPV positive samples from cervical cancer. Together the high risk types (Table 1) constitute 94% of all HPV found in association with invasive cancer (Bosch *et al*, 1995).

Genital HPV types have been divided into high and low risk groups. There are, however, no unambiguous criteria for such a division, which is based on prevalence figures related to in situ/invasive cancer or condyloma/mild dysplasia, respectively. Borders are further blurred if one also takes the possibility into consideration that subtypes and variants may be differently associated with pathologies of different clinical grades of malignancy.

HPV 16 is the prototype "high risk" HPV. Low risk types are represented by types 6 and 11, because of their common occurrence in condyloma.

TABLE 1. HPV types grouped according to their association with precancer/cancer (high risk) and condyloma (low risk)

Risk	HPV types
Low	6, 11, 30, 42, 43, 44
High	16, 18, 31, 33, 35, 39, 45, 52, 58, 59, 68

Types closely related to HPV 16 are underlined. Remaining high risk types are related to HPV 18

The HPV Genome

The viral genome is outlined in Fig. 2. It is present either in free episomal form or as an integrated sequence of nucleotides.

The E6 and E7 gene products are considered crucial for the disturbed growth control. The genes have been labeled "oncogenes" because of their transforming capacity in vitro. E6 protein will, via binding of intermediate cellular proteins, activate and direct the ubiquitin pathway towards destruction of TP53—an event which, by analogy with other human cancers, is believed to relax DNA repair and thus facilitate accumulation of mutations (Huibregtse and Beaudenon, 1996; Liu *et al*, 1997). E6 would then only be an indirectly working "oncogene".

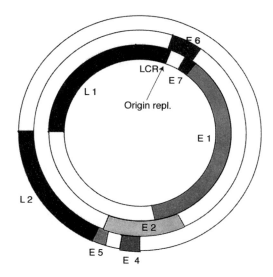

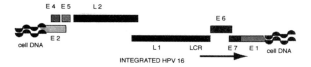

Fig.2. Genome of HPV 16. The long control region (LCR) contains enhancers and other control elements. E = early and L = late viral genes. The integrated genome is depicted with disrupted E2 and E1 genes

E7 forms inactivating complexes with RB, which in turn releases transcription factors important for cell cycle stimulation. Additionally E7 interacts with the cyclin/cyclin dependent kinase system, further enhancing deregulation of the cell cycle (Funk *et al*, 1997; Jones *et al*, 1997; Morozov *et al*, 1997; Ruesch and Laimins, 1997). E6 and E7 proteins from HPV 16 bind much more strongly to their respective targets than the corresponding gene products from low risk HPV 6, which could be the important explanation for the difference in oncogenic risk profile.

Another line of inquiry stems from the observation that permanent upregulation of the transcripts for E6 and E7 is a common phenomenon in HPV associated cancer. Since this is accompanied by reduced capacity for differentiation, including synthesis of infectious virus, it is a dead end that the virus must avoid. Control is exerted from the LCR region (Fig. 2), where four identical E2 binding sites exist. E2 from high risk HPV types binds to one or both of the E2 binding sites 2 and 3. Binding represses transcription from an upstream promoter of E6. These events are characteristic of HPV as long as it is present in episomal form. But after integration, which typically disrupts E2, the control chain will be broken.

Low risk types of HPV have an additional promoter for E6, which would permit E2 to regulate E6 and E7 separately.

The picture above is even more complex, since regulation of E6 and E7, separately or in conjunction, is dependent on the stage of squamous cell differentiation and probably also histiogenetic derivation (eg, endocervical, mucosal, epidermal).

A recent study has begun to unwind a very intricate web of binding sites with different affinity for E2 and different potential to influence transcription from E6 and E7. An important conclusion is that HPV 6, in contrast to high risk HPV, is equipped with the necessary molecular machinery to double check regulation of E6 and E7. As a consequence, HPV 6 is able to sustain cell differentiation required for viral synthesis and avoid the virological disaster of non-productive malignant transformation, fully in keeping with the rarity with which HPV 6 is associated with cervical cancer (Rapp *et al*, 1997). But it still remains to be explained why most HPV 16 infections do not lead to any disruption of cell cycle control and why HPV 6 efficiently induces proliferation in the form of papillomatous condylomata.

No proof exists that any HPV genes are independently and directly capable of transforming human keratinocytes in vivo. Their association with and expression in precancer and cancer may depend on some rare cellular event, such as integration at specific sites and/or fortuitous mutations in cellular genes.

Integration of HPV, which is possible at multiple cellular sites, typically involves partial deletion of E1 and E2 (Sanchez Perez, 1997) but with no direct effect on E6 and E7. The impact of integration on the cell can be manifold: (a) cellular genes at the integration site may be silenced or unduly stimulated, (b) recombination of cellular and viral DNA may lead to abnormal transcription products, (c) E6 and E7 may be expressed in an uncontrolled manner, (d) multiple integrated HPV copies may have bewildering effects via interference with cellular genes and increased E6/E7 gene dosage and (e) the viral gene will persist in the cell lineage arising from the HPV carrier cell, ie it can potentially serve as a marker of clonality.

The Infectious Cycle

The application of classical virological methods to human HPV has not been possible owing to lack of a suitable in vitro system. Bovine papillomavirus has been used instead as the preferred virological model. Extrapolation to humans is, however, risky, firstly, because established rodent rather than bovine target cells have been used and, secondly, because fibroblasts rather than epithelial target cells have been studied (Leptak *et al*, 1991; Riese and DiMaio, 1995). Interesting observations about the platelet derived growth factor beta receptor as a target for papillomavirus mitogenic signalling (Nilson and DiMaio, 1993) and the E5 protein as a transforming factor are therefore not immediately applicable to human biology (Petti *et al*, 1997).

In human epithelium infection is believed to occur via microabrasions. Basally located stem cells are thought of as the important target cells. Few if any infectious HPV copies are produced by these cells, but as they mature during migration towards the mucosal surface, infectious virus particles are produced in abundance (Parker *et al*, 1997), as shown by immunohistochemistry. Some of the virus producing cells undergo a typical cytological change termed "koilocytosis" (Koss and Durfee, 1956; Koss *et al*, 1963). At this stage HPV seems to exist exclusively as episomes, and there is ample opportunity for spread to other people via genital contact and for infection of new genital mucosa and probably also other organs.

Persistent Infection

When no morphological responses are noted, HPV infection seems to subside within a fairly short time. A recent study of 20 year old college women based on repeated sampling during 36 months revealed important facts. About 60% of the 608 participants had become positive at the end of the study period. The number of women who became positive declined as time went by, but during the last 12 months 9% were still added to the already infected cohort. Extension of the observation period would therefore have yielded a higher total than 60% positive. The important conclusion is that a very high proportion of sexually active women will acquire an HPV infection (Ho *et al*, 1998). The usual risk factors connected to sexual behaviour increased the likelihood of infection, which incidentally was not diminished by the use of condoms. The other side of the coin was that HPV positivity subsided within 7–10 months, confirming a previous direct observation of elimination of HPV in two thirds of HPV positive women after one year (Velasco *et al*, 1996). High risk types persisted longer than low risk types (Hildesheim *et al*, 1994).

The mechanism behind the disappearance of HPV may be partly immunological, because antibodies and cellular immunity against viral proteins are known to be elicited (Dillner *et al*, 1989; Dillner, 1992; Müller *et al*, 1992; Olsen *et al*, 1996). It may also reflect a physiologically limited lifespan of the infected epithelial cells.

Some reports have claimed that HPV can persist in and even transform (Shiga *et al*, 1997) mesenchymal cells in humans, but this aspect of the infection has not been well studied. Bovine fibroblasts will, on the other hand, without difficulty support growth of bovine papillomavirus.

Taken together these observations suggest that prevalence studies are bound to give a very incomplete and often misleading picture of the natural history of HPV infection (Svare *et al*, 1998). In reality a very large proportion of women are probably infected, and the longer after infection that the analysis for HPV is performed the more likely it is that no signs of a past infection are picked up.

HPV in Human Populations

Genital HPV is present in all human populations, with broadly similar prevalence in both sexes even including different types.

In females an abundance of studies have been published comparing prevalence of HPV, usually in vaginal smears, in women with cytological abnormalities indicative of dysplasia or CIS and matched controls.

The results have been similar enough to form a basis for consensus about increased prevalence of HPV in dysplasia/CIS and invasive cancer groups compared with women without pathological findings. Almost 100% of women with dysplasia/CIS have HPV genomes present in their smears. A worldwide survey of invasive cervical cancer in 22 different regions demonstrated an average prevalence of 93%, with only little variation from population to population. Type 16 (52%) and HPV 18 (15%) dominated. The HPV 16 related group (16, 31, 33, 35, 52, 58) represented 67% and the type 18 related group (18, 39, 45, 59, 68) 27%, leaving only 6% for all other 14 types sought (Bosch *et al*, 1995).

Age matched controls for women with dysplasia/CIS or invasive cancer have, with one notable exception (a comparison between Denmark and Greenland [Kjær *et al*, 1989; Kjær and Jensen, 1992; Sebbelov *et al*, 1994]), a lower prevalence, the magnitude of which has been very differently reported. The lower prevalence of HPV DNA in healthy females has generally been ascribed to less exposure to virus, mainly because of a low number of male partners. Prevalence of HPV should critically depend on the time since last exposure to effective transmission of HPV. Since signs of infection in the form of detectable HPV DNA may peak and subside differently even comparisons between populations of the same age may be meaningless (Svare *et al*, 1998) and could explain the exceptional data referred to above (Kjær and Jensen, 1992).

Few studies have examined males not selected because of their partnership with HPV infected women. HPV DNA was present in 16.5% of Finnish conscripts (Hippelainen *et al*, 1994a) and in about 30–60% of men attending a clinic for sexually transmitted diseases (Strand *et al*, 1995). Sexual promiscuity was associated with increased risk of being an HPV carrier.

Men selected because of dysplasia/CIS/invasive cancer in their female partners have consistently shown a higher prevalence of HPV than men with female partners who have no morphological signs of HPV infection. One could expect that sexual partners would share the same types of HPV, but, surprisingly, concordance for HPV typing between sexual partners has generally been low or moderate (Hippelainen *et al*, 1994b; Bar Am *et al*, 1995; Strand *et al*, 1995; Gomousa *et al*, 1997). Results are, however, hard to evaluate, because intercourse with multiple partners outside of the index relationship may have occurred.

The long term fate of HPV in males is virtually unknown. Persistence is possible, as evidenced by isolation of viral DNA in penile squamous cell cancer, but the natural history of common asymptomatic infections over time remains to be elucidated. One small study showed essentially the same decrease in prevalence among men as in women as a function of time after first intercourse (Svare *et al*, 1998).

Condylomata and dysplasia have been actively looked for in symptom free men with virologically diagnosed HPV infection. After peniscopy flat condyloma like lesions and dysplasia of various degrees have been established, including the presence of koilocytosis. Such lesions had a high prevalence of HPV DNA compared with the surrounding normal epithelium (Hippelainen *et al*, 1993). Correlative studies of morphology versus the presence of HPV have demonstrated a high prevalence of HPV in condylomata and dysplasia but have also highlighted the impossibility of relating non-neoplastic papular and macular lesions to presence of HPV (Hippelainen *et al*, 1993; Strand *et al*, 1996).

An interesting comparison (Castellsague *et al*, 1997) was made between males in areas with low (Spain) and high (Colombia) incidence of cervical cancer. Husbands of control women defined by absence of cervical neoplasia in the high risk area had a fivefold higher penile HPV DNA prevalence than the corresponding husbands in the low risk area. In the low risk area men, who presumably had acquired their high risk types of HPV by promiscuous sexual practices, were prone to increase risk of their wives for developing cervical neoplasia (Bosch *et al*, 1996). On the other hand, in the high risk area it was not possible to correlate male sexual behaviour and presence of HPV with risk among wives to develop cervical neoplasia (Munoz *et al*, 1996).

Sexual contacts are essential for transmission of genital HPV. Promiscuity has a central role, especially in maintaining a male reservoir. Genital HPV has presumably adapted to this kind of human behaviour by restricting its target cell range to the genital sphere and keeping cytopathogenicity to a minimum. If rare lifelong mono- or oligogamous relations are excepted, a large majority of humans will be infected by HPV mainly during a few crucial years after their sexual debut. Regardless of HPV types, infections will be transient but last long enough to ensure that viruses persist in the population. Prevalence of HPV differs between different populations, but not to the same degree as incidence of cancer or precancer (Munoz *et al*, 1993; Gustafsson *et al*, 1997a). Since all types of HPV seem to be represented in roughly equal proportions regardless of geographical location and since intertype recombinations are unknown, each type can be assumed to have its own "miniepidemic sphere". In a small proportion of females and males low risk types represented by HPV 6 and 11 will cause fibropapillomas (condyloma accuminata) or flat condylomata. These are hot spots of synthesis of HPV, as suggested by intense koilocytosis, which, however, decreases as the lesions regress. In an even lower proportion of infected women dysplasia and/or carcinoma in situ will develop. In these lesions HPV will persist, probably with retention of some infectivity. Type 16 and 18 and their relatives dominate this development. In men dysplasia and CIS may also occur, but at much lower rates than in females, making males a symptom free reservoir of all HPV types.

In the interest of viral maintenance, development of condyloma would be advantageous. It is not life threatening and probably does not impair sexual activity. The common asymptomatic transient mucosal infection may not be sufficient to maintain HPV 6/11 and therefore needs "help" from more infectious condylomata. This scheme, centred around the importance of condylomata, could be sufficient for HPV 6/11 but will leave persistence of the common type 16 less well explained. Its association with in situ and invasive cancer in integrated form is obviously a virological dead end. It is currently unclear whether HPV 16 and other high risk types are maintained by being contagious in subclinical infections under very long periods or whether periodically they are produced in large copy numbers. This question is particularly relevant for males.

By around age 40–50 detection of HPV has declined to low levels. Most infections seem to have vanished, and new infections are uncommon—reflecting altered sexual habits, acquired immunity and possibly a decline in the number of stem cells susceptible to HPV. This apparent cure does not exclude the persistence of HPV in latent undetected form in a few scattered stem cells, which after a long latent time may start to grow as precursors of invasive cervical cancer or remain dormant for the rest of the woman's life.

DEVELOPMENT OF MORPHOLOGICAL ABNORMALITIES

Condylomata have been studied ultrastructurally and immunohistochemically for the presence of HPV capsid antigens and recognizable virions. Many studies have concentrated on koilocytes as indicators of viral maturation. Most reports have shown over 50% prevalence of viral particles and/or capsid antigen in koilocytes (Ferenczy *et al*, 1981; Sato *et al*, 1986; Yun and Sherwood, 1992). The point was made that condylomata, as they persist or recur, tend to have less koilocytosis and visible viral antigen in spite of persistence of HPV DNA, as revealed by molecular methods (Sato *et al*, 1986; Yun and Sherwood, 1992).

Koilocytosis should not be regarded as atypia in the sense used for precancers (see introductory chapter by Pontén) but rather as a viral cytopathic effect. This does not preclude that, as has been claimed by keen observers, one may find combinations of "genuine" atypia and koilocytosis in dysplasia. But interobserver variation is too large to make such subtle distinctions reliable, and "koilocytes" combined with dysplasia tend not to contain viral antigens (McCluggage *et al*, 1996).

The mechanism by which low risk (and occasionally also high risk) HPV drives mesenchymal and squamous epithelial cells to self limited but often intense proliferation is unknown, but papillomata are the only indisputable common morphological response to papillomaviruses from all species, hence the name of this class of virus is most appropriate.

The Transformation Zone

Microscopical scrutiny has convinced students of cervical cancer that the originally transformed cell is located at the transformation zone, that is precancer takes its origin from only a small region of the entire cervix.

The origin of precancer from a very small area poses tumour biological problems, which have not been sufficiently considered. The multistep clonal theory of cancer requires that one target cell (usually a stem cell) has suffered a number of mutations, after which it transforms, possibly via intermediate precancer stages, to begin clonal expansion as malignant neoplasia. The transformation zone is small, with a surface area of perhaps 0.1 cm². From microscopical inspection, basal cell density seems similar to that of adult skin—1.4×10^5 basal cells/cm² (Weinstein, 1984). By analogy with skin, only a proportion of basal cells, perhaps 10% (Heenen and Galand, 1997), are stem cells. This will give only approximately $0.1 \times 0.1 \times 1.4 \times 10^5 = 1400$ stem cells per transformation zone. If three or more independent genetic hits are required for neoplasia to commence in a multihit scenario this number is far too small (Loeb, 1996) to be compatible with spontaneous somatic mutation. A low number of stem cells in the transformation zone and the fact that dysplasia and its presumed sequelae are common in females strongly suggest that spontaneous background rate of mutation, conventional endogenous abrogation of DNA repair and physicochemical exogenous mutagenic hits will never explain cervical precancer. The only biologically reasonable mechanism would be viral or bacterial infection, which results in excessive mutability in a large number of target cells. This could be caused by cycles of intra- and extracellular reinfection, multiple points of viral insertion, mobilization of movable cellular genetic elements or a high mutation/recombination rate of a causative virus.

Nobody has attempted to closely characterize the target cell for neoplasia in the transformation zone. One would suspect a stem cell with capacity to differentiate in direction of squamous and/or glandular cells, because (a) combinations of adenocarcinoma and squamous cell carcinoma are common, (b) atypia in squamous cells is often accompanied by atypia also in glandular cells and (c) metaplasia—a common response to trauma and/or inflammation—has features of both squamous and glandular cell differentiation compatible with origin from a "bipotential" stem cell (Fig. 3).

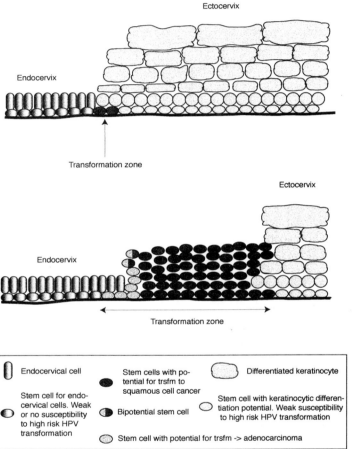

Fig. 3. Schematic drawing of a likely structure of the human transformation zone. The suggested composition is conjectured from morphological evidence, histopathology of HPV associated lesions and knowledge about the restricted host range of HPV. It can only be regarded as a model, still without sufficient experimental backing. The non-traumatized, non-inflamed transformation zone (above) has a sharp border between endocervical cylindrical epithelium and multi-layered ectocervical squamous epithelium. Each type of epithelium is thought to be maintained by its own kind of stem cells, possibly with addition of some bipotential stem cells capable of differentiation either to cylindrical mucus producing endocervical cells or to squamous cells covering the ectocervix. The compartment of stem cells susceptible to HPV infection is small. The lower panel shows the transformation zone after childbirth and/or chronic non-specific infections. It is broadened and populated by an increased number of stem cells susceptible to HPV infection and to the development of dysplasia, CIS and invasive cancer

The strange feature that milder forms of dysplasia tend to involve peripheral parts of the cervix in contrast to centrally placed CIS and invasive cancer has never received a satisfactory explanation. Speculatively, different subsets of stem cells could be involved, or the growth pattern could depend on differences at the level of the infecting HPV genome. For condyloma there is an even more striking preference for peripherally located squamous epithelium, because these lesions often locate to the ectocervix and vagina.

Alternatives for Development of Precancer

Two major hypotheses are outlined in Fig. 4. Morphological progression (upper panel) postulates a stepwise one way progression from slight → moderate → severe dysplasia → CIS → invasive cancer. This scheme does not imply that all precursors of cancer progress, only that lesions of higher grade have generally been preceded by lesions of lower grade. There is both direct and indirect evidence that only a minority of low grade precursors progress to higher grades and CIS that does not inevitably progress to invasive cancer. By longitudinal follow-up Nasiell showed 16% progression from slight dysplasia to severe dyspla-

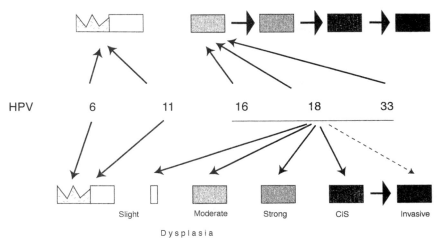

Fig. 4. Two hypotheses for the interrelations between precancer and invasive cervical cancer. The upper panel postulates no important biological difference between slight dysplasia and condyloma. Both are the result of infection by low risk HPV, usually type 6 or 11. They represent, presumably polyclonal, proliferative-cytopathic lesions (CIN1), which gradually regress and have no increased likelihood of progression into moderate dysplasia (CIN2), strong dysplasia/CIS (CIN3) or invasive cancer. The high risk types exemplified by 16, 18, and 33 produce moderate dysplasia, which will either regress or because of poorly characterized co-factors progress to invasive cancer via strong dysplasia/CIS to invasive cancer. The lower panel postulates that each lesion is independently induced by a given type. Type 16 is then, for example, capable of directly inducing anything from slight dysplasia to CIS or even (as suggested by the interrupted arrow) invasive cancer. Only CIS can be regarded a precursor of invasive cancer—dysplasias do not generally progress from low to high grade. The likelihood of progression of CIS to invasive cancer may be governed by differences in the viral genome (eg variant DNA sequences) or the presence of co-carcinogens

sia/CIS (Nasiell *et al*, 1986) and 30% from moderate dysplasia to severe dysplasia/CIS (Nasiell *et al*, 1983). The time from slight/moderate dysplasia to severe dysplasia/CIN was 3.5–4.5 years. Epidemiological data (Gustafsson and Adami, 1989), as well as a small series of direct observations of CIS without interference (Kottmeier, 1955), have indicated that 15–70% of CIS progress to invasive cervical cancer after a period of some 10 years.

Data of the type above, reviewed by Pontén *et al* (1994), provide evidence that regression or at least absence of progression of precursors of invasive cervical cancer is common. For unexplained reasons the likelihood of progression has scored lower in epidemiological than in clinicocytopathological studies. No data have revealed anything about the mechanism, where at least three alternatives are possible. First, immunological defence eliminates precursors either by attacking the cells themselves or by hindering intercellular spread of HPV. There is no direct evidence of immunological elimination. The fact that precursors are more common in immunosuppressed women (Petry *et al*, 1996) only indicates that development of dysplasia/CIS is facilitated by compromised immunity, not that the immune response is capable of erasing already present lesions. Second, diagnostic and/or therapeutic interference. Although this may have played a part in some studies, the ones quoted above do not suffer from any bias due to removal of lesions. Third, time dependent "physiological" elimination of lesions before progression. The dynamics of precursors of cervical cancer are imperfectly known. There is a possibility that putative stem cells from which the lesions take their origin may not be immortal but rather have a limited lifespan measured in number of possible cell cycles. Once this potential is exhausted, stem cells would irreversibly enter terminal differentiation and be eliminated. HPV 16 is capable of immortalizing human keratinocytes (Pirisi *et al*, 1988; Steenbergen *et al*, 1996)—a process that is accompanied by pronounced activation of CDKN2A, an inhibitor of the CDK-cyclin/RB cascade. This event was not coupled to malignant transformation (Nakao *et al*, 1997). It has also been observed that telomerase was activated in connection with immortalization and that invasive cancers, in contrast to normal epithelium, had high levels of telomerase (Anderson *et al*, 1997). Although these experiments hint at immortalization as an important prerequisite for invasive cancer to develop, they do not prove that the difference between regressors and progressors among invasive cervical cancer precursors is linked to immortalization and/or activation of telomerase. The reason for the common occurrence of regression among cervical cancer precursors is as obscure as the reason for total absence of regression once the step to invasiveness has been taken.

The stepwise theory makes the strong prediction that the same stable marker should be present in the cell populations as they traverse the different precursor stages. The hypothesis for this type of genetic progression is that it occurs by selection of more and more "fit" subclones and that the progression continues also when invasive cancer has finally developed. Theoretically, the earliest precursor lesion could either be monoclonal, ie it originates from one cell, or polyclonal, ie it starts from several cells that have more or less simultaneously undergone the phenotypic change which defines, for instance, slight dysplasia. But the subclones that subsequently by selection form more advanced stages of precancer would be expected to be clonal in the sense that they arose from a single cell, which because of genetic progression was able to take one further step towards cancer.

Ideally the marker for clonality should be neutral, that is it should carry no selective advantage or disadvantage. So far the presence of a paternally or maternally inactivated X chromosome has been most useful in human studies (Lyon, 1992).

X chromosome inactivation as a marker of monoclonality ideally requires that normal stem cells from which a given neoplasm is assumed to originate are randomly spread as single units. Such a fine mosaic of "cell tiles" with inactivation of either the paternal or maternal X chromosome cannot be expected in all (or any?) tissues. Therefore the derivation of a monoclonal pattern of any cell population from a field of stem cells with identical X chromosome inactivation usually cannot be excluded. It may thus be spurious (see Fig. 5).

Apart from genetic linkage an argument in favour of morphological progression is simply that removal of precursors should protect against subsequent development of higher degrees of dysplasia or cancer. The strength of this argument is not, however, absolute in cervical pathology, because any treatment of dysplasia or CIS will inevitably also remove a large part of normal cervix, including the transformation zone. It cannot be excluded that removal of target cells for transformation, rather than removal of the precursors themselves, is responsible for a beneficial therapeutic effect of screening (Gustafsson *et al*, 1997b).

Independent development of precancer implies that each lesion has developed separately and then lives its own life. The hypothesis predicts that (a) if multiple lesions exist in the same cervix there would be no genetic link between them and (b) progression, as inferred from emergence of for instance CIS in a case of mild dysplasia followed for many years, is not real but rather depends on de novo development of a second lesion.

Cervical precancer would in this scenario be regarded as lesions developing in a field with multiple foci of HPV infection, which independently of each other develop their own morphological form. The latent time until dysplasia would then be shorter than that for CIS to explain slight but significant differences in peak age incidence (Storm *et al*, 1989).

In its pure form the theory does not make predictions about clonality. Lesions could be polyclonal or monoclonal, depending on the conditions behind a transformation to precancer or cancer. There will be no requirement for selection of "fit" subclones.

Stepwise Progression versus Independent Development of Precancer

Using the X chromosome as marker (Enomoto *et al*, 1997), in situ and invasive cancer have consistently scored as monoclonal ie they were likely derived from a single transformed cell. Recently we have begun to analyse concomitantly pre-

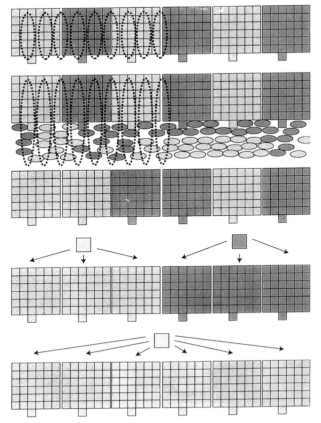

Fig. 5. Clonality analysis by X chromosome inactivation. Each 6 **x** 6 square denotes an epithelial proliferative unit. All cells are derived from a single stem cell (small square at the bottom of the unit). Only the stem cell is capable of self renewal, the other cells and their progeny disappear in terminal differentiation after a variable number of cell divisions. Panel 2 from top also contains a number of mesenchymal stroma cells. Cells are shaded according to the inactivated X chromosome (light, paternal; dark, maternal). Dotted ovals indicate samples removed for molecular analysis of X chromosome inactivation. The uppermost panel shows the ideal state of an alternating 1:1 mixture of paternally or maternally inactivated units. Small samples will then, with exception of those which by chance include parts of two adjacent units, faithfully indicate monoclonality of the units. Panel 2 from top shows how inclusion of stroma inevitably will obscure a monoclonal pattern because the cells will not be distributed in conformity with the epithelial distribution. Virtually all reports about clonality have not considered this source of error. Panel 3 shows adjacent units with identical X chromosome inactivation. Even a large sample, for instance from the two units to the left, will score monoclonal in spite of being derived from two different stem cells. Panels 4 and 5 are probably more realistic, since they show a situation where X chromosome inactivation has taken place already before creation of the proliferative units. In both, monoclonal signals will obtain from the two units at the left, giving the erroneous impression that the sample has been derived from a single cell, an impression which extends to even larger sizes of samples removed for X chromosome inactivation analysis

sent strong dysplasia/CIS and invasive cancer to establish a genetic link (Guo *et al*, 1998b). In 5 of 8 cases the same X chromosome was inactivated in both lesions, indicating that they belong to the same cell clone (Table 2). In several instances the conclusion of monoclonality was reinforced by finding a polyclon-al X chromosome inactivation pattern in normal epithelium, which at least shows that mixtures of cells with paternally or maternally inactivated X chro-mosomes are present in the human cervix. The impression of monoclonality was further substantiated by analysis of pattern of loss of heterozygosity (LOH), which was similar in CIS and invasive cancer. If any difference occurred it always had the form of addition of LOH at a new site. Fig. 6 shows LOH on

TABLE 2. Clonality was investigated by X chromosome inactivation in formalin fixed cervical specimens from preinvasive lesions only (Group A) or invasive lesions with concomitant precancers (Group B)

Case No.	type of tissue	X inactivation pattern	I	II	III	IV	V
Group A							
C34	SCE	M1				M2	
C36	SCE	M1		M2			
C40	Mixed	P			M1		
C43	Mixed	P		M1			
C44	SCE	P		P	P		
C45	SCE	M2		M2*			
C50	Mixed	P		P	P		
C51	SCE	M1			M1*	M1*	
C53	Mixed	P	P				
C54	SCE	P		M2			
C57	SCE	P			M1		
C60	Mixed	M1		M2			
Group B							
C04	Mixed	P				M1	M1
C26	Mixed	P				M1	M2
C27	SCE	M1				M2	M2
C28	Mixed	M1				M1*	M1*
C58	Mixed	P			M1	M1	M1
C76	SCE	M2				M2	M1
C82	SCE	P		M1			M1
C83	Mixed	M1			M2	M1*	M1*
C88	Mixed	P	M1				M1
C89	SCE	M1				M1	M1

Polyacrylamide gel electrophoresis after *Hha*1 digestion and PCR amplification of a polymorphic site in the androgen receptor gene retrived from microdissected areas was employed. Retention of both alleles after enzyme digestion indicated a polyclonal pattern (P), whereas retention of either the larger (M1) or the small-er (M2) allele was interpreted as monoclonality.

chromosome 3 in cervical squamous carcinoma and simultaneously present pre-cancers detected by fluorescence-dUTP-labelled microsatellite markers derived from the Genethon map. Allelic deletion of one or more loci on 3p was present in 8 of 10 cases. In the majority identical patterns of allelic loss were seen in invasive cancers and synchronous precancers, compatible with stepwise selection of cells of increasingly "high grade". Findings also indicate that LOH is an early event, since it was observed in moderate (but not slight) dysplasia (Guo *et al*, 1998a; Guo Z, Hu X, Afink G, Wilander E and Pontén J, unpublished).

Taken together these data provide strong evidence that in situ cancer is clonal neoplasia, which by genetic and morphological progression acquires the additional property of invasiveness.

Studies of low grade precancer are still preliminary but suggest a more complicated picture than with CIS/invasive cancer.

One case of CIN 2 (Enomoto *et al*, 1997) was shown to be polyclonal. In our own series (Guo Z, Pontén F, Wilander E, Sällström J and Pontén J, unpublished) we found 1/2 mild, 2/8 moderate and 2/9 strong dysplasias to be polyclonal (Table 2). As elaborated in Fig. 5, these figures are minimal. The conclusion is that a proportion of dysplasias, the magnitude of which remains to be determined, are polyclonal cell proliferations.

In 3 of 8 cases of coexisting dysplasia, CIS and/or invasive cancer different patterns have emerged with either independent dysplasias or dysplasias with the same X chromosome inactivation as in situ or invasive cancer (Table 2). This demonstrates that a proportion of CIS/invasive cancers have not been derived from coexisting dysplasia, which then must have been initiated as independent precancers (Guo Z, Pontén F, Wilander E, Sällström J and Pontén J, unpublished).

All facts taken together suggest that cervical cancer and precursors can use both paths of Fig. 4. At the end of development stepwise progression is employed at least for CIS → invasive cancer. The beginning of a possible development towards CIS can only partly be linked to stepwise progression from dysplasia. Mild and moderate dysplasias can to an unknown extent arise as independent and even polyclonal lesions (Fig. 7). Some, particularly those with aneuploid DNA content (Kashyap *et al*, 1990), may undergo stepwise progression to higher grades of precancer, but this is far from proven because genetic marker studies are lacking. Current data support the rationality of removing CIS and strong dysplasia, but provide no definite clue as to how to prevent considerable overtreatment (Bergström *et al*, 1993; Adami *et al*, 1994).

Role of HPV Genome in Precancer and Cancer

The two outstanding questions are: (a) How does the HPV genome participate in the creation of the various phenotypes that characterize cervical precancer and cancer and (b) What is the role of HPV for the genetic and morphological

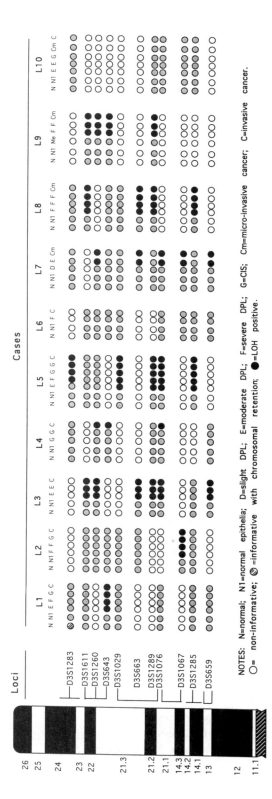

Fig. 6. LOH on chromosome 3 in cervical squamous carcinoma and simultaneously present precancers was detected by fluorescence-dUTP-labelled microsatellite markers derived from the Genethon map. Allelic deletion of one or more loci on 3p was present in 8/10 cases. In the majority identical patterns of allelic loss were seen in invasive cancers and synchronous precancers compatible with stepwise selection of cells of increasingly high grade. Findings also indicate that LOH is an early event, since it was observed in moderate (but not slight) dysplasia

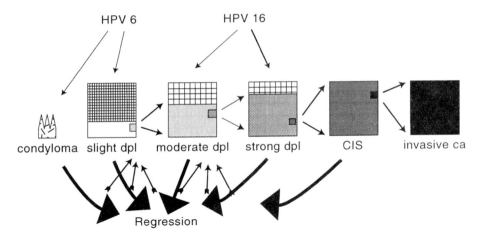

Fig. 7. Hypothesis for the pathogenesis of cervical cancer. HPV 6 and 16, as examples of low and high risk types, respectively, will infect stem cells in the transformation zone. In the majority of instances HPV either disappears or remains undetected in a few cells. The target cells are probably epigenetically different; cells infected with type 6 have the exclusive capacity for squamous cell differentiation and tend to occupy a wide zone peripheral to the transformation zone in contrast to the stem cells susceptible to HPV 16, which can differentiate in both adenomatous and squamous cell directions from the narrow transformation zone. Type 18 may be slightly more likely than type 16 to drive cells in the first direction (Toshima et al, 1997). The stem cells will, in the case of HPV 6, form fibropapillomata or flat condylomata probably as a direct result of the virus infection without any need for a second hit. The prediction is that all condylomata and a large proportion of slight dysplasias will be polyclonal proliferations of cells (hatched pattern) multiplying under the influence of viral genomes. A few cells in slight dysplasias may, after long latent times, mainly because of genetic instability caused by HPV but possibly reinforced (arrows with tail flights) by extraneous mutagens (cigarette smoking?), acquire critical mutations, which involve growth/differentiation control and permit clonal expansion. Moderate and strong dysplasias may be caused by HPV 16, originally possibly as polyclonal proliferations exclusively driven by viral genomes. An occasional cell will, because of selection from a genetically unstable background, begin clonal expansion and progress to a higher grade. CIS is exclusively derived by clonal expansion of a single cell from previous dysplasia. Invasive cancer is similarly by selection derived from a single subclone of pre-existing CIS. The model predicts considerable heterogeneity within the dysplasia categories. Moderate dysplasia may for example be composed of (a) polyclonally multiplying cells directly driven by the HPV 16 genome (hatched area), (b) clonally expanding cells derived by somatic mutation/selection from a previous slight dysplasia (light shaded area) and (c) a subclone (small dark shaded area) prepared to start severe dysplasia after selection and settlement in another part of the cervix. Immortalization is regularly present only in invasive cancer

progression, which now seems firmly established at least for CIS/severe dysplasia → invasive cancer?

The aetiological role of HPV implies that infection is a necessary part of the creation of a precancerous or a malignant phenotype. The evidence that supports this is very strong. Cervical precancer and cancer behave as sexually transmissible diseases. No agent other than HPV meets the epidemiological and virological criteria of being causative. But in view of the high general prevalence of HPV infection it cannot formally be excluded that other factors or influences connected with sexual behaviour are necessary or could even substitute for HPV. Stringent proof of the necessity of HPV for precancer and cancer can probably not be delivered until the virus can be eliminated with vaccination and a sharp reduction in the incidence of precancer and cancer of the cervix subsequently observed.

If one accepts the necessary aetiological role of HPV, several questions remain. For HPV 6, 11 and other types capable of giving papillomatous or flat overgrowth of squamous epithelium, it remains to be shown which viral genes are instrumental for a well balanced disturbance of proliferation and differentiation control. Most studies have been molecular or virological, concentrating on mechanisms of viral reproduction, which seems similar in all species with elaborate control from the LCR region (Fig. 2). There is an indication that RNA splicing in papilloma is different, depending on the state of differentiation of infected squamous cells (Barksdale and Baker, 1995). It also seems as if cells separately infected with two different types of HPV segregate in sectors within the same lesion (Christensen *et al*, 1997). The rare event of papillomas undergoing transformation to cancer apparently depends on secondary events (Gaukroger *et al*, 1993), including activation of EJ-RAS in Shope rabbit papilloma (Peng *et al*, 1996).

In attempts to understand progression, the prevailing approach has been to tackle the problem only indirectly, ie to analyse virological properties of different lesions in situ or as established cell lines. This essentially static approach makes it difficult to distinguish strictly between a role for progression on one hand and a mere association with a given morphology, which is only conjectured to have arisen by progression from a precursor, on the other. The key to any understanding is to elucidate the mechanism by which subclones with selective advantage are created.

One fruitful approach has been to examine the difference between low and high risk genital HPV. Why do high risk types persist longer than low risk types even in the absence of any induction of precancer or cancer? Why do low risk types predominantly induce papillomas without tendency to develop into precancer? Why do high risk types induce such a broad spectrum of morphological responses, ranging from dysplasia to CIS? How do high risk HPV types operate to cause such profound phenotypic disturbances as in invasive cancer and CIS?

The important original finding was that HPV would interfere differently with TP53 depending on type (Tervahauta *et al*, 1993; Kurvinen *et al*, 1994; Ranki *et al*, 1995; Hachisuga *et al*, 1996). The thesis that HPV 16 owes its potential to transform cells malignantly to inactivation of TP53 protein received indirect support from data, which showed that TP53—in contrast to most other human cancers and especially all other squamous cell cancers—was only rarely mutated (Kurvinen *et al*, 1994). This could be explained if functional inactivation by high risk HPV gave the same "push" towards malignant transformation and/or progression as a mutation would. But the issue is far from closed. The role of TP53 in malignant transformation has not been clarified, and it remains to be explained why most cells infected with HPV 16 do not transform in spite of the postulated inactivation of TP53.

A recent study (Zehbe, 1998) suggests that cells carrying a variant of HPV 16 that differs from the prototype by encoding valine instead of leucine because of a base substitution at residue 83 in E6 could be involved in progression from CIS to invasiveness. This report is compatible with other reports (Song *et al*, 1997; Wheeler *et al*, 1997; Xi *et al*, 1997) showing that non-prototype variant HPV 16 may be more strongly associated with cancer than the prototype. Variants show considerable geographical variations in prevalence (Fig. 8), but it is still not known if this also will result in differences in risk of progression of cervical precancer.

As pointed out in the discussion of the small size of the target cell population of the cervix (Fig. 3), and if the hypothesis of stepwise genetic progression (Fig. 7) is correct, it follows that high risk HPV must be an extraordinarily strong risk factor for malignant transformation of individual cells, which far exceeds anything known in human tumour pathology. The virus either activates some extraordinarily effective "gain-of-function" oncogene, or more likely, causes extreme genetic instability with rapid creation of new genotypes. General mechanisms and the importance of such features are discussed in the introductory chapter by Pontén. The only clue of such instability is given by the very common occurrence of LOH (Wistuba *et al*, 1997) (Fig. 6) and aneuploidy even in precancer (Rihet *et al*, 1996), but these features are not unique, since they are found in all other types of squamous cell cancer and in most adenocarcinomas in man. Many elaborate studies have concentrated on lack of control of transcription from HPV E6 and E7, but the link to putative genetical instability remains to be discovered.

SUMMARY

The tumour biology of cervical precancer is unusual. A large variety of individually distinct forms crudely divided into slight, moderate, severe dysplasia and carcinoma in situ exist. Virtually all contain genital human papillomavirus (HPV) either as infectious virions or as episomal or integrated DNA. HPV, which occurs as hundreds of types, subtypes and variants, has a high prevalence in all human populations. Most males are symptomless reservoirs, whereas a proportion of infected women develop condyloma, precancer and subsequently, in a minority, invasive cancer. HPV has unequivocal features of a sexually transmitted infectious agent. Risk of precancer is statistically related to infection with genital HPV, but differences in risk between populations with high and low prevalence of HPV are larger than expected from a direct correlation. Findings fit with HPV as a major risk factor, but other factors must also be oper-

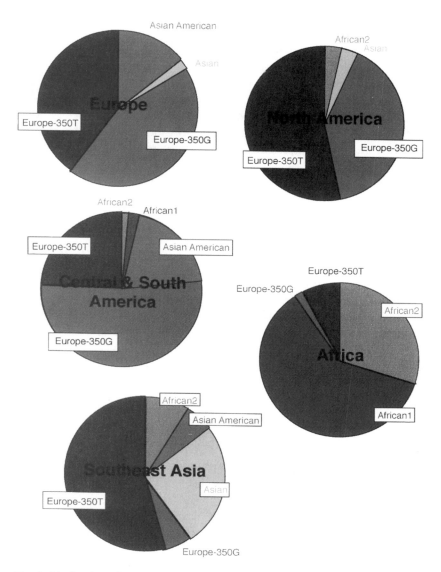

Fig. 8. Distribution of variants of HPV 16 in different continents. Two European variants (350G and 350T) have common polymorphism at codon 350. The European variants dominate in all continents except Africa, where two different African variants together comprise almost 80% (modified from Yamada et al, 1997)

ative. These may include shifts in number of target cells, depending on regeneration and infection by various micro-organisms, hormones, smoking and immunity. Final proof of necessity of HPV infection for precancer can probably be delivered only after its elimination by successful vaccination. Genital condyloma, which is not precancerous, is caused by HPV low risk types, typically 6 or 11, in analogy with papilloma formation in skin and mucosa in a large variety of species. This benign lesion is the hallmark of mammalian HPV pathology and a source of interindividual spread of virus. Slight dysplasia is heterogeneous. Many lesions seem to be polyclonal, self limited cell proliferative responses to infection with low grade HPV. A small proportion are associated with either simultaneous presence or subsequent development of higher grades of dysplasia, in situ or invasive cancer. Evidence exists for two mechanisms: clonal selection of cells with increasingly undifferentiated phenotypes, and independent development of different morphological types of precancer. The relative importance of the two is unknown. High risk HPV, typically 16 or 18, is preferentially associated with high grade dysplasia and in situ cancer, either because it increases risk of clonal progression to these forms or induces them de novo. Severe dysplasia, in situ and invasive cancer always present as monoclonal lesions. Genetic links indicate that these pathologies arise by clonal selection from less advanced precursors. The number of potential target cells for precancer confined to a narrow transformation zone is small. Risk of precancer and malignant transformation per target cell is therefore probably far higher than in any other human tissue subject to cancer. Spontaneous mutation rate and physicochemical carcinogens seem insufficient for the creation of a malignant phenotype in cells of the transformation zone. Currently HPV is the only strong candidate for such a feat. Any or all of the following mechanisms may play a role: overexpression of viral *E6* and *E7* genes, often triggered by disruption of control elements upon integration of viral DNA into the cellular genome, activity of specific (*E6?*) configurations in certain HPV variants, inactivation of *TP53* with decreased capacity for DNA repair and enhanced likelihood of accumulation of "transforming" mutations and viral integration at sites controlling function of cellular oncogenes and/or suppressor genes. Target cells within the transformation zone have the capacity for bidirectional (squamous and/or glandular) differentiation. HPV types seem to drive cells preferentially in different directions after infection/transformation. Low risk types are almost always associated with squamous differentiation, HPV 16 usually also with squamous differentiation and HPV 18 with adenosquamous or adenomatous differentiation. The viral features that determine these subtle differences in performance are unknown, as are all details about how (and if) HPV determines the phenotypes of infected cells, including the reasons for a choice between harmless synthesis of virions and deep persistent disruption of growth and differentiation control. Cervical precancer remains an important and accessible challenge for future understanding of precursors of a common human cancer.

References

Adami H-O, Pontén J, Sparén P, Bergström R, Gustafsson L and Friberg L-G (1994) Survival trend after invasive cervical cancer diagnosis in Sweden before and after cytologic screening. *Cancer* **73** 140–147

Anderson MC, Brown CL, Buckley CH *et al* (1991) Current views on cervical intraepithelial neoplasia. *Journal of Clinical Pathology* **44** 969–978

Anderson S, Shera K, Ihle J *et al* (1997) Telomerase activation in cervical cancer. *American*

Journal of Pathology **151** 25–31

Bar Am A, Niv J, Jaffo A and Peyser RM (1995) Prevalence of human papillomavirus infection and HPV DNA among male partners of Israeli women with genital premalignant and human papillomavirus lesions. *Israel Journal of Medical Science* **31** 349–352

Barksdale S and Baker CC (1995) Differentiation-specific alternative splicing of bovine papillomavirus late mRNAs. *Journal of Virology* **69** 6553–6556

Berard H-U, Chan S-Y, Manos MM *et al* (1994) Identification and assessment of known and novel human papillomaviruses by polymerase chain reaction amplification, restriction fragment length polymorphism, nucleotide sequence, and phylogenetic algorithms. *Journal of Infectious Diseases* **170** 1077–1085

Bergström R, Adami HO, Gustafsson L, Pontén J and Sparén P (1993) Detection of preinvasive cancer of the cervix and the subsequent reduction in invasive cancer incidence: a study based on Swedish county data. *Journal of the National Cancer Institute* **85** 1050–1057

Bosch FX, Manos MM, Muñoz N *et al* (1995) Prevalence of human papillomavirus in cervical cancer: a worldwide perspective. *Journal of the National Cancer Institute* **87** 796–802

Bosch FX, Castellsague X, Muñoz N *et al* (1996) Male sexual behavior and human papillomavirus DNA: key risk factors for cervical cancer in Spain. *Journal of the National Cancer Institute* **88** 1060–1067

Burghardt E (1973) *Early Histological Diagnosis of Cervical Cancer*. Georg Thieme Verlag and WB Saunders Company, Philadelphia, Pensylvania

Burghardt E and Ostor AG (1983) Site and origin of squamous cervical cancer: a histomorphologic study. *Obstetrics and Gynecology* **62** 117–127

Castellsague X, Ghaffari A, Daniel RW, Bosch FX, Muñoz N and Shah KV (1997) Prevalence of penile human papillomavirus DNA in husbands of women with and without cervical neoplasia: a study in Spain and Colombia. *Journal of Infectious Diseases* **176** 353–361

Christensen ND, Koltun WA, Cladel NM *et al* (1997) Coinfection of human foreskin fragments with multiple human papillomavirus types (HPV-11, -40, and -LVX82/MM7) produces regionally separate HPV infections within the same athymic mouse xenograft. *Journal of Virology* **71** 7337–7344

Crum CP and McLachlin CM (1995) Cervical intraepithelial neoplasia. *Journal of Cellular Biochemistry* **23** 71–79

Dillner J (1992) Immunobiology of papillomavirus: prospects for vaccination. *Cancer Journal* **5** 181–186

Dillner L, Bekassy Z, Jonsson N, Moreno-Lopez J and Blomberg J (1989) Detection of IgA antibodies against human papillomavirus in cervical secretions from patients with cervical intraepithelial neoplasia. *International Journal of Cancer* **43** 36–40

Enomoto T, Haba T, Fujita M *et al* (1997) Clonal analysis of high-grade squamous intra-epithelial lesions of the uterine cervix. *International Journal of Cancer* **73** 339–344

Ferenczy A, Braun L and Shah KV (1981) Human papillomavirus (HPV) in condylomatous lesions of cervix. *American Journal of Surgical Pathology* **5** 661–670

Funk JO, Waga S, Harry JB, Espling E, Stillman B and Galloway DA (1997) Inhibition of CDK activity and PCNA-dependent DNA replication by p21 is blocked by interaction with the HPV-16 E7 oncoprotein. *Genes and Development* **11** 2090–2100

Gaukroger JM, Bradley A, Chandrachud L, Jarrett WF and Campo MS (1993) Interaction between bovine papillomavirus type 4 and cocarcinogens in the production of malignant tumours. *Journal of General Virology* **74** 2275–2280

Gomousa MM, Deligeorgi PH, Condi PA, Rammou KR, Ghionis J and Belca HK (1997) Human papillomavirus identification and typing of both sexual partners. *Acta Cytologica* **41** 244–250

Guo Z, Wilander E, Sällström J and Pontén J (1998) Deletion of chromosome 3p is an early event in malignant progression of cervical cancer. *Anticancer Research* **18** 707–712

Gustafsson L and Adami H-O (1989) Natural history of cervical neoplasia: consistent results obtained by an identification technique. *British Journal of Cancer* **60** 132–141

Gustafsson L, Pontén J, Bergstrom R and Adami HO (1997a) International incidence rates of invasive cervical cancer before cytological screening. *International Journal of Cancer* **71** 159–165

Gustafsson L, Pontén J, Zack M and Adami H-O (1997b) International incidence rates of invasive cervical cancer after introduction of cytological screening. *Cancer Causes and Control* **8** 755–763

Hachisuga T, Matsuo N, Iwasaka T, Sugimori H and Tsuneyoshi M (1996) Human papilloma virus and P53 overexpression in carcinomas of the uterine cervix, lower uterine segment and endometrium. *Pathology* **28** 28–31

Heenen M and Galand P (1997) The growth fraction of normal human epidermis. *Dermatology* **194** 313–317

Hildesheim A, Schiffman MH, Gravitt PE *et al* (1994) Persistence of type-specific human papillomavirus infection among cytologically normal women. *Journal of Infectious Diseases* **169** 235–240

Hippelainen MI, Syrjänen S, Hippelainen MJ, Saarikoski S and Syrjänen K (1993) Diagnosis of genital human papillomavirus (HPV) lesions in the male: correlation of peniscopy, histology and in situ hybridisation. *Genitourinary Medicine* **69** 346–351

Hippelainen MI, Hippelainen M, Saarikoski S and Syrjänen K (1994a) Clinical course and prognostic factors of human papillomavirus infections in men. *Sexually Transmitted Diseases* **21** 272–279

Hippelainen MI, Yliskoski M, Syrjänen S *et al* (1994b) Low concordance of genital human papillomavirus (HPV) lesions and viral types in HPV-infected women and their male sexual partners. *Sexually Transmitted Diseases* **21** 76–82

Ho GYF, Bierman R, Beardsley L, Chang CJ and Burk RD (1998) Natural history of cervico-vaginal papillomavirus infection in young women. *New England Journal of Medicine* **338** 423–428

Huibregtse JM and Beaudenon SL (1996) Mechanism of HPV E6 proteins in cellular transformation. *Seminars in Cancer Biology* **7** 317–326

Jones DL, Alani RM and Munger K (1997) The human papillomavirus E7 oncoprotein can uncouple cellular differentiation and proliferation in human keratinocytes by abrogating p21Cip1-mediated inhibition of cdk2. *Genes and Development* **11** 2101–2111

Kashyap V, Das DK and Luthra UK (1990) Microphotometric nuclear DNA analysis in cervical dysplasia of the uterine cervix: its relation to the progression to malignancy and regression to normalcy. *Neoplasma* **37** 497–500

Kjær SK and Jensen OM (1992) Comparison studies of HPV detection in areas at different risk for cervical cancer, In: Muñoz N, Bosch FX, Shah KV and Meheus A (eds). *The Epidemiology of Cervical Cancer and Human Papillomavirus*, pp 243–249, International Agency for Research on Cancer, Lyon

Kjær SK, Teisen C, Haugaard BJ *et al* (1989) Risk factors for cervical cancer in Greenland and Denmark: a population-based cross-sectional study. *International Journal of Cancer* **44** 40–47

Koss LG and Durfee GR (1956) Unusual patterns of squamous epithelium of the uterine cervix. *Annals of the New York Academy of Science* **63** 1245–1261

Koss LG, Stewart FW and Foote FW (1963) Some histological aspects of behavior of epidermoid carcinoma in-situ and related lesions of the uterine cervix: a long-term prospective study. *Cancer* **16** 1160–1211

Kottmeier HL (1955) Evolution et traitement des épithéliomas. *Revue français Gynécologie* **56** 821–825

Kurvinen K, Tervahauta A, Syrjänen S, Chang F and Syrjänen K (1994) The state of the p53 gene in human papillomavirus (HPV)-positive and HPV-negative genital precancer lesions and carcinomas as determined by single-strand conformation polymorphism analysis and sequencing. *Anticancer Research* **14** 177–182

Leptak C, Ramon R, Kulke R *et al* (1991) Tumorigenic transformation of murine keratinocytes by the E5 genes of bovine papillomavirus type 1 and human papillomavirus type 16. *Journal of Virology* **65** 7078–7083

Liu X, Han S, Baluda MA and Park NH (1997) HPV-16 oncogenes E6 and E7 are mutagenic in normal human oral keratinocytes. *Oncogene* **14** 2347–2353

Loeb LA (1996) Many mutations in cancer. *Cancer Surveys* **28** 329–342

Lyon MF (1992) Some milestones in the history of X-chromosome inactivation. *Annual Reviews in Genetics* **26** 16–28

McCluggage WG, Bharucha H, Caughley LM *et al* (1996) Interobserver variation in the reporting of cervical colposcopic biopsy specimens: comparison of grading systems. *Journal of Clinical Pathology* **49** 833–835

Morozov A, Shiyanov P, Barr E, Leiden JM and Raychaudhuri P (1997) Accumulation of human papillomavirus type 16 E7 protein bypasses G1 arrest induced by serum deprivation and by the cell cycle inhibitor p21. *Journal of Virology* **71** 3451–3457

Müller M, Viscidi RP, Sun Y *et al* (1992) Antibodies to HPV-16 E6 and E7 proteins as markers for HPV-16 associated invasive cervical carcinoma. *Virology* **187** 508–514

Muñoz N, Bosch FX, de Sanjosé S *et al* (1993) Risk factors for cervical intraepithelial neoplasia grade III/carcinoma in situ in Spain and Colombia. *Cancer Epidemiology, Biomarkers and Prevention* **2** 423–431

Muñoz N, Castellsague X, Bosch FX *et al* (1996) Difficulty in elucidating the male role in cervical cancer in Colombia, a high-risk area for the disease. *Journal of the National Cancer Institute* **88** 1068–1075

Nakao Y, Yang X, Yokoyama M *et al* (1997) Induction of p16 during immortalization by HPV 16 and 18 and not during malignant transformation. *British Journal of Cancer* **75** 1410–1416

Nasiell K, Nasiell M and Vaclavinkova V (1983) Behavior of moderate cervical dysplasia during long term follow-up. *Obstetrics and Gynecology* **61** 609–614

Nasiell K, Roger V and Nasiell M (1986) Behavior of mild cervical dysplasia during long term follow-up. *Obstetrics and Gynecology* **67** 665–669

National Cancer Institute Workshop (1989) The 1988 Bethesda system for reporting cervical/vaginal cytological diagnoses. *Journal of American Medical Association* **262** 931–934

Nilson LA and DiMaio D (1993) Platelet-derived growth factor receptor can mediate tumorigenic transformation by the bovine papillomavirus E5 protein. *Molecular and Cellular Biology* **13** 4137–4145

Olsen AO, Dillner J, Gjoen K, Sauer T, Orstavik I and Magnus P (1996) A population-based case-control study of human papillomavirus-type-16 seropositivity and incident high-grade dysplasia of the uterine cervix. *International Journal of Cancer* **68** 415–419

Ong CK, Chan SY, Campo MS *et al* (1993) Evolution of human papillomavirus type 18: an ancient phylogenetic root in Africa and intratype diversity reflect coevolution with human ethnic groups. *Journal of Virology* **67** 6424–6431

Papanicolaou GN and Traut HF (1943) *Diagnosis of uterine cancer by the vaginal smear.* Commonwealth Fund, New York, N Y

Parker JN, Zhao W, Askins KJ, Broker TR and Chow LT (1997) Mutational analyses of differentiation-dependent human papillomavirus type 18 enhancer elements in epithelial raft cultures of neonatal foreskin keratinocytes. *Cell Growth and Differentiation* **8** 751–762

Parkin DM, Pisani P and Ferlay J (1993) Estimates of the worldwide incidence of eighteen major cancers in 1985. *International Journal of Cancer* **54** 594–606

Peng X, Lang CM and Kreider JW (1996) Immortalization of inbred rabbit keratinocytes from a Shope papilloma and tumorigenic transformation of the cells by EJ-*ras*. *Cancer Letters* **108** 101–109

Petry KU, Kochel H, Bode U *et al* (1996) Human papillomavirus is associated with the frequent detection of warty and basaloid high-grade neoplasia of the vulva and cervical neoplasia among immunocompromised women. *Gynecologic Oncology* **60** 30–34

Petti LM, Reddy V, Smith SO and DiMaio D (1997) Identification of amino acids in the transmembrane and juxtamembrane domains of the platelet-derived growth factor receptor required for productive interaction with the bovine papillomavirus E5 protein. *Journal of Virology* **71** 7318–7327

Pirisi L, Creek KE, Doniger J and Dipaolo JA (1988) Continuous cell lines with altered growth and differentation properties originate after transfection of human keratinocytes with human papillomavirus type-16 DNA. *Carcinogenesis* **9** 1573–1579

Pontén J, Adami H-O, Bergström R *et al* (1994) Strategies for global control of cervical cancer. *International Journal of Cancer* **58** 1–26

Ranki A, Lassus J and Niemi KM (1995) Relation of p53 tumor suppressor protein expression to human papillomavirus (HPV) DNA and to cellular atypia in male genital warts and in premalignant lesions. *Acta Dermato-Venerologica* **75** 180–186

Rapp B, Pawellek A, Kraetzer F *et al* (1997) Cell-type-specific separate regulation of the E6 and E7 promoters of human papillomavirus type 6a by the viral transcription factor E2. *Journal of Virology* **71** 6956–6966

Riese DJ II and DiMaio D (1995) An intact PDGF signaling pathway is required for efficient growth transformation of mouse C127 cells by the bovine papillomavirus E5 protein. *Oncogene* **10** 1431–1439

Rihet S, Lorenzato M and Clavel C (1996) Oncogenic human papillomaviruses and ploidy in cervical lesions. *Journal of Clinical Pathology* **49** 892–896

Ruesch MN and Laimins LA (1997) Initiation of DNA synthesis by human papillomavirus E7 oncoproteins is resistant to p21-mediated inhibition of cyclin E-cdk2 activity. *Journal of Virology* **71** 5570–5578

Sanchez Perez AM, Soriano S, Clarke AR and Gaston K (1997) Disruption of the human papillomavirus type 16 E2 gene protects cervical carcinoma cells from E2F-induced apoptosis. *Journal of General Virology* **78** 3009–3018

Sato S, Okagaki T, Clark BA *et al* (1986) Sensitivity of koilocytosis, immunocytochemistry, and electron microscopy as compared to DNA hybridization in detecting human papillomavirus in cervical and vaginal condyloma and intraepithelial neoplasia. *International Journal of Gynecological Pathology* **5** 297–307

Sebbelov AM, Svendsen C, Jensen H, Kjær SK and Norrild B (1994) Prevalence of HPV in premalignant and malignant cervical lesions in Greenland and Denmark: PCR and *in situ* hybridization analysis on archival material. *Research in Virology* **145** 83–92

Shiga T, Shirasawa H, Shimizu K, Dezawa M, Masuda Y and Simizu B (1997) Normal human fibroblasts immortalized by introduction of human papillomavirus type 16 (HPV-16) E6-E7 genes. *Microbiology and Immunology* **41** 313–319

Song YS, Kee SH, Kim JW *et al* (1997) Major sequence variants in E7 gene of human papillomavirus type 16 from cervical cancerous and noncancerous lesions of Korean women. *Gynecologic Oncology* **66** 275–281

Steenbergen RD, Walboomers JM, Meijer CJ *et al* (1996) Transition of human papillomavirus type 16 and 18 transfected human foreskin keratinocytes towards immortality: activation of telomerase and allele losses at 3p, 10p, 11q and/or 18q. *Oncogene* **13** 1249–1257

Storm HH, Manders T, Friis S and Bang S (1989) *Cancer Incidence in Denmark*, Danish Cancer Society, Copenhagen

Strand A, Rylander E, Wilander E and Zehbe I (1995) HPV infection in male partners of women with squamous intraepithelial neoplasia and/or high-risk HPV. *Acta Dermato-Venereologica* **75** 312–316

Strand A, Rylander E, Wilander E, Zehbe I and Kraaz W (1996) Histopathologic examination of penile epithelial lesions is of limited diagnostic value in human papillomavirus infection. *Sexually Transmitted Diseases* **23** 293–298

Svare EI, Kjær SK, Worm A-M *et al* (1998) Risk factors for HPV infection in women from sexually transmitted disease clinics: comparison between two areas with different cervical cancer incidence. *International Journal of Cancer* **75** 1–8

Tervahauta AI, Syrjänen SM, Vayrynen M, Saastamoinen J and Syrjänen KJ (1993) Expression of p53 protein related to the presence of human papillomavirus (HPV) DNA in genital carcinomas and precancer lesions. *Anticancer Research* **13** 1107–1111

van Ranst MA, Tachezy R, Delilus H and Burk RD (1993) Taxonomy of the human papillomavirus group. *Papillomavirus Reports* **4** 61–65

Velasco J, Fernandez Blanco C, Lopez Carrascosa I, Cueto Espinar A and Sampedro A (1996) Disappearance of DNA HPV in sequential specimens of occult cervical infection in a "normal" population. *European Journal of Gynaecological Oncology* **17** 372–377

Weinstein GD, McCullough JL and Ross P (1984) Cell proliferation in normal epidermis. *Journal of Investigative Dermatology* **82** 623–628

Wheeler CM, Yamada T, Hildesheim A and Jenison SA (1997) Human papillomavirus type 16 sequence variants: identification by E6 and L1 lineage-specific hybridization. *Journal of Clinical Microbiology* **35** 11–19

WHO (1995) IARC Monographs on the evaluation of carcinogenic risks to humans. Human papillomaviruses. *International Agency for Research on Cancer* **64** p. 378. Lyon, France

Wieland U and Pfister H (1997) Papillomaviruses in human patholgoy: Epidemiology, pathogenesis and oncogenic role, In: Barasso GEGaR (ed). *Human Papilloma Virus Infection: A Clinical Atlas*, pp 1–16, Ullstein Mosby GmbH & Co, KG, Berlin/Wiesbaden

Wistuba II, Montellano FD, Milchgrub S *et al* (1997) Deletions of chromosome 3p are frequent and early events in the pathogenesis of uterine cervical carcinoma. *Cancer Research* **57** 3154–3158

Xi LF, Koutsky LA, Galloway DA *et al* (1997) Genomic variation of human papillomavirus type 16 and risk for high grade cervical intraepithelial neoplasia. *Journal of the National Cancer Institute* **89** 796–802

Yamada T, Manos MM, Peto J *et al* (1997) Human papillomavirus type 16 sequence variation in cervical cancers: A worldwide perspective. *Journal of virology* **71** 2463–2472

Yun K and Sherwood MJ (1992) In situ hybridization at light and electron microscopic levels: identification of human papillomavirus nucleic acids. *Pathology* **24** 91–98

Zehbe I, Wilander E, Delius H and Tommasino M (1998) Human papillomavirus 16 E6 variants are more prevalent in invasive cervical carcinoma than the prototype. *Cancer Research* **58** 829–833

zur Hausen H (1977) Human papillomaviruses and their possible role in squamous cell carcinomas. *Current Topics in Microbiology and Immunology* **78** 1–30

zur Hausen H (1987) Papillomaviruses in human cancer. *Cancer* **59** 1692–1696

The authors are responsible for the accuracy of the references.

Biographical Notes

Charles W Boone, MD, PhD, FCAP, obtained his MD degree from the University of California San Francisco in 1951. His activities in basic science include a graduate year in physical chemistry with Dr Linus Pauling, a PhD in biochemistry from UC Los Angeles and 14 years as chief, cell biology section, laboratory of carcinogenesis, National Cancer Institute, NIH. He became American Board Certified in pathology and five years later was elected fellow of the College of American Pathologists in 1984. In clinical medicine, he trained for two years in community and family medicine at the University of Maryland and UC Irvine. Since 1988, he has been a programme director in the chemoprevention branch at the NCI.

Douglas E Brash is professor of therapeutic radiology and genetics at Yale School of Medicine. His past research has focused on DNA photoproducts made by ultraviolet light, the mutations they cause and genes mutated by sunlight in human skin cancers. His findings in these areas led to the laboratory's current interest in ultraviolet light induced apoptosis and the contribution of apoptosis to the clonal expansion or regression of early cancers.

Christer Busch, professor of pathology at University Hospital, Tromsø, Norway, graduated in medicine from the University of Uppsala, Sweden, in 1968, and obtained his PhD in 1974. He has been active in vascular biology and urological research. Dr Busch has been president of the International Society of Urological Pathology since 1997.

V. Peter Collins, a graduate of the National University of Ireland, received his doctorate from the Karolinska Institute, Stockholm, and trained in histopathology and cytology at the Karolinska Hospital. His major interests have been the diagnosis, biology and genetics of human brain tumours. He was appointed head of clinical research at the Stockholm branch of the Ludwig Institute in 1985 and professor of neuropathology at the University of Gothenburg in 1990. He returned to the Karolinska Institute as professor of tumour pathology in 1994 and has recently been elected to the chair of histopathology, University of Cambridge.

Carlos Cordon-Cardo, who graduated MD from the Autonomous University, Barcelona, is director of the division of molecular pathology at Memorial Sloan-Kettering Cancer Center, New York, and associate professor of pathology at Cornell University Medical College. His research focuses on molecular alterations of tumour suppressor genes in human cancer, including the proposal of a model defining two distinct pathways for tumour progression of human bladder cancer. His current work is aimed at understanding the co-operative effects of mutations of cell cycle regulators and the development and characterization of animal models for loss of function of specific cell cycle regulators.

Lars Egevad graduated in medicine from Umeå University, Sweden, in 1988. He has specialized in genitourinary pathology and is now a cytopathologist at the Karolinska Hospital, Stockholm. His main research interest is prostate pathology.

Zhongmin Guo graduated from Guangdong Medical Institute, People's Republic of China, in 1983. He received a master's degree in pathology and oncology from Guandong Medical Institute and was appointed lecturer in 1986 and associate professor in 1993 in the institute's department of pathology. He is now a PhD student in pathology in the department of genet-

231

ics and pathology, Uppsala University, Sweden. His work mainly concerns clonal evolution and genetic mechanisms in cervical carcinogenesis.

Michael Haggman, PhD, graduated in medicine from the Karolinska Institute, Stockholm, and was certified as a specialist in urology in 1987. He is now a senior registrar in the department of urology, University Hospital, Uppsala, Sweden. His main research field is prostate cancer.

Pierre Hainaut, PhD, is a scientist at the International Agency for Research on Cancer, WHO, Lyon. He trained in zoology and received his PhD at the University of Liège in Belgium in 1987. As a postdoctoral fellow in 1991–1995, he worked in the group of Dr J Milner at the Universities of Cambridge and of York on the regulation of the *TP53* tumour suppressor gene. He joined IARC in 1995 and is developing a research project on the involvement of *TP53* and other cell cycle regulatory genes in oesophageal cancers. He is also responsible for the IARC *TP53* mutation database.

Gary J Kelloff received his BS in 1964 and MD in 1976 from the University of Colorado, followed by postgraduate training at Grady Memorial Hospital, Atlanta, Georgia. His early research focused on oncogenes, particularly oncogenic retroviruses, at the National Cancer Institute (NCI) in the laboratory of cellular and molecular biology, laboratory of viral carcinogenesis and the viral carcinogenesis branch. Since 1983 he has been directing chemoprevention research and is currently chief of the chemoprevention branch, division of cancer prevention at NCI. His primary focus is designing and managing a chemoprevention research and drug development programme, encompassing all aspects of drug discovery through clinical trials.

Ruggero Montesano obtained an MD at the University of Turin, Italy, in 1965 and a PhD in 1974 at the Courtauld Institute of Biochemistry, University of London. He joined the International Agency for Research on Cancer (Lyon, France) in 1972 and since 1980 has been chief of the unit of mechanisms of carcinogenesis, responsible for the IARC fellowships programme since 1982 and co-ordinator of the Gambia hepatitis intervention study since 1993. His main contributions have been in the area of environmental carcinogenesis and mechanisms of carcinogenesis with emphasis on studies on the role of DNA damage and repair. In recent years he has also investigated the occurrence of genetic changes in oncogenes and tumour suppressor genes in human cancer (oesophagus, liver) and the value of the implementation of such approaches to molecular cancer epidemiological studies.

Jan Pontén, professor of pathology at the University of Uppsala, graduated from the Karolinska Institute, Stockholm. His early research concerned transformation by Rous sarcoma virus and SV 40, and his later studies explored several aspects of tumour biology including, latterly, cervical cancer and the carcinogenetic effect of ultraviolet light on human skin. He was chairman of the research committee of the Swedish Cancer Research Foundation, 1983–1993.

Daryl Shibata is a graduate of the University of California at Los Angeles and San Diego. He obtained his medical degree and pathology training at the University of Southern California School of Medicine. Currently his laboratory is in the University of Southern California/Norris Comprehensive Cancer Center. Recent research efforts are focused on further dissecting multistep human tumour progression through phylogenetic approaches.

Index

LIST OF PREVIOUS ISSUES

VOLUME 21 1994

Palliative Medicine: Problem Areas in Pain and Symptom Management
Guest Editor: G W Hanks

VOLUME 22 1995

Molecular Mechanisms of the Immune Response
Guest Editors: W F Bodmer and
M J Owen

VOLUME 23 1995

Preventing Prostate Cancer: Screening versus Chemoprevention
Guest Editors: R T D Oliver, A Belldegrun
and P F M Wrigley

VOLUME 24 1995

Cell Adhesion and Cancer
Guest Editors: I Hart and N Hogg

VOLUME 25 1995

Genetics and Cancer: A Second Look
Guest Editors: B A J Ponder,
W K Cavenee and E Solomon

VOLUME 26 1996

Skin Cancer
Guest Editors: I M Leigh, J A Newton
Bishop and M L Kripke

VOLUME 27 1996

Cell Signalling
Guest Editors: P J Parker and T Pawson

VOLUME 28 1996

Genetic Instability in Cancer
Guest Editor: T Lindahl

VOLUME 29 1997

Checkpoint Controls and Cancer
Guest Editor: M B Kastan

VOLUME 30 1997

Lymphoma
Guest Editor: A C Wotherspoon

VOLUME 31 1998

Bladder Cancer
Guest Editors: R T D Oliver and
M J Coptcoat